FINANCIAL ANALYSIS AND DECISION MAKING FOR HEALTHCARE ORGANIZATIONS

A Guide for the Healthcare Professional

LOUIS C. GAPENSKI

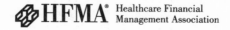

HFMA® Healthcare Financial Management Association

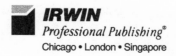

IRWIN
Professional Publishing®
Chicago • London • Singapore

McGraw-Hill
   A Division of The McGraw-Hill Companies

FINANCIAL ANALYSIS AND DECISION MAKING FOR HEALTHCARE
ORGANIZATIONS: A GUIDE FOR THE HEALTHCARE PROFESSIONAL

1 2 3 4 5 6 7 8 9 0 DOC DOC 9 0 9 8 7 6

ISBN 0-7863-1033-2

This publication is designed to provide accurate and authoritative information in regard to
the subject matter covered. It is sold with the understanding that neither the author nor the
publisher is engaged in rendering legal, accounting,or other professional service. If legal
advice or other expert assistance is required, the services of a competent professional person
should be sought.

From a Declaration of Principles jointly adopted by a Committee
of the American Bar Association and a Committee of Publishers.

Library of Congress Cataloging-in-Publication Data
Gapenski, Louis C.
   Financial analysis and decision making for healthcare
organizations : a guide for the healthcare professional / Louis C.
Gapenski.
      p. cm.
   Includes index.
   ISBN 0-7863-1033-2
   1. Health facilities—Business management. 2. Health facilities—
Finance. I. Title.
RA971.3.G369 1997
362.1'068'1—dc21   96–45343

PREFACE

After years of teaching corporate financial management and writing corporate finance textbooks and casebooks, I began teaching the healthcare financial management course in the University of Florida's graduate program in Health and Hospital Administration. The first thing that struck me was that no textbook was available that truly focused on healthcare financial management. To me, financial management is primarily concerned with analysis and decision making, yet the books available covered a lot of accounting and institutional detail (the third-party payer system, Medicare cost reports, and so on), with only a little bit of financial management thrown in here and there. To meet the needs of academic programs, I created a healthcare financial management text for use in on-campus master's programs that emphasized analysis and decision making.

At that point, I became involved in several healthcare executive training programs. It again quickly became clear that no suitable text was available for these programs, including my healthcare financial management text, which was written for master's-level students rather than practitioners. Thus, I set about the task of writing this book.

My goal in writing *Financial Analysis and Decision Making for Healthcare Organizations* was to create a book that provides healthcare managers with an operational knowledge of financial management theory and concepts so that they may use this information to enhance their own financial decision making.

Many people at the University of Florida and elsewhere provided inspiration as well as more tangible support for the book. In particular, the staff at Irwin Professional Publishing, especially Kristine Rynne and Patrick Muller, deserve a great deal of credit for helping to bring the book to fruition.

Good financial decision making is vital to the economic well-being of the healthcare industry. Because of its importance, finan-

cial analysis and decision making should be thoroughly understood, but this is easier said than done. I hope that this book will
provide guidance in how to make better financial decisions in the
highly competitive healthcare industry of today.

    To make the book the best that it can be, I need comments and
recommendations from you, its readers. Please don't hesitate to write
if you have any suggestions for improving the value of this book.

Louis C. Gapenski, PhD
Department of Health Services Administration
Box 100195 Health Science Center
University of Florida
Gainesville, Florida 32610-0195

ABOUT THE AUTHOR

Dr. Louis C. Gapenski is a leading academic in health services administration and financial management. He is currently an associate professor in the Department of Health Services Administration at the University of Florida in Gainesville and an affiliate associate professor at the Department of Finance, Insurance, and Real Estate. In addition, Dr. Gapenski is a visiting associate professor at the Medical School of the University of Wisconsin and a faculty member of the University of Wisconsin Nonresident Administrative Medicine Program.

Dr. Gapenski is the author of over 50 books and articles, as well as a reviewer for many leading healthcare services journals such as *Healthcare Financial Management, Hospitals & Health Services Administration, Health Services Management Research,* and *The Journal of Health Administration Education.* His financial management textbooks, including *Understanding Health Care Financial Management: Text, Cases, and Models* (AUPHA/Health Administration Press, 1996), are used at leading institutions worldwide.

Dr. Gapenski received a B.S. degree from the Virginia Military Institute, an M.S. degree from the U.S. Naval Postgraduate School, and M.B.A. and Ph.D. degrees from the University of Florida. Dr. Gapenski is highly active in professional organizations and executive education programs.

CONTENTS

Chapter 3

Required Rates of Return   71

Chapter 6

The Cost of Capital   173

Chapter 8

Capital Investment Decisions: Risk Considerations   245

Chapter 9

Capital Investment Decisions: Mergers and Acquisitions   273

1

CHAPTER

The Basics of Financial Analysis and Decision Making

It was a brisk fall day in Chicago, so both George Atkinson and Beth Zalenski felt a rush of exhilaration as they began their daily noontime jog through Lincoln Park. George, the administrator of an investor-owned physician group practice, and Beth, the vice president for operations of a not-for-profit hospital, often pass the time by "comparing notes" and discussing issues relating to the healthcare industry. As usual, they hadn't passed the quarter-mile mark before their conversation turned to work.

Beth had attended an executive committee meeting the day before, and she was disturbed by the fact that the committee refused to forward to the board of trustees a proposal to construct an ambulatory care clinic in a poor neighborhood about two miles from the hospital. "They just don't understand," she said emphatically. "Our mission is to serve the public, and this clinic would provide healthcare access to some of the most underserved people in Chicago." Although George suspected what the answer might be, he went ahead and asked Beth why the committee had turned the proposal down. Her response was, "It's always the same: money, money, money. They want new initiatives to return at least 10 percent, and the clinic doesn't pass muster. It seems like financial considerations dominate everything we do these days. What do they think we are, a for-profit institution?"

1

*At the one-mile mark, after Beth had worked out some of her frus-
tration, they began to discuss the differences between the healthcare
industry and other businesses, and between for-profit and not-for-profit
organizations. Further, they discussed how these differences affect financial analysis and decision making.*

*Business ownership is one of the topics covered in this chapter,
which provides essential background material related to financial analysis
and decision making in healthcare organizations. At the end of the jog,
Beth reached some conclusions about the importance of financial analysis
and decision making to both not-for-profit and for-profit businesses. They
appear at the end of this chapter. After you read the chapter, see if your
conclusions agree with hers.*

INTRODUCTION

Financial analysis and decision making involve using numerical
analysis to help healthcare managers make better decisions regarding the future of their organizations. Managers in the healthcare
industry face a vast array of decisions. Many of these decisions
have little or no influence on the financial well-being of the organization. However, some decisions, such as those relating to capital
investments, can have a profound impact on an organization's
financial condition. Since a sound financial condition is critical to
the ability of any organization to provide goods or services, and
even to organizational survival, it is important that healthcare
managers at all levels have the knowledge and skills necessary to
properly assess the financial impact of their decisions.

This book focuses on the basics of financial analysis and decision making. Its goal is to familiarize readers with the most important concepts and techniques used regularly by finance professionals. When you have finished the book, you will be thoroughly
familiar with many concepts—such as financial risk, opportunity
costs, and asset valuation—that contribute to good financial analysis and decision making. More importantly, you will know how to
apply these concepts, so the concepts can be used to make better
decisions within your organization. As an added benefit, you will
gain insights that will help you better manage your personal
finances because many financial decision-making concepts and
techniques are applicable to both business and personal decisions.

ROAD MAP TO LEARNING

The text was designed specifically to promote the learning process. To begin, the material is organized so that principles and concepts build upon and reinforce one another. Chapter 1 gets you started by introducing the key concepts of financial analysis and decision making and presenting some background material that influences financial decision making within healthcare organizations. Chapters 2 and 3 discuss risk and return, concepts that underlie all financial decisions. Chapter 4 introduces discounted cash flow analysis, or time value of money, another cornerstone of financial decision making.

Chapters 5 through 9 focus on asset valuation, first from the standpoint of investors who supply capital to businesses and then from the perspective of managers who make capital investment decisions within firms. The bridge between investors' and managers' decisions is the cost of capital, which is covered in Chapter 6.

Chapters 10 and 11 cover financing decisions. Chapter 10 examines the capital structure decision, which involves the appropriate mix of debt and equity capital. Chapter 11 discusses lease financing, an alternative source of capital to healthcare firms.

Chapter 12, which concludes the body of the book, discusses capitation. Although not one of the key elements of financial analysis and decision making, capitated reimbursement has had a profound impact on the way providers must think about financial analysis and decision making. Thus, a chapter devoted to capitation (and risk sharing) is a logical way to conclude the book.

In addition to the chapter presentations, the text contains three other features to assist the learning process. First, each chapter contains a set of self-assessment exercises designed to help you review key concepts. Completion of these exercises will reinforce the material and confirm your understanding of the key concepts as you move through the book. Appendix A contains the solutions to the self-assessment exercises, so you can gain immediate feedback regarding your comprehension of the key concepts.

Second, each chapter contains selected references. Some of these references provide additional readings on foundation material, but most of the references guide you to articles written by healthcare professionals, including academics, consultants, and practitioners, so the referenced articles focus on topics of most interest to healthcare managers.

Finally, technology has spawned many tools that aid in financial analysis and decision making, but the most widely accepted and beneficial byproducts are the personal computer and spreadsheet software. Spreadsheet models permit healthcare managers to gain insights into the financial implications of the decisions at hand that they would simply miss in the old pencil-and-calculator environment. To help readers appreciate the value of spreadsheets in financial decision making, the text includes a diskette containing spreadsheet models for selected financial decisions. The models, which can be easily accessed by IBM-compatible personal computers with or without spreadsheet software, are tied to selected self-examination exercises. Appendix B contains instructions for using the diskette. All readers who are not familiar with the power of spreadsheets should spend at least some time working with the spreadsheet models.

THE IMPORTANCE OF FINANCIAL MARKETS AND INSTRUMENTS TO HEALTHCARE MANAGERS

About half of the material in Chapters 2 and 3 and all of the material in Chapter 5 pertains to financial markets and instruments. In essence, these chapters discuss the types of debt and equity, how interest rates and required rates of return on equity are established, and how investors value stocks and bonds. A very logical question is this: Why does a book on financial analysis and decision making for healthcare managers devote so many pages to stocks and bonds? There are three reasons why it is important for healthcare managers to understand financial markets and instruments. First, many healthcare organizations are investor owned, so managers must consider the impact of managerial decisions on the firm's stock price. To do this, managers must be aware of the types of common stock and how investors value stock. Also, virtually all healthcare organizations, regardless of ownership, use one or more forms of debt financing; so healthcare managers must be familiar with the different forms of debt, how interest rates are set, and how managerial decisions affect the firm's cost of debt.

Second, when healthcare managers make capital investment decisions, such as whether or not to buy an MRI system, they need to consider the cost of the funds used to make the purchase. Funds are not free, and part of the costs of new plant and equipment are the "capital costs" inherent in using the firm's funds. To fully understand and measure such capital costs, healthcare managers, including those at not-for-profit organizations, need to have a basic understanding of financial markets and instruments.

Finally, the same general techniques used to value securities are used to judge the value of capital investments, so securities valuation provides an introduction to the more complex world of real asset valuation.

The bad news is that some foundation material needs to be covered before the book can move into the more interesting aspects, those related to managerial analysis and decisions within healthcare organizations. But the good news is that a knowledge of financial markets and instruments will not only make you a better healthcare manager but also a better manager of your own personal finances!

THE FIVE MOST IMPORTANT FINANCIAL CONCEPTS

At a recent meeting of finance academics and practitioners, a panel session was devoted to identifying the five most important concepts in finance. After much discussion, the panelists agreed on the following list, which is a good way to briefly introduce readers to the primary concepts that will be covered in detail in the remaining chapters. By the time you finish reading this book, these five concepts should be second nature to you. If they are, you will have gained a great deal from your effort.

Cash Is King

It is easy for someone to be blinded by accounting statements such as the income statement and balance sheet. After all, they are constructed in a precise manner according to an extensive set of rules called generally accepted accounting principles (GAAP). It seems only reasonable that mangers should focus on accounting data when making financial decisions within the firm.

But there is a catch. The true profitability of a business, and hence its true financial condition, is not a function of the income reported on its income statement but rather the actual cash that flows into and out of the business. Small business owners recognize this concept intuitively: If you have more money in the bank at the end of the month, you are better off than if you have less money, regardless of what the income statement reports. It's not that accounting statements aren't important or useful, it's just that they do not—except for the cash flow statement—focus on what is truly important for financial decision making. All financial decisions, and especially investment decisions, must focus on cash flows. The important point to remember is that "cash is king."

Time Value of Money

A dollar in hand today is worth more than a dollar to be received in the future, say, one year from today. Having a dollar today permits immediate consumption, as well as the alternative of putting the dollar away (perhaps in a mattress) and spending it at some time in the future; whereas, a dollar to be received in the future cannot be used for immediate consumption. In the words of one economist, "I'd rather have a Big Mac today than tomorrow." Another way to consider the time value of money is to recognize that a dollar received today could be invested in a savings account (or any other investment), generate a return, and presumably be worth more than a dollar in the future.

The implication of the differential value of money over time is that future dollars (future cash flows) must somehow be adjusted to reflect the fact that they are worth less than current dollars. The process of making this adjustment is called *discounted cash flow analysis.* The book devotes an entire chapter (Chapter 4) to discounted cash flow analysis, and these concepts will be used again and again in following chapters.

Risk and Return

All financial decisions involve two elements: risk and return. The return is the amount you expect to earn on some investment. Risk arises because there is usually some chance that you might not earn the expected return. Since investment returns are rarely certain, it is important that healthcare managers view investment decisions as a joint risk and return decision. The correct question to ask when making investment decisions is not which alternative has the best return but rather which investment has the best return *relative to its riskiness.*

The concept of risk and return has profound implications for financial analysis and decision making. First, we must be able to define financial risk; and once defined, we must be able to measure it. As important, once risk is measured, we must be able to incorporate differential risk into the decision process: Higher risk alternatives must somehow be assessed a penalty vis-à-vis lower risk alternatives.

Opportunity Costs

A wise person once said, "There is no free lunch." (He or she apparently attended many of the same luncheons I did.) The rough financial translation of this saying is that no resource (including time) is free because the use of a resource for one purpose automatically deprives the user of the opportunity to use the resource for another purpose. The resource may be cash, or it may be land, buildings, or equipment, but in almost all situations use of a resource implies an opportunity cost.

To illustrate, suppose a hospital receives an unrestricted contribution of $100,000. The hospital's managers are evaluating using the funds to buy state-of-the-art X-ray equipment. Since the money was obtained at no cost to the hospital, shouldn't it be treated as "free" in the analysis? The answer is no! By using the $100,000 to purchase X-ray equipment, the hospital is losing the opportunity to use the funds for other purposes, and hence there is an opportunity cost associated with the funds. What is the amount of this opportunity cost? Many alternative uses might be proposed for the $100,000, but for financial analysis purposes, the next best use is to invest the funds in securities that have the same financial risk as the X-ray equipment. Thus, the return available on investments in similar-risk securities must be charged as an opportunity cost against the X-ray project, even though there was no explicit cost to the funds that would be used to make the purchase.

Don't Put All Your Eggs in One Basket

This is probably the best bit of advice ever passed on from one generation to the next. The implication is that diversification reduces risk. In the finance sense, this advice means that investors, whether managers saving for their retirement or HMOs deciding what to do with excess cash, should hold portfolios of assets (many assets) rather than just a single asset. It is less risky for Mary Mitchell to hold a diversified portfolio of stocks and bonds in her retirement fund than it is to hold one stock. Similarly, it is less risky for BestCare HMO to diversify its investments by offering many different products in many different geographic areas than it is to offer a single product in one market.

The fact that diversification reduces risk has important implications for financial analysis and decision making. When assets are held in portfolios, as opposed to individually, the way risk is defined and measured is changed. Since risk is an important element in all decisions, portfolio effects must be explicitly considered in financial analysis and decision making.

CONCEPT OF A BUSINESS

There are many ways to describe a business. For example, from an accounting perspective, a business may be characterized by its financial statements; while from a legal perspective, a business may be thought of in terms of its legal organization—its charter and bylaws. However, for financial decision-making purposes, it is often useful to think of businesses in the following way.

A business is an entity—the form of organization makes no difference here—that (1) obtains funds from the capital markets, such as the bond and stock markets; (2) uses the funds acquired to purchase assets; and (3) operates the assets to provide goods or services and, for an investor-owned business, to make profits. This simple model of a business immediately focuses attention on two very important financial decisions that must be made by all businesses.

First, businesses raise funds in two primary forms: debt capital and equity capital. One important financial decision is the financing mix, or the proportion of debt and equity capital. Should firms use mostly debt capital, mostly equity capital, or some balanced mix of the two? This decision, called the capital structure decision, is discussed in detail in Chapter 10. Here, you will see that the capital structure decision involves a risk/return trade-off: The greater the use of debt financing, the higher the expected return to the firm's owners, but the greater the risk.

Our simple concept of a business points out a second important financial decision. Once funds are raised in the capital markets, they must be invested in real, or physical, assets. (Financial businesses invest their funds in financial assets such as mortgages, but this book focuses on the healthcare industry, so we are concerned with businesses that invest in real assets such as hospitals, nursing homes, clinics, information systems, and diagnostic equipment.) What capital investments should the business make? In other words, which investments should be selected from the almost unlimited number of choices available? This decision, which is critical to both a business's strategic direction and its financial well-being, is discussed in Chapters 7, 8, and 9. You will see that, from a financial perspective, businesses should invest in capital assets that return at least as much as the return available on alternative investments of similar risk.

Often, when befuddled with the detail of some financial decision, it is useful to "go back to the basics" and think about businesses in terms of their three primary activities: raising capital, investing capital in real assets, and operating those assets to provide goods or services. Keeping these ideas in mind forces managers to stay focused on business essentials.

FORMS OF BUSINESS ORGANIZATION

Financial decision making does not occur in isolation, but rather within some organizational context. Furthermore, the organizational context influences how financial decisions are made. Thus, managers must be familiar with the forms of business organization and how they affect financial decision making. There are three primary forms of business organization: the sole proprietorship, the partnership, and the corporation. Because most healthcare managers work for corporations, including not-for-profit corporations, this book concentrates on that form of organization. However, many individual professional practices are organized as proprietorships, and partnerships are also common in group practices and joint ventures.

Sole Proprietorship

A sole proprietorship is a business owned by an individual. Going into business as a sole proprietor is easy—one merely begins business operations. However, most cities require even the smallest businesses to be licensed, and state licensure is required for most healthcare professionals.

The sole proprietorship form of organization has three important advantages: (1) It is easily and inexpensively formed; (2) it is subject to few governmental regulations; and (3) the business pays no corporate income taxes—all earnings of the business, whether they are reinvested in the business or withdrawn by the owner, are taxed as personal income to the proprietor. In general, a sole proprietorship results in lower total taxes because corporate profits are taxed twice, once at the corporate level and again at the personal level, when the profits are distributed as dividends.

Sole proprietorships also have three important disadvantages: (1) Unless the proprietor is very wealthy, it is difficult for a proprietorship to obtain large sums of capital; (2) the proprietor has unlimited personal liability for the debts of the business, which can result in losses greater than the amount put into the business; and (3) the life of the business is limited to the life of the proprietor. For these reasons, the sole proprietorship form of organization is restricted primarily to relatively small businesses, such as sole practices by healthcare professionals.

Partnership

A partnership is formed whenever two or more individuals (or organizations) associate to conduct a noncorporate business. Partnerships may operate under different degrees of formality, ranging from informal, oral understandings to formal agreements filed with the state in which the partnership does business. Like a sole proprietorship, the major advantage of the partnership form of organization is its low cost and ease of formation. The disadvantages are also similar to those of a sole proprietorship: (1) unlimited liability, (2) limited life of the business entity, (3) difficulty of transferring ownership, and (4) difficulty in raising large sums of capital.

As to liability, partners risk all of their personal assets, even those not invested in the business, because each partner is personally liable for all the partnership's debts. Also, the tax treatment of a partnership is similar to that of a sole proprietorship: The partnership's earnings are allocated to the partners and taxed as personal income, regardless of whether the earnings are actually paid out to the partners or retained in the business. Many group practices are organized as partnerships, although the corporate form of organization is also popular.

The first three disadvantages—unlimited liability, impermanence of the business, and difficulty in transferring ownership—lead to the fourth: the difficulty that partnerships (and sole proprietorships) have in attracting substantial amounts of capital. This is no particular problem in a slow-growing business, but if a business needs to expand rapidly to take advantage of market opportunities, the difficulty of attracting capital becomes a real handicap. Thus, many growth companies start out as sole proprietorships or partnerships but then ultimately convert to a corporate form of organization.

Note that some specialized types of partnerships have somewhat different characteristics than the "plain vanilla" kind. First, it is possible to limit the liabilities of some of the partners by establishing a limited partnership, wherein certain partners are designated general partners and others limited partners. In a limited partnership, the limited partners are liable only for the amount of their investment in the partnership, while the general partners have unlimited liability. However, the limited partners typically have no control, which rests solely with the general partners. Limited partnerships are quite common in real estate and mineral investments, but they are not widely used in the healthcare industry because one partner is usually unwilling to accept the majority of the business's risk, while the other is unwilling to forgo control.

The limited liability partnership (LLP), sometimes called a limited liability company (LLC) (although it is not a corporation) is a relatively new type of partnership that is now available in many states. In a regular or limited partnership, at least one partner is liable for the debts of the partnership. However, in an LLP, all partners enjoy limited liability, just as if they were shareholders in a corporation. In effect, as we discuss in the next section, the LLP form of organization combines the limited liability advantage of a corporation with the tax advantages of a partnership.

Corporation

A corporation is a legal entity created by a state, which is separate and distinct from its owners and managers. The creation of a separate business entity gives the corporation three primary advantages: (1) A corporation has unlimited life: It can continue in existence after its original owners and managers have died or left the company; (2) it is easy to transfer ownership in a corporation because ownership is divided into shares of stock that can be easily sold, at least for large corporations; and (3) owners of a corporation have limited liability.

Most large healthcare organizations are corporations. Some examples are Columbia/HCA Healthcare in the hospital industry, Beverly Enterprises in the nursing home industry, United HealthCare in the managed care industry, and Bristol-Myers Squibb in the pharmaceutical industry.

To illustrate the limited liability feature, suppose you invested $25,000 in a partnership that went bankrupt with assets having a liquidation value of $100,000 and debts totaling $500,000. Since the partners are liable for the debts of the partnership, you could be assessed for a share of the partnership's debt in addition to losing your initial $25,000 contribution. In fact, if your partners are unable to pay their shares of the indebtedness, you could be held liable for the entire $400,000 deficiency. However, had your $25,000 been invested in a corporation that went bankrupt, your potential loss would be limited to the original $25,000 investment. Note, though, that the limited liability feature of ownership is often fictitious for small, financially weak corporations because bankers and other lenders will require personal guarantees from the stockholders.

The three factors—unlimited life, ease of ownership transfer, and limited liability—make it much easier for corporations to raise money in the capital markets than for sole proprietorships or partnerships. Additionally, corporations historically have been able to provide more generous insurance and retirement plans to their managers than have sole proprietorships or partnerships, although this advantage has been reduced in the last few years.

A type of corporation that is common among physicians and other individual and group practice healthcare professionals is the professional corporation (PC) or, in some states, the professional association (PA). All 50 states have statutes that prescribe the requirements for such corporations, which provide the usual benefits of incorporation but do not relieve the participants of professional liability.

The corporate form of organization does have two primary disadvantages: (1) Corporate earnings of taxable entities are subject to double taxation—once at the corporate level and then again at the personal level when dividends are paid to stockholders; and (2) setting up a corporation—which requires drawing up a charter and bylaws, and then filing the required periodic state and federal reports—is more costly and time-consuming than for a sole proprietorship or partnership.

FORMS OF OWNERSHIP

One of the major differences between the healthcare industry and other industries is the variety in forms of ownership. Most industries consist entirely of investor-owned (for-profit) corporations. However, in the healthcare industry, not-for-profit corporations play a major role. For example, about 60 percent of the hospitals in the United States are private, not-for-profit hospitals; 25 percent are governmental; and only 15 percent are investor owned. Furthermore, not-for-profit ownership is common in the nursing home, home healthcare, and managed care industries. Since the form of ownership affects the way decisions are made, it is essential for managers in the healthcare industry to understand the differences among the forms of ownership and how these differences impact financial decision making. (The financial management of governmental entities is fundamentally different from the financial management of private businesses. This book is designed for financial decision making in private businesses, although the basic concepts presented are applicable in all situations.)

Investor-Owned (For-Profit) Corporations

When the average person thinks of a corporation, he or she thinks of an investor-owned, or for-profit, corporation. The IBMs and General Motors of this world, along with Columbia/HCA Healthcare and Beverly Enterprises, are investor-owned corporations. Investors become owners of such companies by buying the firm's common stock. Investors may buy the common stock of the firm when it first sells its shares to the public, which is called an initial public offering (IPO). Funds raised from new shareholders in an IPO generally go to the issuing corporation. However, in some situations, shares can be sold to the public for the first time by the company's original owners rather than by the company itself. In this case, the proceeds from the sale go to the original owners, not to the company.

Once shares are initially sold in an IPO, they are traded in the secondary market, either through exchanges such as the New York Stock Exchange (NYSE) and the American Stock Exchange (AMEX) or in the over-the-counter (OTC) market. When shares are bought and sold in the secondary market, the corporations whose stock is traded receive no funds from the trades; corporations only receive funds when the shares are initially sold. For example, Beverly Enterprises, the largest operator of nursing homes in the United States, has about 98 million shares of common stock outstanding, owned by about 8,000 stockholders, including mutual and pension funds that, in turn, are owned by thousands of individuals. In 1995, 157,740,000 shares of Beverly were traded on the NYSE; so, on average, a share was sold more than once during the year. These transactions were solely between investors, and Beverly Enterprises did not receive a nickel from the trades.

As the owners of investor-owned companies, shareholders have three basic rights:

1. *The right of control.* Common stockholders, and no one else, have the right to vote for the corporation's board of directors. The board of directors, in turn, elects the management team that runs the day-to-day operations of the corporation. Each year, a company's shareholders receive a proxy ballot, which they use to vote for directors as well as for other issues that require shareholder approval. In this way, shareholders exercise control.

2. *The right to residual earnings.* Shareholders have claim to the residual earnings, or net income, of the firm. A corporation sells products or services and realizes revenues from the sales. To produce these revenues, the corporation must incur expenses for materials, labor, insurance, debt capital, and so on. Any excess (or loss) of revenues over expenses belongs to the owners—the shareholders—of the firm. Management may elect to retain some of the earnings in the firm rather than pay them out to the shareholders as dividends, but this is presumably done with the owners' blessing, since the funds belong to the shareholders.

3. *The right to residual liquidation proceeds.* In the event of bankruptcy and liquidation, the shareholders are entitled to any proceeds that remain after all other claimants are satisfied. However, since

shareholders are last on the priority list of liquidation claimants, shareholders often receive nothing when corporations go bankrupt.

There are three key features of investor-owned corporations that impact managerial decision making: (1) The owners of the firm are well defined, and they exercise control of the firm by the proxy process; (2) the residual earnings of the firm belong to the owners, so management is responsible to a single, well-defined group (the stockholders) for the profitability of the firm; and (3) investor-owned corporations are subject to taxation at the local, state, and federal levels.

Not-for-Profit (Tax-Exempt) Corporations

If a corporation meets a set of stringent requirements, it can qualify for tax-exempt status. Such businesses are called not-for-profit corporations or tax-exempt corporations. Tax-exempt corporations are sometimes called nonprofit corporations, but since such businesses need profits to sustain operations, most industry participants prefer the term not-for-profit corporation. Tax-exempt status is granted to organizations that meet the tax definition of a charitable organization and hence qualify under Internal Revenue Service (IRS) Tax Code Section 501(c)(3) or 501(c)(4). Thus, such corporations are also known as 501(c)(3) or 501(c)(4) corporations.

Not-for-profit corporations can be pure charities, such as the American Heart Association, or can be not-for-profit businesses that produce services for sale, such as not-for-profit hospitals. Financial decision making is somewhat different for pure charities than for businesses. This book, which focuses on financial decision making within revenue-generating entities, concentrates on not-for-profit businesses.

The key to tax-exempt status is charitable activity. The tax code defines a charitable organization as any corporation, community chest, fund, or foundation that is organized and operated exclusively for religious, charitable, scientific, public safety, literary, or educational purposes. Since the promotion of health is commonly considered a charitable activity, a corporation that provides healthcare services, provided it meets other requirements, can qualify for tax-exempt status. In addition to the charitable purpose, a not-for-profit corporation must be organized and operated so that (1) it operates exclusively for the public, rather than private, interest; (2) none of the profits are used for private gain; (3) no political activity is conducted; and (4) if liquidation occurs, the assets will continue to be used for a charitable purpose. Since individuals cannot benefit from not-for-profit corporations' profits, such organizations cannot pay dividends. Note, however, that prohibition of private gain does not prevent parties to not-for-profit corporations, such as managers, from benefiting through salaries, perquisites, and the like.

Not-for-profit corporations differ significantly from investor-owned corporations. Since not-for-profit firms have no shareholders, there is no single body of individuals who have ownership rights to the firm's residual earnings and who exercise control of the firm. Rather, control is exercised by a board of trustees, which is not constrained by outside oversight. Also, not-for-profit corporations are generally exempt from taxation, including both property and income taxes, and they have the right to issue tax-exempt debt. Finally, individual contributions to not-for-profit organizations can be deducted from taxable income by the donor, so not-for-profit firms have access to tax-favored contribution capital.

The fiscal problems currently facing the federal and most state and local governments have caused some politicians to take a closer look at the tax subsidies provided to not-for-profit hospitals. For example, several bills recently have been introduced in Congress that would require hospitals to meet minimum standards for care to the indigent or lose federal tax-exempt status. Sponsors say the bills are needed because not-for-profit hospitals don't provide sufficient services to indigent patients despite generous tax breaks designed to promote charity care.

Officials in at least 12 states have also been fighting to restrict or strip tax exemptions to hospitals. Indeed, in 1993, Texas passed a law that sets charity care standards that hospitals must meet to maintain tax-exempt status. Furthermore, money-starved municipalities in several states have levied property taxes on not-for-profit hospitals that have neglected their charitable missions. More initiatives to restrict, or even abolish, tax-exempt status for hospitals are bound to appear in the future.

The inherent differences between investor-owned and not-for-profit organizations have profound implications for most elements of financial decision making, including goals of the firm, financing decisions (the choice between debt and equity financing and the types of securities to issue), and capital investment decisions.

These differences will be highlighted as they occur throughout the remainder of the book.

FINANCIAL GOALS

Financial decisions are not made in a vacuum but, rather, with some goal in mind. In general, financial decisions must be consistent with and support the firm's goals. Thus, a firm's goals provide the framework for its financial goals and hence for financial decision making within healthcare organizations.

Investor-Owned Firms

All corporations have a set of stakeholders who have an interest, primarily financial, in the business. For example, a hospital's stakeholders include its stockholders (if investor-owned), board of directors (or trustees), managers, employees, medical staff, creditors, suppliers, patients, and even its potential patients; so corporate managers have a large number of clienteles that could influence financial goals. However, since investor-owned corporations have a well-defined owner's clientele that employs the managers, the primary goal of investor-owned firms for financial decision-making purposes is generally assumed to be shareholder wealth maximization, which translates into stock price maximization. Investor-owned firms do, of course, have other objectives. Managers, who make the actual decisions, are interested in their own personal welfare, in their employees' welfare, and in the good of the community and of society at large. Still, for investor-owned firms such as Columbia/HCA Healthcare and Beverly Enterprises, the goal of stock price maximization is a reasonable operating objective upon which to build financial decision rules.

The primary obstacle to universal acceptance of shareholder wealth maximization as the goal of investor-owned firms is the agency problem. An agency problem exists when one or more individuals (the principals) hire another individual or group of individuals (the agents) to perform some service on their behalf, and then delegate decision-making authority to those agents.

An agency problem between stockholders and managers is created whenever the manager of a firm owns less than 100 percent of the firm's common stock. If a firm is a sole proprietorship managed by the owner, it will be managed to maximize the owner's well-being. Much of the owner's well-being will stem from increased personal wealth, but the owner will also extract well-being from the firm in the form of perquisites or leisure. Since there are no other owners, no one is hurt by those owner/managers who want to take more of their well-being in the form of perquisites and leisure and less in personal wealth.

However, now assume that the owner/manager incorporates the business, sells half of the shares to outside stockholders, and keeps the manager's job. Now, one-half of the wealth created by the business goes to the outside shareholders, so there is less motivation for the owner-manager to take all actions possible to maximize shareholder wealth. Furthermore, half the costs of perquisites and leisure are being borne by the nonmanager owners. Thus, with outside shareholders, managers are less motivated to pursue shareholder wealth maximization as the primary goal of the firm.

In general, the managers of large, investor-owned firms hold only a very small proportion of the firm's stock, so they benefit very little from stock price increases. On the other hand, managers benefit substantially from such actions as increasing the size of the firm to justify higher salaries and more perquisites, awarding themselves excessive retirement plans, and so on, while these actions are often detrimental to shareholders' wealth. It is easy to visualize many situations in which managers are motivated to take actions that are in their best interest rather than in the best interest of the firm's stockholders.

However, there are some actions shareholders can take to mitigate the agency problem, and market forces also act to keep managers focused on shareholders' concerns, including stock price. For example, executive compensation packages usually include some elements that are tied either directly or indirectly to stock price. Also, institutional investors, which now dominate ownership and trading of common stocks, are exercising more and more influence over managerial actions, especially when managers have not been acting in shareholders' interests. Finally, companies that are poor performers are much more subject to hostile takeovers than are companies whose stock price is maximized. In the words of the president of a major managed care corporation, "If you want to keep control, don't let your company's stock sell at a bargain price."

In summary, it is clear that managers of investor-owned firms can have motivations that are inconsistent with shareholder wealth maximization. Still, there are sufficient mechanisms at work to force managers to view shareholder wealth maximization as an important, if not primary, goal. Thus, shareholder wealth maximization is a reasonable goal for financial decision making within investor-owned firms.

Not-for-Profit Firms

The appropriate financial goal for not-for-profit firms is not as clear-cut as for investor-owned firms. Since not-for-profit firms do not have shareholder/owners, it is clear that shareholder wealth maximization is not an appropriate goal for such organizations. While managers of investor-owned companies can ensure job security and good compensation by pleasing only one clientele of stakeholders—the shareholders—managers of not-for-profit firms face a different situation. They have to be responsive to different stakeholder clienteles because there is not a single, well-defined group that exercises control.

Typically, the goal of not-for-profit firms is stated in terms of a mission. For example, the mission statement of Crescent Beach Community Hospital, a 350-bed, not-for-profit, acute care hospital, is as follows:

> Crescent Beach Community Hospital, along with its medical staff, is a recognized, innovative healthcare leader dedicated to meeting the needs of the community. We strive to be the best comprehensive healthcare provider through our commitment to excellence.

Although this mission statement provides the hospital's managers and employees with a framework for developing specific goals and objectives, it does not provide much insight into the hospital's financial goals. For Crescent Beach Community Hospital to accomplish its mission, its managers have identified five financial goals.

1. The hospital must maintain its financial viability.
2. The hospital must generate sufficient profits to permit it to continue to provide the current range of healthcare services to the community. This means that current plant and equipment must be replaced as it becomes obsolete.

3. The hospital must generate sufficient profits to invest in new medical technologies and services as they are developed and needed.
4. Although the hospital has an aggressive philanthropy program in place, it does not want to rely on this program, or government grants, to fund its operations.
5. The hospital will strive to provide services to the community as inexpensively as possible, given the above financial requirements.

In effect, the hospital's managers are saying that to achieve the "commitment to excellence" contained in its mission statement, the hospital must remain financially strong and profitable. Financially weak organizations cannot continue to accomplish their stated missions over the long run.

It is interesting to note that Crescent Beach Community Hospital's financial management practices are probably not much different from the practices of investor-owned hospitals. Of course, for-profit hospitals have to worry about stock price, and they receive only an insignificant number of contributions and grants. But, to maximize shareholder wealth, for-profit hospitals also must retain their financial viability and have the financial resources necessary to offer new services and technologies. Furthermore, competition in the market for hospital services will not permit for-profit hospitals to charge appreciably more for services than their not-for-profit competitors do. Although for-profit and not-for-profit corporations are fundamentally different, day-to-day financial decisions within the two types of businesses are likely to have a common goal: to maintain the financial viability of the enterprise.

BASIC FINANCIAL STATEMENTS

Financial statements provide a means for reporting the financial condition of a business, so it is important for healthcare managers to have a basic understanding of these statements. The two statements that are most important to understanding financial decision making are the income statement and the balance sheet. The next two sections briefly describe these statements. The purpose here is merely to provide the background needed to use these statements in financial decision making.

Income Statement

A firm's income statement provides information about its ability to generate profits over some reporting period, often a year. To illustrate, Table 1–1 contains the 1995 and 1996 income statements (also called statements of revenues and expenses) for Suburban Medical Center, a 650-bed, not-for-profit, acute care hospital.

Some points about the income statements are worth noting:

1. *General format.* The income statements in Table 1–1 reflect the general format specified by the accounting profession, although there is some flexibility in presentation. The first line of the income statement gives the hospital's patient services revenues, net of all allowances and bad debt losses. Then, the expenses incurred by the hospital in producing those revenues are reported and deducted from net revenues. Note that income is segregated into operating

TABLE 1–1

Suburban Medical Center: Income Statements for Years Ending December 31 (Thousands of Dollars)

	1996	1995
Net patient services revenue	$108,600	$ 97,393
Other operating revenue	6,205	9,364
Total operating revenue	$114,805	$106,757
Operating expenses:		
Nursing services	$ 58,285	$ 56,752
Dietary services	5,424	4,718
General services	13,198	11,655
Administrative services	11,427	11,585
Employee health and welfare	10,250	10,705
Provision for uncollectibles	3,328	3,469
Provision for malpractice	1,320	1,204
Depreciation	4,130	4,025
Interest expense	1,542	1,521
Total operating expenses	$108,904	$105,634
Income from operations	$ 5,901	$ 1,123
Contributions and grants	$ 2,253	$ 874
Investment income	418	398
Nonoperating gain (loss)	$ 2,671	$ 1,272
Net income (revenues over expenses)	$ 8,572	$ 2,395

and nonoperating so that it is easy to distinguish between income derived from the sale of products and services and income derived from other sources. (Note, though, that proposed changes in format may blur the distinction between operating and nonoperating income, at least in the body of the income statement.)

2. *Earnings*. Suburban had an excess of revenues over expenses (or net income) of $8,572,000 in 1996. Of course, being not-for-profit, the hospital paid no dividends, so it retained all of its $8,572,000 in net income. It is important to recognize that the earnings (excess of revenues over expenses, or net income) reported on a firm's income statement do not represent cash generated by operations but, rather, earnings as defined by generally accepted accounting principles.

3. *Cash flow*. A firm's net cash flow from operating and nonoperating sources is approximately equal to its net income plus any noncash expenses. (That is, any expense deducted from revenues that is not a cash expense must be added back to convert income to cash flow.) In 1996, Suburban's cash flow was $8,572,000 net income plus $4,130,000 depreciation (a noncash expense), for a total net cash flow of $12,702,000. Depreciation does not really provide funds; it is simply a noncash charge that is added back to net income to obtain an estimate of the firm's net cash flow from operating and nonoperating sources. Another statement, the statement of cash flows, provides clearer insights into Suburban's net cash flows, but a discussion of this statement is better left to accounting books.

Balance Sheet

Whereas the income statement reports on revenues and expenses over some period of time, the balance sheet provides a "snapshot" of a business's assets and liabilities at a single point in time. Any business must have assets if it is to operate; and in order to acquire assets, firms must obtain capital, which creates liabilities for the firm. Table 1–2 contains Suburban's 1995 and 1996 balance sheets.

Again, here are some pertinent points:

1. *General format*. The balance sheet is divided into two sections: the assets section and the liabilities and equity section.

2. *Assets*. The top, or assets, section of the balance sheet shows that Suburban needed $151,278,000 in total assets to generate its 1996 net patient services revenue of $108,600,000.

TABLE 1–2

Suburban Medical Center: Balance Sheets for December 31
(Thousands of Dollars)

	1996	1995
Assets:		
Cash and securities	$ 6,263	$ 5,095
Accounts receivable	21,840	20,738
Inventories	3,177	2,982
Total current assets	$ 31,280	$ 28,815
Gross plant and equipment	$145,158	$140,865
Accumulated depreciation	25,160	21,030
Net plant and equipment	$119,998	$119,835
Total assets	$151,278	$148,650
Liabilities and Equity:		
Accounts payable	$ 4,707	$ 5,145
Accrued wages	5,650	5,421
Notes payable	2,975	6,237
Total current liabilities	$ 13,332	$ 16,803
Long-term debt	30,582	33,055
Fund balance	107,364	98,792
Total liabilities and funds	$151,278	$148,650

Assets are grouped into two categories: current and fixed. Current assets are assets, such as inventories, that have a relatively short life, usually less than one year, before they are converted into cash. Fixed assets are long-term assets such as land, buildings, and equipment. Of Suburban's 1996 total assets of $151,278,000, $31,280,000 were in current, or short-term, assets. Cash and securities, which represents actual cash and commercial checking accounts as well as short-term securities holdings, totaled $6,263,000; accounts receivable, which represents services provided but revenues not yet collected, totaled $21,840,000; and inventories of supplies totaled $3,177,000. The gross plant and equipment (fixed assets) amount of $145,158,000 represents the initial cost of Suburban's land, hospital, and equipment, but wear and tear (depreciation) over time has reduced the value of the fixed assets by $25,160,000. Consequently, the accounting value of the firm's long-term assets at the end of 1996 was $119,998,000.

3. *Liabilities and equity.* The bottom, or liabilities and equity, section of the balance sheet lists a firm's sources of capital. Capital comes in two basic forms: debt and equity. There are many different types of debt capital: long-term and short-term, interest-bearing and non-interest-bearing, secured and unsecured, taxable and tax-exempt, and so on. Similarly, there are different types of equity capital. For example, in investor-owned corporations, equity is represented by preferred stock and common stock, while the equivalent capital in not-for-profit corporations is called "fund capital."

Suburban obtained the funds, or capital, used to purchase its $151,278,000 in assets (1) by buying supplies on credit from its suppliers (accounts payable); (2) by paying its employees' wages periodically rather than daily (accrued wages); (3) by borrowing from banks (notes payable); (4) by borrowing from institutions such as insurance companies and mutual funds, as well as from individuals (long-term debt); and (6) by retaining earnings in the firm (fund balance). Accounts payable, accrued wages, and notes payable are liabilities that must be paid off (satisfied) within one year, so they are classified as current liabilities. Long-term debts have maturities over one year, so they are classified as long-term liabilities, while fund capital represents the cumulative profitability of the hospital.

4. *Cash versus other assets.* Although the hospital's assets are all stated in terms of dollars, only cash represents actual money. We see that Suburban could—if it liquidated any securities held—write checks at the end of 1996 for a total of $6,263,000 (versus current liabilities of $13,332,000 coming due during 1997). The non-cash current assets (accounts receivable and inventories) will presumably be converted to cash within a year, but they do not represent cash on hand.

5. *Retentions.* A firm's fund (equity) account is built up over time by retentions (retained earnings). Note that in 1996 Suburban reported on its income statement an $8,572,000 excess of earnings over expenses. Since none of this amount can be paid out in dividends, the entire excess is retained in the firm. Thus, barring any asset sales or revaluations, Suburban's fund account should increase from year to year by the amount of net income (excess of revenues over expenses).

1996 Fund balance = 1995 Fund balance + 1996 Net income
$107,364,000 = $98,792,000 + $8,572,000

6. *Accumulated depreciation.* Accumulated depreciation reported on the balance sheet is subtracted from gross fixed assets, so the larger a firm's accumulated depreciation, all else the same, the smaller the reported value of its total assets. Note that accumulated depreciation on the balance sheet increases each year by the amount of depreciation expense reported on the income statement.

1996 Accumulated depreciation = 1995 Accumulated depreciation + 1996 Depreciation expense
$25,160,000 = $21,030,000 + $4,130,000

SOME IMPORTANT FINANCIAL MEASURES

It is often useful to combine some of the elements of a firm's income statement and balance sheet to create ratios that summarize various aspects of financial performance. This section, which uses 1996 data from Tables 1–1 and 1–2, presents several such ratios.

Total Margin (Total Profit Margin)

The total margin, or total profit margin, is computed by dividing net income (excess of revenues over expenses) by revenues, and it gives the overall profit per dollar of sales.

$$\text{Total margin} = \frac{\text{Net income}}{\text{Revenues}} = \frac{\$8,572}{\$114,805} = 7.5\%$$

The total margin tells us that Suburban made 7.5 cents on every dollar of revenue in 1996. Note, however, that the total margin includes profits made on both operating and nonoperating activities.

Operating Margin

The operating margin is computed by dividing operating income (excess of operating revenues over operating expenses) by revenues, and it gives the operating profit per dollar of sales.

$$\text{Operating margin} = \frac{\text{Operating income}}{\text{Revenues}} = \frac{\$5,901}{\$114,805} = 5.1\%$$

Suburban's operating margin indicates that the hospital generated 5.1 cents of operating profits on each dollar of net revenue.

Note that the operating margin removes the influence of nonoperating gains and losses and hence focuses on the profitability of the hospital's primary line of business. Margin measures indicate how much of revenues flow through to profits. Since expenses take away from profits, margin measures give a good indication of how well a firm is managing its expenses.

Return on Assets (ROA)

The ratio of net income to total assets measures the return on assets (ROA).

$$\text{Return on assets} = \frac{\text{Net income}}{\text{Total assets}} = \frac{\$8,572}{\$151,278} = 5.7\%$$

ROA measures how well a firm's assets are generating profits. The higher the ROA, the better the firm's assets are performing. In 1996, Suburban generated 5.7 cents for each dollar invested in assets.

Return on Equity (ROE)

The ratio of net income to total equity (fund capital) measures the return on equity (ROE).

$$\text{Return on equity} = \frac{\text{Net income}}{\text{Total equity}} = \frac{\$8,572}{\$107,364} = 8.0\%$$

ROE focuses on the return to stockholders' total investment for investor-owned firms and on the return on fund capital for not-for-profit firms. Thus, Suburban's fund capital investment generated 8.0 cents for each dollar invested in 1996. Note that ROA and ROE could be calculated on the basis of operating income rather than net income to remove the impact of nonoperating gains and losses.

Total Debt to Total Assets (Debt Ratio)

The ratio of total debt to total assets, generally called the debt ratio, measures the percentage of total funds provided by creditors.

$$\text{Debt ratio} = \frac{\text{Total debt}}{\text{Total assets}} = \frac{\$43,914}{\$151,278} = 0.290, \text{ or } 29.0\%$$

Debt is defined here to include both current liabilities and long-term debt. Creditors prefer low debt ratios since the lower the ratio, the greater the cushion against creditors' losses in the event of liquidation. The owners, on the other hand, may seek higher debt usage either to magnify earnings or because selling new stock would mean giving up some degree of control. In not-for-profit firms, managers may use high amounts of debt to fund services that cannot be supported by profit retentions.

TAXES

The values of financial assets, such as a share of stock issued by Beverly Enterprises or a municipal bond issued by the Alachua County Health Facilities Authority for Shands Hospital, as well as the values of many real assets such as medical office buildings, hospitals, and MRI systems, depend on the stream of usable cash flows that the asset is expected to produce. Since taxes can reduce the cash flows that are usable to an asset's owners, financial decisions must include the impact of local, state, and federal taxes.

Local and state tax laws vary widely, and federal tax laws change often. On average, there have been major changes to the federal tax code every three to four years since 1913, when the federal tax system was initiated. Furthermore, certain aspects of the tax code are tied to inflation, so changes automatically occur each year based on the previous year's inflation rate. For these reasons, it is not practical to provide a thorough discussion of tax laws in this book. It is necessary, though, to present some tax law concepts that will be used in later chapters.

Individual (Personal) Income Taxes

Individuals pay personal taxes on wages and salaries; on investment income such as dividends, interest, and profits from the sale of securities; and on the profits of sole proprietorships and partnerships. Federal income taxes are progressive; that is, the higher one's income, the larger the marginal tax rate. (The marginal rate is the rate on the last dollar earned.) Currently (1996), the highest marginal federal tax rate for individuals is 39.6 percent, and Medicare taxes and deduction disallowances can raise this rate to over 40 percent. When state and local income taxes are factored in, individual income tax marginal rates can climb to 50 percent.

Individuals can receive dividend income on stocks and mutual funds that they own and interest income on savings accounts, certificates of deposit, bonds, and the like. Such income from securities is taxed as ordinary income and hence is taxed at rates going up to 50 percent. Since corporations pay dividends out of earnings that have already been taxed, there is double taxation on corporate income.

Note, however, that under federal tax laws, interest on most state and local government bonds, called municipals, or munis, is not subject to federal income taxes. Such bonds include bonds issued by municipal healthcare authorities on behalf of not-for-profit healthcare organizations. Thus, investors get to keep all of the interest received from municipal bonds but only a portion of the interest received from bonds issued by the federal government or by corporations. This means that a lower interest rate muni bond can provide the same after-tax return as a higher-yielding corporate or Treasury bond.

For example, consider a taxpayer in the 39.6 percent federal tax bracket who could buy a taxable corporate bond that yielded 10 percent interest ($10 of interest per year per $100 of investment). What yield would a similar risk muni bond have to offer to make the investor indifferent between the muni and the corporate? (For simplicity, assume there is no state income tax. If state income taxes apply, the after-tax return on the corporate bond is reduced even further. Municipal bond income is exempt from state taxes in the state of issuance.)

Here's how to think about this problem. If an individual owns a $1,000 bond, the annual interest payment is $0.10(\$1,000) = \$100$ per year. (Bonds typically pay interest semiannually, so the annual payment actually would consist of two $50 payments.) The after-tax yield, or return, on the corporate bond is found as follows:

$$
\begin{aligned}
\text{After-tax return} &= \text{Pretax yield} - \text{Yield lost to taxes} \\
&= \text{Pretax yield} - \text{Pretax yield(Tax rate)} \\
&= \text{Pretax yield}(1 - T) \\
&= 10\%(1 - 0.396) = 10\%(0.604) = 6.04\%
\end{aligned}
$$

where T is the investor's marginal tax rate. The investor would have to pay income taxes of $39.60 on the $100 interest received. Under these conditions, the investor would be indifferent between a corporate bond with a 10 percent yield and a municipal bond with a 6.04 percent yield, assuming that the bonds had similar risk.

If the investor wanted to know what yield on a taxable bond is equivalent to a 6.04 percent yield on a muni bond, he or she would follow this procedure:

$$\text{Equivalent yield on taxable bond} = \frac{\text{Yield on muni}}{1-T}$$

$$= \frac{6.04\%}{1-0.396} = \frac{6.04\%}{0.604} = 10.0\%$$

The exemption of municipal bonds from federal taxes stems from the separation of power of federal and state and local governments, and its primary effect is to allow state and local governments—and hence not-for-profit healthcare providers—to borrow at lower rates than otherwise possible.

Corporate Income Taxes

Income generated by for-profit corporations is taxed at the federal level at marginal rates that run from 15 percent to 39 percent.

Interest and Dividends Received by an Investor-Owned Corporation

Interest income received by a taxable corporation is taxed as ordinary income. However, in general, 70 percent of the dividends received by one corporation from another is excluded from taxable income, while the remaining 30 percent is taxed at the ordinary tax rate. Thus, a corporation paying a 34 percent marginal tax rate would have an effective tax rate of only $0.30(0.34) = 0.102 = 10.2\%$ on its dividend income. If this company had \$10,000 in pretax dividend income, its after-tax dividend income would be \$8,980.

$$
\begin{aligned}
\text{After-tax income} &= \text{Pretax income} - \text{Taxes} \\
&= \text{Pretax income} - \text{Pretax income} \\
&\quad \text{(Effective tax rate)} \\
&= \text{Pretax income}(1 - \text{Effective tax rate}) \\
&= \$10,000[1 - 0.30\,(0.34)] \\
&= \$10,000(1 - 0.102) = \$10,000(0.898) \\
&= \$8,980
\end{aligned}
$$

If a taxable corporation has surplus funds that can be temporarily invested in securities, the tax laws favor investment in stocks, which pay dividends, rather than in bonds, which pay interest. For example, suppose Superior Home Health Services has $100,000 to invest temporarily, and it could buy either bonds that paid interest of $8,000 per year or preferred stock that paid dividends of $7,000 per year. Since Superior's marginal tax rate is 34 percent, its tax on the interest if it bought the bonds would be 0.34($8,000) = $2,720, so its after-tax income would be $8,000 − $2,720 = $5,280. If it bought the preferred stock, its tax would be 0.34[0.30($7,000)] = $714, resulting in an after-tax income of $6,286. Other factors might lead Superior to invest in the bonds; but, for taxable corporate investors, the tax laws clearly favor stock investments.

Interest and Dividends Received by a Not-for-Profit Corporation

Interest and dividend income received from securities purchased by not-for-profit corporations with temporary surplus cash is not taxable. Note, however, that not-for-profit firms are prohibited from issuing tax-exempt bonds for the specific purpose of investing the proceeds in other securities. If not-for-profit firms could engage in such tax arbitrage operations, they could, in theory, generate an unlimited amount of income by issuing tax-exempt bonds that require, say, a 5 percent interest rate, and then use the proceeds to purchase higher-yielding securities that are taxable to most investors, say, Treasury bonds with a 6 percent interest rate.

Interest and Dividends Paid by an Investor-Owned Corporation

A firm's assets can be financed either with debt or equity capital. If a firm uses debt financing, it must pay interest on that debt; whereas, if a taxable firm uses equity financing, it will usually pay dividends to its stockholders. Corporate interest paid is deducted from operating income to obtain taxable income, but dividends are not tax deductible. Put another way, dividends are paid from after-tax income. Therefore, Superior Home Health Services, which is in the 34 percent tax bracket, needs only $1 of pretax earnings to pay $1 of interest expense, but it needs $1.52 of pretax earnings to pay $1 in dividends.

$$\text{Dollars of pretax income} = \frac{\$1}{1 - \text{Tax rate}} = \frac{\$1}{0.66} = \$1.52$$

The implication here is that the government subsidizes debt financing by making interest payments tax deductible, but it grants no such benefit to equity financing. This differential taxation of interest and dividend payments has a profound impact on the choice between debt and equity financing, as you will see in Chapter 10.

At the three-mile mark of their jog, George and Beth reached some conclusions about the similarities and differences between healthcare and other businesses, and between for-profit and not-for-profit organizations. First, they concluded that a business is a business is a business. In essence, healthcare firms must operate just like firms in other industries, especially service industries. Capital must be raised and invested in assets, and then those assets must be operated efficiently.

Also, Beth finally agreed that the ability of a not-for-profit business to provide services to the community depends on its financial viability. Thus, proposed investments must be evaluated for profitability, and unprofitable investments must be carefully scrutinized to ensure that the benefit to the community outweighs their negative financial impact.

As their jog wound down, George and Beth concluded that, from a financial perspective, neither industry nor ownership has a significant impact on financial analysis and decision making. Those financial characteristics that lead to stock price maximization for investor-owned firms also contribute to financial flexibility for not-for-profit firms. To be competitive in the market for healthcare services, the two types of firms must operate in much the same way.

SELF-ASSESSMENT EXERCISES

Each chapter contains a set of self-assessment exercises. These exercises cover the key points of the chapter, and they give you the opportunity to assess your understanding of the material. Solutions to the self-assessment exercises are contained in Appendix A.

1–1 a. What are the three primary forms of business organization (as opposed to ownership)?

b. Briefly describe the advantages and disadvantages of each form.

1–2   The two major types of ownership are investor-owned (for-profit) and not-for-profit businesses.

   a. Who are the owners of investor-owned corporations? How do they exercise control? Who has claim to the profits (residual earnings) of investor-owned firms?

   b. Who are the owners of not-for-profit corporations? Who exercises control over a not-for-profit firm's managers? Who has claim to the profits (excess of revenues over expenses) of not-for-profit firms?

   c. What requirements must be met for a corporation to qualify for not-for-profit status?

   d. What are the differences in tax treatment between investor-owned and not-for-profit businesses?

1–3   Financial management decisions are not made in a vacuum but, rather, with some objective(s) in mind.

   a. What is the primary goal of investor-owned firms?

   b. Do managers of investor-owned firms always act in the best interests of their firms' owners? What is the name of the managerial self-interest problem? What factors tend to influence managers to act in the best interests of their firms' owners?

   c. Who are a firm's stakeholders? Do both investor-owned and not-for-profit firms have stakeholders?

   d. Regardless of the overall mission of a not-for-profit firm, what might be some of its financial manage-ment goals? Are the financial management goals of investor-owned and not-for-profit firms appreciably different?

1–4   Suppose an individual is considering buying a $1,000 U.S. Treasury bond (T-bond) that pays $80 in interest annually. Thus, the rate of return (yield) on the bond is 8.0 percent.

   a. What is the after-tax yield on this bond to an indi-vidual investor in the 28 percent tax bracket?

   b. As an alternative, assume that the investor could buy a $1,000 municipal (tax-exempt) hospital rev-enue bond that pays $70 in interest annually. What yield would a taxable T-bond have to offer to make the investor indifferent to the two alternatives? (Assume that the two bonds are similar in all other respects, including risk.)

1–5   Consider the following questions related to the taxation of investor-owned corporations.

    a. Generally, taxable corporations pay interest expense on their debt financing and dividends on their equity financing. Explain the difference in tax consequences to the paying firm between interest and dividends. Do the U.S. tax laws favor one form of financing (debt or equity) over the other?

    b. Now assume that a taxable firm has excess cash to invest and that it can invest the funds in either bonds (and earn interest) or preferred stock (and earn dividends) of the XYZ Company. Both investments have the same pretax yield. From a tax standpoint alone, which of the two investments makes the most sense? Why?

    c. Now assume that the pretax yield on XYZ's bonds is 10 percent and that the pretax yield on its preferred stock is 9 percent. What is the after-tax rate of return (yield) on each investment to a taxable corporation in the 34 percent tax bracket? What is the after-tax rate of return on each investment to an individual investor in the 28 percent tax bracket?

1–6   Briefly explain the following five important finance concepts.

    a. Cash is king.

    b. Time value of money.

    c. Risk and return.

    d. Opportunity costs.

    e. Don't put all your eggs in one basket.

1–7   a. What is the purpose and structure of an income statement?

    b. What is the purpose and structure of a balance sheet?

c. What is the definition and interpretation of the following financial measures?

(1) Total margin.

(2) Operating margin.

(3) Return on assets.

(4) Return on equity.

(5) Debt ratio.

SELECTED REFERENCES

Blair, John D., Grant T. Savage, and Carlton J. Whitehead. "A Strategic Approach for Negotiating with Hospital Stakeholders." *Healthcare Management Review,* Winter 1989, pp. 13–23.

Clement, Jan P., Dean G. Smith, and John R. C. Wheeler. "What Do We Want and What Do We Get from Not-for-Profit Hospitals?" *Hospital and Health Services Administration,* Summer 1994, pp. 159–78.

Fallon, Robert P. "Not-For-Profit Does Not Equal No Profit: Profitability Planning in Not-For-Profit Organizations." *Health Care Management Review,* Summer 1991, pp. 47–59.

Fottler, Myron D., John D. Blair, Carlton J. Whitehead, Michael D. Laus, and Grant T. Savage. "Assessing Key Stakeholders: Who Matters to Hospitals and Why?" *Hospital and Health Services Administration,* Winter 1989, pp. 525–46.

Herzlinger, Regina E., and William S. Krasker. "Who Profits From Nonprofits." *Harvard Business Review,* January–February 1987, pp. 93–105.

McLean, Robert A. "Agency Costs and Complex Contracts in Healthcare Organizations." *Health Care Management Review,* Winter 1989, pp. 65–71.

Nauert, Roger C., A. Beckwith Sanborn, II, Charles F. MacKelvie, and James L. Harvitt. "Hospitals Face Loss of Federal Tax-Exempt Status." *Healthcare Financial Management,* September 1988, pp. 48–60.

Pink, George H., and Peggy Leatt. "Are Managers Compensated for Hospital Financial Performance?" *Health Care Management Review,* Summer 1991, pp. 37–45.

Umbdenstock, Richard J., Winifred M. Hageman, and Bruce Amundson. "The Five Critical Areas for Effective Governance of Not-for-Profit Hospitals." *Hospital and Health Services Administration,* Winter 1990, pp. 481–92.

Walker, C. Langford, and L. Wade Humphreys. "Hospital Control and Decision Making: A Financial Perspective." *Healthcare Financial Management,* June 1993, pp. 90–96.

Wolfson, Jay, and Scott L. Hopes. "What Makes Tax-Exempt Hospitals Special?" *Healthcare Financial Management,* July 1994, pp. 57–60.

2

CHAPTER

Investment Returns and Financial Risk

The board of trustees at South Mesa Regional Medical Center, a not-for-profit hospital, faced a big decision at their most recent meeting. The main agenda item was whether or not to approve a proposed expansion into home healthcare. At the meeting, the financial staff presented an analysis of the proposed project, indicating that they thought the project would be profitable under the most likely scenario regarding number of home visits, types of services provided, and reimbursement levels. On the basis of this analysis, several of the board members favored approval.

However, just before a vote was taken, Paul Vogel, a board member and president of a local bank, asked the CFO if the staff had conducted a risk analysis. Somewhat sheepishly, the CFO admitted that the financial staff did not think a risk analysis was necessary. "Besides," he added, "none of the board would understand what it was all about, so it would just be a big waste of time."

Needless to say, many of the board members were less than enthusiastic about the CFO's response to Mr. Vogel's question, so they quickly agreed to table the agenda item until the next meeting, at which time the CFO was directed to present a risk analysis of the project. With nothing significant remaining on the agenda, the meeting ended much earlier than normal. However, several of the board members stayed on to discuss the entire concept of risk as it relates to healthcare investment decisions. Since most of the board members were professionals who had to deal with financial risk in their own businesses, just about everyone had some ideas on the subject.

After over an hour of discussion, the late-stayers decided to call it a day. Nothing really had been resolved, but they all agreed on three points. First, financial risk is too important to ignore when making business decisions, especially in those decisions that will have a profound impact on the future financial condition of the business. Second, risk means many things to many people; so to feel comfortable about incorporating risk into business decision processes, it is necessary to develop a formal definition of risk. Finally, to be usable in business decisions, financial risk must be quantitatively measurable, so decision makers can judge which alternatives are riskier than others.

At the following board meeting, the CFO presented a risk analysis of the hospital's proposed expansion into home healthcare. After you read the chapter, you should have a much better understanding of what financial risk is all about. Read the CFOs comments at the end of the chapter and see if you agree with his analysis and the ultimate decision.

INTRODUCTION

Two of the most important concepts in healthcare financial analysis and decision making are investment returns and financial risk. How are financial returns measured? What is financial risk, how is it measured, and what impact does it have on managerial decisions? In all honesty, it would be great if we could just gloss over financial risk, and its related concept of returns, and quickly move on to more applied topics such as capital investment and financing decisions. Unfortunately, it is just not possible to gain a solid understanding of healthcare financial analysis and decision making without having a solid appreciation of risk and return concepts.

If investors—both individuals and businesses—viewed risk as a benign fact of life, there would be little problem. However, decision makers are, for the most part, averse to risk. Risk is to be avoided, and if it is to be taken on, there must be some reward for doing so. Thus, decision makers view risk as a "four-letter word." Investments of higher risk, whether they be stock investments of an individual or diagnostic equipment investments of a radiology group, must offer higher returns to make them financially worthwhile. It is this characteristic of good financial decision making that makes risk concepts so important.

Two factors come into play that complicate any discussion of financial risk. First, financial risk is seen both by businesses and the investors in businesses. There is some risk inherent in the business itself that depends on the type of business. For example, pharmaceutical firms are generally acknowledged to face a great deal of risk, while healthcare providers typically have less risk. Then, the investors in any business (the stockholders and creditors) must bear the riskiness inherent in the business but as modified by the nature of the securities they hold. For example, the stock of Beverly Enterprises is more risky than the debt of the firm, although the risk of both securities depends on the inherent risk of the long-term care industry. Not-for-profit firms have the same partitioning of risk with debtholders, but now the inherent riskiness of the business is split between debtholders and noncreditor stakeholders, including managers, employees, suppliers, and other parties to the firm.

The second complicating factor results because the riskiness of any asset changes with the context in which the asset is held. For example, a stock held in isolation is riskier than the same stock held as part of a large portfolio (collection) of stocks. Similarly, an MRI system that is operated independently is more risky than one that is operated by a large, geographically-dispersed company that owns numerous types of diagnostic equipment.

In this chapter, basic risk concepts are presented from both the standpoint of individual investors and businesses. It is necessary for healthcare managers to be familiar with both contexts because investors supply the capital that businesses need to function. But, before beginning the discussion of financial risk, it is necessary to understand the concept of investment returns.

INVESTMENT RETURNS

In most investments, an individual or a business spends money today with the expectation of receiving money in the future. To illustrate, suppose you buy 10 shares of stock for $1,000. The stock pays no dividends, but at the end of one year, you sell the stock for

$1,100. What is the return on your $1,000 investment? One way of expressing an investment return is in dollar terms. The dollar return is simply the total dollars received from the investment less the amount invested.

$$\text{Dollar return} = \text{Amount received} - \text{Amount invested}$$
$$= \$1,100 - \$1,000$$
$$= \$100$$

If, at the end of the year, you sold the stock for only $900, your dollar return would be –$100.

Although expressing returns in dollars is simple to do, there are two problems: (1) To make a meaningful judgment about the adequacy of the return, you need to know the amount invested—a $100 return after one year on a $100 investment is a very good return, while a $100 return on a $10,000 investment is a poor return. (2) You also need to know the timing of the return—a $100 return in one year on a $100 investment is a very good return, but a $100 return in 50 years is a poor return.

The solution to the problem of interpreting dollar returns is to express investment returns as a rate of return, or percentage return. For example, the rate of return on the stock investment, assuming the stock is sold for $1,100, is 10 percent.

$$\text{Rate of return} = \frac{\text{Amount received} - \text{Amount invested}}{\text{Amount invested}}$$
$$= \frac{\$1,100 - \$1,000}{\$1,000} = \frac{\$100}{\$1,000} = 0.10 = 10\%$$

Rate of return "normalizes" the return by considering the return per unit of investment. In this example, the return of 0.10, or 10 percent, indicates that each dollar invested will earn 0.10 ($1.00) = $0.10, which amounts to 10 cents on the dollar. A negative rate of return indicates that the original investment will not even be recovered. For example, selling the stock for only $900 results in a –10 percent rate of return, which means that only 90 cents of every dollar invested will be returned. Note that a $10 return on a $1,000 investment results in a rate of return of only 1 percent, so percentage return takes into consideration the size of the investment.

Expressing rate of return on an annual basis, which is typically done in practice, also solves the timing (holding period) problem. A $10 return after one year on a $100 dollar investment results in a 10 percent annual rate of return, while a $10 return after five years only yields a 1.9 percent annual rate of return. You will learn the techniques necessary to calculate annual rates of return on investments of more than one year in Chapter 4.

INTRODUCTION TO FINANCIAL RISK

With the concept of financial return in mind, let's now turn our attention to financial risk. Risk is defined in most dictionaries as "a hazard; a peril; exposure to loss or injury." Thus, risk refers to the chance that some unfavorable event will occur. If you engage in skydiving, you are taking a chance with your life—skydiving is risky. If you gamble at roulette, you are not risking your life, but you are taking a financial risk. Even when you invest in stocks or bonds, you are taking a risk in the hope of earning a positive rate of return. Similarly, when a healthcare business invests in new assets such as diagnostic equipment, it is taking a financial risk.

To illustrate financial risk, consider two potential personal investments. The first investment consists of a one-year, $1,000 face value U.S. Treasury bill that you buy for $950. Treasury bills are sold at discount (less than face value) and return face, or par, value at maturity. You expect to receive $1,000 at maturity in one year, so your expected rate of return on the T-bill investment is ($1,000 − $950)/$950 = $50/$950 = 0.053 = 5.3%. Since the $1,000 return is fixed by contract (the T-bill promises to pay this amount), and since the U.S. government is certain to make the payment (the only exception would be a national disaster, a very improbable event), there is virtually a 100 percent probability that your investment will actually earn the 5.3 percent rate of return that you expect. In this situation, the investment is defined as being riskless, or risk free. (Note that the T-bill does have some purchasing power risk. Embedded in the 5.3 percent expected rate of return is some inflation expectation, and if actual inflation exceeds that expected, the real, or inflation adjusted, return will be less than expected. In many situations, however, purchasing power risk is not considered because it tends to affect all investments in a similar way.)

Now assume that your $950 is invested in a biotechnology partnership that will be terminated in one year. If the partnership develops a new commercially valuable product, its rights will be sold and you will receive \$2,000 from the partnership, for a rate of return of (\$2,000 − \$950)/\$950 = \$1,050/\$950 = 1.1053 = 110.53%. If nothing worthwhile is developed, the partnership will be worthless, you would receive nothing, and your rate of return would be (\$0 − \$950)/\$950 = −1.00 = −100%. Now assume there is a 50 percent chance that a valuable product will be developed. In this admittedly unrealistic situation, your expected rate of return (in the statistical sense) is the same 5.3 percent as on the T-bill investment: 0.50 (110.53%) + 0.50 (−100%) = 5.3%. However, the biotechnology partnership is a far cry from being riskless. If things go poorly, your realized rate of return will be −100 percent—you will lose the entire \$950 investment. Because there is a significant chance of actually earning a return that is considerably less than you expect to earn, the partnership investment is described as being very risky.

Financial risk, then, is related to the probability of earning a return less than expected. The greater the chance of low (or even negative) returns, the greater the amount of financial risk.

Note that we have taken a somewhat narrow view of financial risk, defining it as the probability of earning a return far below that expected. There are many different ways of viewing financial risk. For example, for a person saving for retirement, financial risk could be defined as the probability of not achieving some specified standard of living at retirement. However, the narrow definition presented here is most relevant to the types of business investment decisions made within healthcare organizations.

RISK AVERSION

Why is it so important to define and measure financial risk? The reason is that both individual and business investors, for the most part, dislike risk. Suppose you were given the choice between a sure one million dollars and the flip of a coin for either zero or two million dollars. You, and just about everyone else, would "take the million and run." Those people who take the sure million dollars are said to be "risk averse"; a person who is indifferent between the two alternatives (views them as the same) is risk neutral; and an individual who prefers the gamble over the sure thing is a risk seeker.

Of course, people and businesses do gamble and take other chances, so all of us typically exhibit some risk-seeking behavior at one time or another. However, most individual investors would never put a sizable proportion of their wealth at risk, and most business executives would never "bet the business" because most people are risk averse when it really matters.

What are the implications of risk aversion for financial decision making? First, given two investments with similar returns but differing risk, investors will favor the lower-risk alternative. Second, investors will require higher returns on higher-risk investments. These simple outcomes of risk-averse behavior have a significant impact on many facets of financial decision making, and hence these results will appear time and time again in later chapters.

PROBABILITY DISTRIBUTIONS

The chance that an event will occur is called its probability of occurrence, or just probability. For example, a weather forecast might predict a 40 percent chance of rain. Or, when rolling a single die (one of a pair of dice), the probability of rolling a two is one out of six, or $1/6 = 0.1667 = 16.67\%$. If all possible outcomes related to a particular event are listed, and a probability is assigned to each outcome, the result is a probability distribution. In the example of the role of a die, the probability distribution of outcomes looks like this:

Outcome	Probability
1	0.1667 = 16.67%
2	0.1667 = 16.67%
3	0.1667 = 16.67%
4	0.1667 = 16.67%
5	0.1667 = 16.67%
6	0.1667 = 16.67%
	1.0000 = 100.00%

The possible outcomes (the number of dots showing after the roll) are listed in the left column, while the probability of each outcome is listed in the right column, expressed as both decimals and percentages. For a complete probability distribution (one that includes all possible outcomes for the event), the probabilities must sum to 1.0, or 100 percent.

Probabilities can also be assigned to possible outcomes (in this case, returns) on both financial and real asset investments. If you buy a stock, the return will usually come in the form of dividends and capital gains (selling the stock for more than you paid for it) or losses (selling the stock for less than you paid for it). Since all stock returns are uncertain, there is some chance that the dividends will not be as high as expected or that the stock price will not increase as much as expected or that it will even decrease. The higher the probabilities of dividends and stock price well below those expected, the greater the risk.

For an example of a real asset investment, consider a hospital evaluating the purchase of an MRI system. The cost of the system is an investment, and the net cash inflows that stem from patient usage is the return. Thus, it is possible to estimate the expected return on the MRI investment. The return, however, is a function of the net cash inflows, which, in turn, are a function of the number of procedures, charge per procedure, negotiated discounts, operating costs, and so on. These values typically are not known with certainty, but rather depend on factors such as patient demographics, physician acceptance, HMO penetration, reimbursement levels, wage rates, and so on. Thus, the hospital actually faces some probability distribution of returns, rather than a return known with certainty, and the greater the probability of returns well below those anticipated, the greater the risk of the MRI investment.

EXPECTED RATE OF RETURN

We know now that financial risk is associated with returns less than those anticipated, but it is useful at this point to define the concept more precisely. Table 2–1 contains the estimated returns distribution developed by the financial staff of Crescent Beach Community Hospital for two proposed projects: an MRI system and a walk-in clinic. Here, the economic state reflects a combination of factors that affect each project's profitability. For example, for the MRI project, the very poor economic state signifies very low physician acceptance and hence very low usage, very high discounts on reimbursements, very high operating costs, and so on. The economic states are defined in a similar fashion for the walk-in clinic project.

The expected rate of return on any investment is the weighted average of the return distribution, where the weights are the probabilities of occurrence. For example, the expected rate of return on the MRI system is 10.0 percent.

TABLE 2–1

Estimated Returns for Two Proposed Investment Projects

Economic State	Probability of State Occurring	Rate of Return if State Occurs	
		MRI	Clinic
Very poor	0.10	−10%	−20%
Poor	0.20	0	0
Average	0.40	10	15
Good	0.20	20	30
Very good	0.10	30	50
	1.00		

Expected rate of return = Probability of Return 1 × Return 1
+ Probability of Return 2 × Return 2
+ and so on
= 0.10 (−10%) + 0.20 (0%) + 0.40(10%)
+ 0.20 (20%) + 0.10 (30%)
= 10.0%

Calculated in a similar manner, the expected rate of return on the walk-in clinic is 15.0 percent. In some situations, the expected rate of return may not even be realizable, but it is the best single-value measure of return when there is uncertainty and hence a return distribution.

STAND-ALONE RISK

We can look at the two distributions in Table 2–1 and intuitively con-clude that the clinic is more risky than the MRI system because the clinic has a chance of a 20 percent loss, while the worst possible loss on the MRI system is 10 percent. This intuitive risk assessment is looking at the stand-alone risk of the two investments. That is, we are focusing on the riskiness that is relevant assuming that the MRI system or the walk-in clinic would be the business's only asset (oper-ated in isolation). In the next section, portfolio effects will be intro-duced, but for now, let's continue our discussion of stand-alone risk.

We can see that stand-alone risk depends on the "tightness" of the investment's return distribution. If an investment has a tight return distribution, with returns falling close to the expected return, it has relatively low stand-alone risk. Conversely, an investment with a return distribution that is "loose," and hence that has values well below the expected return, is relatively risky.

Note that risk and return are two separate attributes of an investment. An investment might have a very tight distribution of returns, and hence very low risk, but its expected rate of return might be only 2 percent. In this situation, the investment probably would not be financially attractive, in spite of its low risk. Similarly, a high-risk investment with a sufficiently high expected rate of return would be attractive.

To be truly useful, any measure of risk should have a definite value, so we need some way to measure the "degree of tightness" of an investment's return distribution. One such measure is standard deviation, which is often given the symbol σ (Greek lower-case sigma). Standard deviation is a common statistical measure of the dispersion of a distribution about its mean—the smaller the standard deviation, the tighter the distribution, and hence the lower the riskiness of the investment. To illustrate the calculation of standard deviation, consider the MRI project's estimated returns listed in Table 2–1.

1. Calculate the expected rate of return, E(Rate of return).

$$
\begin{aligned}
\text{E(Rate of return)} &= \text{Sum of all } P_i(\text{Rate of return}_i) \\
&= 0.10(-10\%) + 0.20(0\%) + 0.40(10\%) \\
&\quad + 0.20(20\%) + 0.10(30\%) \\
&= 10.0\%
\end{aligned}
$$

2. Calculate the variance of the rate of return distribution.

$$
\begin{aligned}
\text{Variance} &= \text{Sum of all } P_i[\text{Rate of return}_i - \text{E(Rate of return)}]^2 \\
&= 0.10(-10\% - 10\%)^2 + 0.20(0\% - 10\%)^2 \\
&\quad + 0.40(10\% - 10\%)^2 + 0.20(20\% - 10\%)^2 \\
&\quad + 0.10(30\% - 10\%)^2 \\
&= 120.00
\end{aligned}
$$

3. Finally, take the square root of the variance to obtain the standard deviation.

$$
\text{Standard deviation} = \sigma = \sqrt{\text{Variance}} = \sqrt{120.00} = 10.95\% \approx 11\%
$$

Using the same procedure, the clinic project listed in Table 2–1 was found to have a standard deviation of returns of about 18 percent. Since the clinic project's standard deviation of returns is larger than that of the MRI project, the clinic project has more stand-alone risk than the MRI project.

Investments with higher expected returns often have larger standard deviations than investments with smaller expected returns. To illustrate, suppose Project X has a 30 percent expected rate of return with a standard deviation of 10 percent, while Project Y has a 10 percent expected rate of return with a standard deviation of 5 percent. According to their standard deviations, Project X is twice as risky as Project Y. However, if the returns on Projects X and Y are approximately normal (follow a bell-shaped distribution), then Project X would have a very small probability of a negative return in spite of its higher standard deviation, while Project Y, even with a standard deviation only half as large as that of Project X, would have a much higher probability of a loss. Therefore, standard deviation does not give a good picture of one investment's stand-alone risk relative to other alternatives if the investments' expected rates of return differ substantially.

The coefficient of variation (CV), which is defined as the standard deviation divided by the expected value, measures the risk per unit of return and hence standardizes the measurement of risk.

$$\text{Coefficient of variation} = CV = \frac{\sigma}{E(\text{Value})}$$

$$\text{Project X: } CV = 10\% / 30\% = 0.33$$
$$\text{Project Y: } CV = 5\% / 10\% = 0.50$$

Thus, Project Y actually has more risk per unit of expected return than Project X, and Project Y is riskier than Project X in spite of the fact that Project X's standard deviation is twice as large. When investments are likely to have expected rates of return that are substantially different from one another, the coefficient of variation is the preferred measure of stand-alone risk, although the standard deviation is often used as the stand-alone risk measure when investments have about the same expected profitability.

RISK IN A PORTFOLIO CONTEXT

The preceding section developed two risk measures—standard deviation and coefficient of variation—that apply to investments held in isolation. However, most investments are not held in isolation but, rather, are held as part of a collection, or portfolio, of investments; individual investors hold portfolios of securities, while businesses hold portfolios of projects (different product or service lines). When investments are held as part of portfolios, the primary concern of investors is not the realized rate of return on an individual investment but, rather, the realized rate of return on the entire portfolio. Similarly, the riskiness of each individual asset is not as important to the investor as is the aggregate riskiness of the portfolio. The whole nature of risk and how it is defined and measured changes when we consider that investments are not held by themselves (in isolation) but rather as parts of portfolios.

Portfolio Returns

To help illustrate the concept of portfolio risk and return, consider the returns estimated for the five investment alternatives listed in Table 2–2. The individual investment alternatives (Investments A, B, and C) could be projects under consideration by South West Clinics, Inc., or they could be stocks that you are evaluating for personal investment purposes. The remaining two alternatives in Table 2–2 are portfolios. Portfolio AB consists of 50 percent invested in Investment A and 50 percent in Investment B (say, $10,000 invested in A and $10,000 invested in B), while Portfolio AC is an equal-weighted portfolio of Investments A and C.

TABLE 2–2

Estimated Returns for Three Individual Investments and Two Portfolios

Economic State	Probability of State Occurring	Rate of Return if State Occurs				
		A	B	C	AB	AC
Very poor	0.10	−10%	30%	−25%	10%	−17.5%
Poor	0.20	0	20	−5	10	−2.5
Average	0.40	10	10	15	10	12.5
Good	0.20	20	0	35	10	27.5
Very good	0.10	30	−10	55	10	42.5
	1.00					
Expected rate of return		10.0%	10.0%	15.0%	10.0%	12.5%
Standard deviation		11.0%	11.0%	21.9%	0.0%	16.4%
Coefficient of variation		1.10	1.10	1.46	0.0	1.31

As shown in the bottom of the table, Investments A and B have 10 percent expected rates of return, while the expected rate of return for Investment C is 15 percent. Investments A and B have identical stand-alone risk as measured by standard deviation and coefficient of variation, while Investment C has higher risk.

Turning to Portfolios AB and AC, the expected rate of return on a portfolio is simply the weighted average of the expected returns on the assets that make up the portfolio, with the weights being the proportion of the total portfolio invested in each asset.

E(Portfolio rate of return) = Sum of all w_iE(Rate of return$_i$)

Here, w_i is the proportion of each investment in the overall portfolio, and E(Rate of return$_i$) is the expected rate of return on each investment. Thus, the expected rate of return on Portfolio AB is 10 percent.

$$E(\text{Rate of return}_{AB}) = 0.5(10\%) + 0.5(10\%) = 10\%$$

And the expected rate of return on Portfolio AC is 12.5 percent.

$$E(\text{Rate of return}_{AC}) = 0.5(10\%) + 0.5(15\%) = 12.5\%$$

Alternatively, the expected rate of return on a portfolio can be calculated by looking at the portfolio's return distribution. For example, the return distribution for Portfolio AC contained in Table 2–2 produces the same 12.5 percent expected rate of return as calculated above.

$$\begin{aligned} E(\text{Rate of return}_{AC}) &= 0.10(-17.5\%) + 0.20(-2.5\%) \\ &\quad + 0.40(12.5\%) + 0.20(27.5\%) \\ &\quad + 0.10(42.5\%) \\ &= 12.5\% \end{aligned}$$

Of course, after the fact, the actual, or realized, returns on Investments A and C will probably be different from their expected values, and hence the realized rate of return on Portfolio AC will likely be different from the 12.5 percent expected return.

Portfolio Risk

As just demonstrated, the expected rate of return on a portfolio of investments is simply a weighted average of the expected returns on the individual investments in the portfolio. However, unlike returns, the riskiness of a portfolio is generally not a weighted average of the riskiness of the individual components of the port-folio; the portfolio's riskiness may be smaller than the weighted average of each component's riskiness. Indeed, the riskiness of a portfolio may be less than that of the least-risk component.

A simple example will help make this point clear. Suppose you are given the opportunity to flip a coin once; if it comes up heads, you win $10,000, but if it comes up tails, you lose $8,000. This is a rea-sonable bet; the expected dollar return is 0.5($10,000) + 0.5(–$8,000) = $1,000. However, it is a highly risky proposition because you have a 50 percent chance of losing $8,000. Thus, because of risk aversion, most people would refuse to make the bet, especially if the $8,000 potential loss would result in financial disaster. Alternatively, sup-pose you are given the opportunity to flip the coin 100 times, and you would win $100 for each head but lose $80 for each tail. It is pos-sible, although extremely unlikely, that you would flip all heads and win $10,000, and it is also possible, and also extremely unlikely, that you would flip all tails and lose $8,000, but the chances are very high that you would actually flip about 50 heads and about 50 tails, win-ning a net $1,000. Even if you flipped a few more tails than heads, you would still make money on the gamble.

Although each individual flip is a risky bet, collectively you have a low-risk proposition, because you have diversified away most of the risk. In effect, you have created a portfolio of invest-ments; each flip of the coin can be thought of as one investment, so you have a 100-investment portfolio. Furthermore, the return on each investment is independent of the returns on the other invest-ments—you have a 50 percent chance of winning on each flip of the coin regardless of the results of the previous flips. By combining the flips into a single gamble, that is, into an investment portfolio, you can reduce the risk associated with each individual bet. In fact, if the gamble consisted of a very large number of flips, you could totally eliminate the risk inherent in the gamble because the probability of a near-equal number of heads and tails would be extremely high, and the result would be a sure profit. The key to the benefits of a portfolio of coin tosses is that the negative consequences of tossing a tail can be offset by the positive consequences of tossing a head.

To examine portfolio effects in more depth, it is easiest to focus on portfolios composed of two investments. You will see that it is possible to combine two risky investments with special properties into a portfolio that is completely riskless; that is, a portfolio with a standard deviation and coefficient of variation of returns of zero. To illustrate, consider Portfolio AB in Table 2–2. Each individual investment (A and B) is quite risky when held in isolation, but a portfolio of the two investments has a rate of return of 10 percent in every possible state of the economy, and hence it offers a riskless 10 percent return. (This result is verified by the values of zero for Portfolio AB's standard deviation and coefficient of variation of returns.)

The reason Investments A and B can be combined to form a riskless portfolio is that their returns move exactly counter to one another; in economic states when A's returns are low, those of B are high, and vice versa. The fact that gains on one investment in the portfolio exactly offset losses in the other results in a riskless portfolio. The movement relationship of two variables (the tendency to move either together or in opposition) is called correlation, and the correlation coefficient (r) measures this relationship. Investments A and B can be combined to form a riskless portfolio because the returns on A and B are perfectly negatively correlated, which is designated by $r = -1.0$. In every state where Investment A has a return higher than its expected return, Investment B has a return lower than its expected return, and vice versa.

The opposite of perfect negative correlation is perfect positive correlation, with $r = +1.0$. Returns on two perfectly positively correlated investments move up and down together as the economic state changes. When the returns on two investments are perfectly positively correlated, combining the investments into a portfolio will not lower risk; the riskiness of the portfolio is merely the weighted average of the risks of the two components.

To illustrate the impact of perfect positive correlation, consider Portfolio AC in Table 2–2. Here, the standard deviation of the portfolio is simply the weighted average standard deviation of its components.

$$\sigma_{AC} = 0.5(11.0\%) + 0.5(21.9\%)$$
$$= 16.4\%$$

There is no risk reduction in this situation; forming a portfolio does nothing to reduce risk when the returns on the two assets are perfectly positively correlated.

Portfolios AB and AC in Table 2–2 demonstrate that when the returns on two investments are perfectly negatively correlated ($r = -1.0$), all risk can be eliminated by combining the assets, but when the returns on two investments are perfectly positively correlated (r = +1.0), combining them into a portfolio is of no value in reducing risk. The obvious questions at this point are (1) what is the correlation among the returns on "real-world" investments, and (2) what happens to portfolio risk when more than two assets are combined?

It is difficult to generalize about the correlations among investment alternatives, but the correlations among two randomly selected investments—whether they be real assets in a healthcare company's portfolio of projects or financial assets in an individual's investment portfolio—are almost never –1.0 or +1.0. In fact, it is almost impossible to find actual investment opportunities with returns that are negatively correlated with one another or even to find investments with returns that are uncorrelated, or independent (r = 0.0). Since all real asset investment returns (returns on projects owned by businesses) are affected to a greater or lesser degree by general economic conditions, and since the returns on financial assets (stocks and bonds) are usually linked to the performance of real assets, investment returns tend to be positively correlated with one another. However, since investment returns are not affected identically by general economic conditions, returns on most real-world investments are not perfectly positively correlated.

In general, the correlation between the returns of two randomly chosen investments will be in the range of +0.4 to +0.8. Returns on investments that are similar in nature, such as two inpatient projects in a hospital or two stocks in the same industry, will usually have return correlations at the upper end of the range, while the returns on dissimilar real or financial assets tend to have correlations at the low end of the range.

What happens when a portfolio is created with two investments that have positive, but not perfectly positive, returns correlation? Some risk can be eliminated by combining the two investments, but not all risk can be eliminated. That is, the portfolio will be less risky than the weighted-average of each component's risk, or possibly even less risky than the lower-risk component, but some risk will still remain.

Of course, businesses are not restricted to two projects, and individual investors are not restricted to holding two-asset portfolios. Most companies have tens or even hundreds or thousands of individual projects (products or service lines), and most individual

investors hold many different stocks and bonds, or perhaps mutual funds, which themselves may be composed of hundreds of individual securities. Thus, what is most relevant to financial decision
making is not what happens when two investments are combined
into portfolios but, rather, what happens when many investments
are combined.

To illustrate the risk impact of creating portfolios of two, three,
four, or many more investments, consider Figure 2–1. The figure plots
the riskiness inherent in holding randomly selected portfolios of one
asset, two assets, three assets, four assets, and so on. The plot is based
on historical annual returns on common stock traded on the New
York Stock Exchange (NYSE), but the conclusions reached are roughly applicable to portfolios made up of any type of investment, such as
healthcare providers offering many different types of services.

On average, the riskiness inherent in holding a one-stock portfolio is about 35 percent, as measured by the standard deviation of

FIGURE 2–1

Portfolio Size and Risk

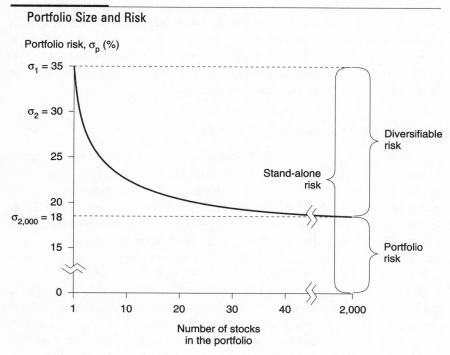

annual returns. (Another way of saying this is the standard deviation of annual returns of an average NYSE stock is about 35 percent.) The average two-stock portfolio has a standard deviation of about 30 percent, so it is less risky to hold an average two-stock portfolio than to hold a single stock of average risk. The average three-stock portfolio has a standard deviation of returns of about 28 percent, so an average three-stock portfolio is even less risky than an average two-stock portfolio. As more and more stocks are randomly added to create larger and larger portfolios, the riskiness of the portfolios decreases. However, (1) as more and more stocks are added, the incremental risk reduction of adding even more stocks decreases, and (2) regardless of how many stocks are added, some risk always remains in the portfolio; even with 2,000 stocks, the standard deviation of portfolio returns is about 18 percent.

The reason all risk cannot be eliminated by creating a very large portfolio is that the returns on investment alternatives, although not perfectly so, are still positively correlated with one another. In other words, all investments are affected to a lesser or greater degree by general economic conditions; if the economy booms, all investments tend to do well, while in a recession all investments tend to do poorly. Note that if there were zero correlation among investment returns, a very large portfolio would be riskless (standard deviation = 0%), or close to it. Since this is not the case, even very large portfolios are risky.

Diversifiable Risk versus Portfolio Risk

Figure 2–1 shows that almost half of the stand-alone risk inherent in an average NYSE stock can be eliminated if the stock is held as part of a large portfolio. If an investor wanted to create the lowest-risk portfolio of NYSE stocks, he or she would have to own all 2,000 or so stocks. Such a portfolio is called the market portfolio because it consists of the entire stock market (or at least one entire segment of the stock market). Fortunately, it is not necessary to own 2,000 stocks to gain the risk-reducing benefit inherent in holding portfolios. Most of the benefit can be obtained by only holding about 50 randomly selected stocks. Such a large, randomly chosen portfolio is called a well-diversified portfolio. (A portfolio of, say, 50 health-care stocks or 50 utility stocks is not well diversified because the stocks are in the same industry and hence not randomly chosen.)

That part of the stand-alone riskiness of an individual invest-ment that can be eliminated by diversification (by holding a well-diversified portfolio) is called diversifiable risk. That part of the riskiness of an individual investment that cannot be eliminated by diversification is called portfolio risk. Thus, every investment, whether it be the stock of Beverly Enterprises held by an individ-ual investor or an MRI system operated by a hospital, has some diversifiable risk that can be eliminated by holding the asset as part of a well-diversified portfolio and some portfolio risk that cannot be diversified away. Of course, some investments benefit more from portfolio risk-reducing effects than others, but, in general, any investment will have some of its stand-alone risk eliminated by holding it as part of a well-diversified portfolio.

Diversifiable risk as seen by individuals investing in stocks is caused by events that are unique to a single firm, such as new product or service introductions, strikes, and lawsuits. Since these events are essentially random, their effects can be eliminated by diversification. When one stock in a portfolio does worse than expected because of a negative event unique to that firm, another stock in the portfolio will do better than expected due to a firm-unique positive event. On average, bad events will be offset by good events; so lower than expected returns will be offset by high-er than expected returns, leaving the investor with an overall port-folio return closer to that expected.

The same logic can be applied to a firm with a well-diversified portfolio of projects (products or services). Perhaps hospital returns generated from inpatient surgery are less than expected because of a faster-than-expected movement to outpatient proce-dures, but this might be offset by returns that are greater than expected on state-of-the-art diagnostic services. (Of course, if the hospital offered both inpatient and outpatient surgery, it would be hedging itself against the trend towards more outpatient proce-dures because reduced demand for inpatient services would be off-set by increased demand for outpatient services.)

The bottom line here is that the negative impact of random events that are unique to a particular firm, or to a particular product or service within a firm, can be offset by positive events in other firms or in other products or services. Thus, the risk due to such ran-dom, unique events can be eliminated by portfolio diversification. Unfortunately, not all risk can be diversified away. Stock portfolio risk, the risk that remains in diversified portfolios, stems from factors that systematically affect all stocks in a portfolio, such as wars, inflation, recessions, and high interest rates. Similarly, when health-care assets form the portfolio, portfolio risk stems from factors such as managed care penetration, which could lower reimbursement levels for all services provided. Portfolio risk cannot be eliminated, so even well-diversified investors, whether they be individuals with large securities' portfolios or diversified health companies with many different service lines, must deal with this type of risk.

Implications for Investors

The ability of investors to eliminate some portion of the stand-alone riskiness inherent in individual investments has two very significant implications for investors, especially individuals buying securities, but also businesses offering products and services.

1. It is not rational to hold a single investment. Much of the stand-alone riskiness inherent in individual investments can be eliminated by holding a well-diversified portfolio; so investors, who are risk averse, should seek to eliminate all diversifiable risk. Individual investors can easily diversify their personal investment portfolios, either by buying many individual stocks and bonds or by buying mutual funds that hold diversified portfolios of stocks and bonds. Businesses cannot diversify their investments as easily as individuals, but businesses that offer a diverse line of products or services are less risky than businesses that rely on a single product or service.

2. Since the portfolio risk of an individual asset, and not its stand-alone risk, is the risk that "counts" to well-diversified investors, traditional stand-alone risk measures such as standard deviation and coefficient of variation of returns are not relevant to most investors. Thus, it is necessary to rethink our definition and measures of financial risk for individual assets. This is done in the following two sections.

THE RISK OF BUSINESS ASSETS TO THE COMPANY: CORPORATE RISK

Firms typically offer many products or services and thus can be thought of as having a large number (hundreds or even thousands) of individual projects. For example, most HMOs offer healthcare services to a large number of diverse groups of enrollees (covered lives) in numerous service areas; and many hospitals (or hospital systems) offer a large number of inpatient, outpatient, and even home health services that cover a wide geographical area and treat a wide range of illnesses and injuries. Thus, healthcare managers in firms that offer a number of individual products or services actually manage a portfolio of projects. Furthermore, when stock investors buy the stock of a single company, they are really buying a portfolio of individual projects, so a well-diversified portfolio of 50 or more stocks is really a portfolio of tens of thousands of individual projects run by the companies whose stock is in the portfolio.

From this description, it is obvious that the individual projects of a business actually reside in two different portfolios. First, a project is part of the firm's overall portfolio of projects. For example, the Women's Center at Columbia North Florida Regional Medical Center is one project of thousands that make up Columbia/HCA's portfolio of projects. Second, for stockholders, a project is one very small part of a well-diversified investment portfolio. Investors who own Columbia/HCA stock own the Women's Center along with thousands of other Columbia/HCA projects at hundreds of hospitals, plus tens of thousands of projects owned by other companies in their stock portfolios.

Thus, the portfolio riskiness of a business project depends on one's perspective. A healthcare manager sees project riskiness from the standpoint of the business's portfolio of projects, while a stock investor sees the riskiness inherent in holding the project as part of a well-diversified stock portfolio. Since the portfolio context is different, the riskiness of a given project is defined and measured in different ways. In this section, the riskiness of business assets to the company is discussed. In the next section, the riskiness of business assets to stockholders is covered.

For now, put on your manager's hat. What is the riskiness of a project to your business? Since the project is part of the business's portfolio of assets, its stand-alone risk is not relevant because the project is not held in isolation. The relevant risk of any project to the business is its contribution to the business's overall risk, or the impact of the project on the firm's overall standard deviation of return. This type of portfolio risk, which focuses on the firm's portfolio of projects, is called corporate risk.

To illustrate corporate risk, assume that Project P represents the expansion into a new service area by AtlanticCare, a for-profit HMO with many existing projects. Table 2–3 contains the estimated rate of return distributions for Project P and for AtlanticCare as a whole. AtlanticCare's rate of return, like that of Project P, is uncertain and depends on future economic events. Overall, AtlanticCare's expected rate of return is 7.0 percent, with a standard deviation of 2.0 percent and a coefficient of variation of 0.3, while Project P has an expected rate of return of 10.0 percent, a standard deviation of 4.0 percent, and a coefficient of variation of 0.4. Thus, looking at the stand-alone risk measures, Project P is riskier than the HMO in the aggregate; that is, Project P is riskier than AtlanticCare's average project.

However, the relevant risk of Project P is not its stand-alone risk but, rather, its contribution to AtlanticCare's overall riskiness. Project P's corporate risk depends not only on its standard deviation of returns but also on the correlation between the returns on Project P and the returns on the HMO's average project (AtlanticCare's rate of return distribution). If Project P's returns were negatively correlated with the returns on AtlanticCare's other projects, then accepting it would reduce the riskiness of the HMO's aggregate returns. And the

TABLE 2–3

Estimated Return Distributions for Project P and AtlanticCare

State of Economy	Probability of Occurrence	Rate of Return	
		Project P	**AtlanticCare**
Very poor	0.05	2.5%	1.0%
Poor	0.20	5.0	6.0
Average	0.50	10.0	7.0
Good	0.20	15.0	8.0
Very good	0.05	17.5	13.0
Expected return		10.0%	7.0%
Standard deviation		4.0%	2.0%
Coefficient of variation		0.4	0.3
Correlation coefficient		0.80	

larger Project P's standard deviation, the greater the risk reduction. (An economic state resulting in a low return on AtlanticCare's average project would produce a high return on Project P, and vice versa, so the returns would offset one another, and AtlanticCare's overall risk would be reduced.) In this situation, Project P would be viewed as a very low-risk project relative to the HMO's average project, in spite of its higher stand-alone risk. In reality, however, Project P's returns are positively correlated with AtlanticCare's aggregate returns, and the project has twice the standard deviation, so accepting it would increase the risk of the HMO's aggregate returns.

The quantitative measure of corporate risk is a project's corporate beta, or corporate b, which is the slope of the regression (scatter plot) line that results when the project's returns are plotted on the Y axis and the returns on the firm's average project are plotted on the X axis. Figure 2–2 contains this regression line, which is often called the corporate characteristic line, for Project P.

The slope (rise over run) of Project P's corporate characteristic line, which is Project P's corporate beta coefficient, is about 1.60; it can be found algebraically as follows:

FIGURE 2–2

Corporate Characteristic Line for Project P

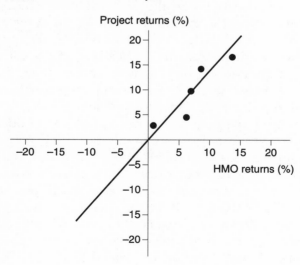

$$\text{Corporate } b_P = (\sigma_P / \sigma_F)\, r_{PF}$$

where

σ_P = standard deviation of Project P's returns,

σ_F = standard deviation of the firm's returns, and

r_{PF} = correlation coefficient between the returns on Project P and the firm's returns.

Thus,

$$\text{Corporate } b_P = (4.0\% / 2.0\%)0.80 = 1.60$$

A project's corporate beta measures the volatility of returns on the project relative to the firm as a whole (or relative to the firm's average project), which has a corporate beta of 1.0. (To estimate the corporate beta of the firm's average project, the firm's aggregate returns are plotted on both the X and Y axes, so the resulting slope of the corporate characteristic line is 1.0.)

If a project's corporate beta is 2.0, its returns are twice as volatile as the firm's returns; thus, adding such a project to the firm would increase the overall volatility of the firm's returns and hence increase the riskiness of the business. A corporate beta of 1.0 indicates that the project's returns have the same volatility as the firm; hence, taking on the project would add identical risk to the firm's existing assets. A corporate beta of 0.5 indicates that the project's returns are less volatile than the firm's returns, so taking on the project would lower the overall risk of the firm. A negative corporate beta, which results when a project's returns are negatively correlated with the firm's returns, indicates that the returns on the project move countercyclically to the returns of the firms. The addition of such a project to the firm's portfolio of projects could reduce a firm's riskiness by a large amount, but such projects are very hard to find because most projects are in a single line of business, or in similar lines, so their returns are highly positively correlated.

With a corporate beta of 1.6, the returns on Project P are 1.6 times as volatile as the returns on AtlanticCare's average project. Economic events that would result in a return 10 percent less than expected on the HMO as a whole would produce a 16 percent less-than-expected return on Project P. Thus, adding project P to AtlanticCare's portfolio of projects would increase the risk of the HMO; hence, Project P would be judged to have more corporate risk than AtlanticCare's average project.

THE RISK OF BUSINESS ASSETS TO STOCKHOLDERS: MARKET RISK

The last section discussed the riskiness of projects to a business. This section discusses the riskiness of business projects to stock investors. Why should a healthcare manager be concerned about how investors view risk? The answer is simple: Stock investors are the suppliers of equity capital to for-profit businesses, so they set the rates of return that such businesses must pay to raise equity capital. These rates, in turn, set the minimum profitability that businesses must earn on the equity portion of their real asset investments. Thus, by understanding how stock investors view risk and set rates of return, managers can better evaluate business investments. Later, we will see that the actions of stock investors are important also to managers of not-for-profit businesses because returns on equity investments in for-profit healthcare firms establish opportunity cost rates for capital investments within not-for-profit firms.

Since stock investors hold well-diversified portfolios of stocks, the relevant riskiness of an individual project undertaken by a company in the portfolio is its contribution to the riskiness of a well-diversified stock portfolio. Thus, the riskiness of the Women's Center at Columbia North Florida Regional Medical Center to an individual investor who has a portfolio of 50 stocks or to a trust officer managing a 150-stock portfolio or to a 500-stock mutual fund owner is the contribution that the project makes to the stock portfolio's riskiness. Some of the stand-alone riskiness of the project will be diversified away by combining the project with all the other projects in the stock portfolio. The remaining risk is called market risk, which is defined as the contribution of a project to the riskiness of a well-diversified stock portfolio.

The next issue is how to measure a project's market risk. A project's market beta measures the volatility of the project's returns relative to the returns on a well-diversified portfolio of stocks. Table 2–4 contains hypothetical estimates of the rate of return on a well-diversified portfolio of stocks, commonly called the market portfolio, or just the market, along with the returns on AtlanticCare's Project P. In practice, some stock index, say the S&P 500 or the NYSE Index, is used as a proxy for the market portfolio. (The Standard & Poor's 500 is an index made up of 500 stocks across many industries, while the New York Stock Exchange Index is made up of the roughly 2,000 stocks listed on the New York Stock Exchange.)

TABLE 2-4

Estimated Return Distributions for Project P and the Market

State of Economy	Probability of Occurrence	Rate of Return	
		Project P	The Market
Very poor	0.05	2.5%	−15.0%
Poor	0.20	5.0	5.0
Average	0.50	10.0	15.0
Good	0.20	15.0	25.0
Very good	0.05	17.5	45.0
Expected return		10.0%	15.0%
Standard deviation		4.0%	11.4%
Coefficient of variation		0.4	0.8
Correlation coefficient		0.94	

The market beta of Project P is found by constructing the market characteristic line for the project, which is the regression (scatter plot) line that results from plotting the returns on Project P against the returns on the market. Project P's market characteristic line, which is shown in Figure 2–3, has a slope of 0.33; hence, Project P's market beta is 0.33. Note that the market characteristic line and corporate characteristic line (discussed in the previous section) are very similar; the sole difference is the return plotted on the X axis. The corporate characteristic line uses the firm's returns, while the market characteristic line uses the market's returns. Thus, the former measures the project's volatility relative to the firm's average project, while the latter measures the volatility relative to the average stock.

Note that Project P's market beta, Market b_P, can be calculated as follows:

$$\text{Market } b_P = (\sigma_P / \sigma_M) r_{PM}$$

where

σ_P = standard deviation of Project P's returns,

σ_M = standard deviation of the market's returns, and

r_{PM} = correlation coefficient of returns between Project P and the market.

Thus, using the data from Table 2–4,

$$\text{Market } b_P = (4.0\% / 11.4\%)0.94 = 0.33$$

FIGURE 2–3

Market Characteristic Line for Project P

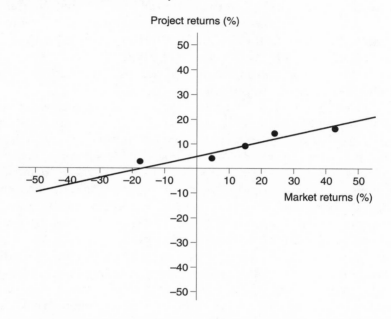

Project P's market beta measures its market risk, which is the risk relevant to AtlanticCare's well-diversified shareholders. Intuitively, a project's market beta measures the volatility of the project's returns relative to the returns on a well-diversified port-folio of stocks (the market portfolio), which has a beta of 1.0.

A project with a market beta of 2.0 has returns that are twice as volatile as the returns on the market, and adding it to a well-diversified stock portfolio would increase the portfolio's risk. A market beta of 1.0 indicates that the project's returns have the same volatility as the market; adding such a project would have no impact on the riskiness of the market portfolio. A market beta of 0.5 indicates that the project's returns are half as volatile as the returns on the market, and so adding such a project to a well-diversified stock portfolio would reduce its risk.

With a market beta of 0.33, Project P has only one-third the riskiness inherent in the market portfolio. If general economic con-ditions resulted in a 10 percent less-than-expected return on the market portfolio, the return on Project P would be only 3.3 percent less than expected. Thus, Project P has below-average market risk.

Since AtlanticCare's stockholders are assumed to hold well-diversified stock portfolios (with a beta of 1.0), the HMO's acceptance of Project P would reduce the riskiness of shareholder portfolios. (As you will see shortly, the beta of a portfolio is merely the weighted average of the betas of the individual components of the portfolio. Thus, adding a component with a lower beta than the portfolio average lowers the beta of the portfolio and, hence, lowers the riskiness of the portfolio.)

Note that a negative market beta, which results when a project's returns are negatively correlated with the market's returns, indicates that the returns on the project move countercyclically to the returns on the market—when the market's return goes up, the project's return goes down and vice versa. Negative beta projects are valuable to stockholders because of their risk-reduction characteristics. However, negative market beta projects are rare since most projects' returns, as well as the market's returns, are positively correlated with the economy as a whole.

In closing, note one important point about the interpretation of project market betas. The comparison that is most relevant to managerial decision making is the market risk of the project relative to the market risk of the firm. Thus, when investor-owned firms conduct project market risk analyses, the question that is relevant to managers is this: How does the project's market risk compare to the market risk of the firm's average project? This question is answered by comparing the project's market beta to the firm's market beta, which is the slope of the market characteristic line formed by regressing the firm's aggregate returns against the market's returns. For example, using the data in Tables 2–3 and 2–4, we find AtlanticCare's market beta to be 0.17; so Project P, with a market beta of 0.33, would have more market risk than the HMO's average project.

PORTFOLIO BETAS

Individual investors hold portfolios of stocks, each with its own market risk as measured by the stock's market beta coefficient; while businesses hold portfolios of projects, each with its own corporate and market betas. What impact does the beta of a portfolio component have on the overall portfolio's beta? The beta of any portfolio of investments is simply the weighted average of the individual investments' betas.

$$b_p = \text{Sum of all } w_i b_i$$

Here, b_p is the beta of the portfolio, which measures the volatility of the entire portfolio, w_i is the fraction of the portfolio invested in one particular asset, and b_i is the beta coefficient of that asset.

To illustrate, Columbia/HCA Healthcare might have a market beta of 1.2, indicating that the returns on its stock are slightly more volatile that the returns on a well-diversified portfolio (with a beta of 1.0); hence, the stock is somewhat riskier than the average stock. But each project within Columbia/HCA Healthcare has its own market risk, as measured by each project's market beta. Some projects may have very high market betas, say, over 1.5; while other projects may have very low market betas, say, under 0.5. When all the projects are combined, the overall market beta of the company is 1.2. For ease, assume that Columbia/HCA Healthcare has only the following three projects:

Project	Market Beta	Dollar Investment	Proportion
A	0.5	$15,000	15.0%
B	1.0	30,000	30.0
C	1.5	55,000	55.0
		$100,000	100.0%

The weighted average of the project market betas, which is the firm's market beta, is 1.2:

$$\begin{aligned} b_p &= \text{Sum of all } w_i b_i \\ &= 0.15(0.5) + 0.30(1.0) + 0.55(1.5) \\ &= 1.20 \end{aligned}$$

Note that each project within Columbia/HCA Healthcare's fictitious portfolio of three projects also has a corporate beta that measures the volatility of the project's returns relative to the corporation as a whole. The weighted average of these project corporate betas must equal 1.00, which is the corporate beta of any business.

RELEVANCE OF THE THREE RISK MEASURES

Thus far, the chapter has discussed in some detail three measures of financial risk—stand-alone, corporate, and market—but it is unclear which is the most relevant risk in financial decision making. It turns out that the risk that is relevant to any financial decision depends on the situation at hand.

When the decision involves a single investment that will be held in isolation, stand-alone risk is the relevant risk. Here, the risk and return on the portfolio is the same as the risk and return on the single asset in the portfolio. In this situation, the riskiness faced by the investor, whether it be an individual considering a stock purchase or a business considering an MRI investment, is defined in terms of returns less than expected, and the appropriate measure is the standard deviation or coefficient of variation of the return distribution.

However, in most real-world investment decisions, the asset under consideration will not be held in isolation but, rather, will be held as part of an investment portfolio. Individual investors normally hold portfolios of stocks, while businesses normally hold portfolios of real asset investments (projects). For individual investors holding stock portfolios, the most relevant risk is the asset's contribution to the overall riskiness of a well-diversified stock portfolio. This risk, called market risk, is measured by the asset's market beta.

For businesses, the most relevant risk depends on whether the business is for-profit or not-for-profit. For investor-owned businesses, the goal is shareholder wealth maximization, so risk must be measured in shareholder terms. Since stockholders tend to hold large portfolios of securities, and hence a very large portfolio of individual projects, the most relevant risk of a project under consideration by a for-profit firm is its contribution to a well-diversified stock portfolio (the market portfolio). Of course, this is the project's market risk.

Not-for-profit firms do not have stockholders, and their goals stem from a mission statement that generally involves service to society. In this situation, market risk is not relevant—the concern to managers is the impact of the project on the riskiness of the business, which is defined as the project's corporate risk. Thus, the risk measure most relevant to projects in not-for-profit firms is a project's corporate beta. We will address the issue of risk relevance again in Chapter 8, where we discuss the risk considerations inherent in capital investment decisions.

A REVIEW OF RISK CONCEPTS

This chapter has covered a lot of ground, and it is easy to lose sight of the major concepts. To help put things into perspective, here is a review of the key concepts.

1. Risk definition and measurement is very important to financial decision making because people, in general, are risk averse and hence require higher returns from investments having higher risk.

2. In general, financial risk is associated with the prospect of returns less than the expected return. The higher the probability of a return being far less than expected, the greater the risk.

3. The riskiness of investments held in isolation (standing alone) can be measured by the dispersion of the rate of return distribution about its expected value. The two most commonly used measures of stand-alone risk are the standard deviation and coefficient of variation of the return distribution.

4. Most investments are not held in isolation but, rather, as part of investment portfolios. Individual investors hold portfolios of securities, and businesses hold portfolios of projects (products or services).

5. When investments with returns that are less than perfectly positively correlated are combined, it is possible to create a portfolio that is less risky than its components. The risk reduction occurs because the less-than-expected returns on some investments are offset by greater-than-expected returns on other investments. However, among real-world investments, it is impossible to eliminate all risk because the returns on all assets are influenced to a greater or lesser degree by changes in overall economic conditions.

6. That portion of the stand-alone risk of an investment that can be eliminated by holding the investment in a well-diversified portfolio is called diversifiable risk, while the risk that remains is called portfolio risk.

7. There are two different types of portfolio risk. Corporate risk is the riskiness of business projects when they are considered as part of a business's portfolio of projects. Market risk is the riskiness of business projects (or of the stocks of entire businesses) when they are considered as part of an individual investor's well-diversified portfolio of securities.

8. Corporate risk is measured by a project's corporate beta, which reflects the volatility of the project's returns relative to the returns of the aggregate business. The corporate risk of a project under consideration is a function of the project's standard deviation of returns, the standard deviation of returns on the business as a whole, and the correlation between the returns on the project and the returns on the business.

9. Market risk is measured by a project's (or stock's) market beta, which reflects the volatility of a project's (or stock's) returns relative to the returns on a well-diversified portfolio of securities. The market risk of a project (or stock) under consideration is a function of the project's (or stock's) standard deviation of returns, the standard deviation of returns on a well-diversified portfolio of securities, and the correlation between the returns on the project (or stock) and the returns on the security portfolio.

10. Stand-alone risk is most relevant to investments held in isolation; corporate risk is most relevant to projects held by not-for-profit firms; and market risk is most relevant to projects held by investor-owned firms.

11. The overall beta coefficient of a portfolio is the weighted average of the betas of the components of the portfolio, where the weights are the proportion of the overall investment in each component. Thus, the weighted average of corporate betas of all projects in a business must equal one, while the weighted average of all projects' market betas must equal the market beta of the firm's stock.

The risk concepts covered in this chapter will be used over and over throughout the book, because defining and measuring risk is critical to conducting sound financial analyses and making good financial decisions. Specifically, risk concepts are used in the next chapter to develop required rates of return on stock investments.

———

In the discussion of the financial risk inherent in the expansion into home healthcare, the CFO made the following points:

1. South Mesa Regional Medical Center is a not-for-profit business, so the relevant risk of the expansion project is its corporate risk or the contribution of the project to the overall riskiness of the hospital's returns.

2. After a thorough project risk analysis (which is covered in Chapter 8), the project was judged to have below-average corporate risk. Thus, the project was judged to be less risky than most of the hospital's other assets.

3. Since the expected rate of return on the project is more than that required on an average-risk project, and since the project is judged to have below-average risk, the project's return is more than that needed to compensate the hospital for its risk.

After the risk analysis, the board voted unanimously to approve the project. The hospital moved aggressively into home healthcare, and the move has had a positive impact on both the hospital's profitability and its riskiness, as increasing home healthcare revenues offset somewhat the hospital's decreasing inpatient revenues.

SELF-ASSESSMENT EXERCISES

The exercises in this section cover the key points of the chapter and give you the opportunity to assess your understanding of the material. Solutions to the self-assessment exercises are contained in Appendix A.

2–1   Assume that you invested $10,000 in the stock of General Medical Corporation with the intention of selling after one year. The stock pays no dividends, so your entire return will be based on the price of the stock when you sell.

a. To begin, assume that the stock sale nets you $11,500. What would be the dollar return on your stock investment? What would be the rate of return?

b. Now assume that the stock price falls, and you net only $9,500 when the stock is sold. Now what would be the dollar return on your stock investment? What would be the rate of return?

2–2   a. What is financial risk? Give a simple example that illustrates the concept of financial risk.

b. What is risk aversion? Why is the concept of risk aversion so important to financial decision making?

2–3   Consider the following probability distributions of returns estimated for a proposed project involving a new ultrasound machine:

State of the Economy	Probability of Occurrence	Rate of Return
Very poor	0.10	−10.0%
Poor	0.20	0.0
Average	0.40	10.0
Good	0.20	20.0
Very good	0.10	30.0

       a. What is the expected rate of return on the project?

       b. What is the project's standard deviation of returns?

       c. What is the project's coefficient of variation of returns?

       d. What type of risk do the standard deviation and coefficient of variation measure?

       e. In what situation is this risk relevant?

2–4   a. Explain why holding investments in portfolios has such a profound impact on our concept of financial risk.

       b. Assume that two investments are combined in a portfolio.

          (1) In words, what is the expected rate of return on the portfolio?

          (2) What condition must be present for the portfolio to have lower risk than the lesser-risk investment?

       c. Explain the difference between portfolio risk and diversifiable risk.

       d. What are the implications of portfolio theory for investors?

2–5   a. What are the two types of portfolio risk?

       b. Consider corporate risk.

          (1) How is it defined?

          (2) How is it measured?

          (3) Write out the formula for a project's corporate beta.

          (4) Explain how each factor in the formula affects a project's corporate risk.

       c. Now, consider market risk.

          (1) How is it defined?

          (2) How is it measured?

          (3) Write out the formula for a project's market beta.

          (4) Explain how each factor in the formula affects a project's market risk.

       d. Under what circumstances are each type of risk—stand-alone, corporate, and market—relevant?

SELECTED REFERENCES

Brigham, Eugene F. and Louis C. Gapenski. *Financial Management: Theory and Practice.* Fort Worth, TX: Dryden Press, 1997, Chapters 4 and 5.

Gapenski, Louis C. "Project Risk Definition and Measurement in a Not-for-Profit Setting." *Health Services Management Research,* November 1992, pp. 216–24.

3

CHAPTER

Required Rates of Return

The Christmas bells rang extra long at Barnett University Hospital — the CEO had just been informed by the Foundation Director that the hospital had received a $10 million gift from the estate of a long-time benefactor. The contribution, along with an additional $10 million to be raised by issuing new debt, was enough to fund a new academic research building, a project that had been envisioned, but unfunded, for some time. Ground breaking could now be scheduled for the spring, and the new facility could be in operation in about two years.

The word spread quickly throughout the hospital, especially among the medical staff who would be using the new research facility. In the staff dining room, two physicians were discussing the hospital's good fortune when the conversation turned to the additional debt financing needed to complete the funding. "I wonder how much we'll have to pay to borrow for the new building," questioned Dr. George Baker, the head of radiology. "If my memory is correct, it cost the hospital over 15 percent to borrow in the early 1980s; whereas, the last debt issue, in 1995, had an interest rate of less than 6 percent. I just don't understand why our borrowing costs fluctuate so much," he concluded.

Fortunately for Dr. Baker, his lunch companion that day was Dr. Elizabeth Brooks, a pediatrician who had just completed an executive MBA program offered by the university's college of business administration. "Well," she said, "I'm no expert, but I do think I can explain why different debt issues have different interest rates and why rates change over time."

Although reading this chapter will not make you an expert in how investors set required rates of return, it will introduce you to the basics. When you finish reading the chapter, you should be able to help Dr. Baker understand how interest rates are set. At the end of the chapter, Dr. Brooks will present her views. See if you agree with her.

INTRODUCTION

Chapter 2 discussed investment returns and financial risk, so we now know how to define risk and, more importantly, how it can be measured. We know also that individual investors and businesses are averse to risk, so investments with higher risk must have higher expected rates of return to attract capital. The next logical question is this: How much return must an investment provide to compensate an investor for a given amount of risk? Put another way: How do investors set required rates of return on investments? Chapter 3 tackles this issue.

The concept of required rates of return is extremely important in financial decision making. First, when businesses go to the financial markets to raise capital, investors must make judgments about the riskiness of the business and then set required rates of return on the basis of their judgments. By understanding how investors set required returns, managers can better structure their businesses to minimize the costs of the firm's debt and equity capital. Second, when businesses make their own investment decisions, whether choosing among securities for temporary investment or among alternative capital investments, it is necessary to set required rates of return to assess the financial values of the investments being analyzed. The emphasis in this chapter is on required rates of return on securities because it is necessary to understand the risk/return relationship for a business's securities before the concept can be extended to a business's real asset investments.

The two primary classes of business securities are debt and equity, so the chapter is divided into two major sections. As a precursor to the discussions of debt and equity required rates of return, it is necessary to understand the basic forms and features of each security because these elements define the riskiness of the securities as seen by investors.

DEBT FINANCING

Debt financing is one of two major types of business financing; the other being equity financing. The two types of financing are quite different from one another because the suppliers of debt capital (a business's creditors) have a fixed, contractual claim against the firm's earnings, whereas the suppliers of equity capital (a business's stockholders, or owners) have a claim against the business's residual earnings. Creditors expect to be paid the interest due on a loan even when earnings are poor or worse yet, when a firm is losing money. Indeed, businesses have a legally binding contractual obligation to make such payments, but no such obligation exists for dividend payments to stockholders.

Debt financing is divided into two types: short-term debt (with maturities of one year or less) and long-term debt. Although the basic characteristics that contribute to the riskiness of debt apply to both types, they tend to be used for different purposes. Long-term debt is typically used to fund capital investments (along with equity or fund capital), while short-term debt is usually employed to finance short-term seasonal or cyclical needs, which often involves current assets such as receivables and inventories. The discussion here focuses on long-term debt because it is most relevant to the book's focus on financial analysis and decision making.

There are many types of long-term debt: amortized and non-amortized, publicly issued and privately placed, taxable and tax exempt, secured and unsecured, callable and noncallable, and so on. In this section, we briefly discuss those long-term debt instruments most commonly used in the healthcare industry.

Term Loans

A term loan is a contract under which a borrower agrees to make a series of interest and principal payments, on specified dates, to a lender. Term loans are usually negotiated directly between the borrowing firm and a financial institution—generally a bank, a mutual fund, an insurance company, or a pension fund. Thus, term loans are private placements as opposed to public offerings, which are typically used on bonds. Although the maturities of term loans vary from 2 to 30 years, most are for periods in the 3- to 15-year range. Also, term loans are usually amortized in equal installments over the life of the loan, so part of the principal of the loan is retired with each payment. For example, Sacramento Cardiology Group has a $100,000 five-year term loan with Bank of America to fund the purchase of new diagnostic equipment. The interest rate on the fixed-rate loan is 10 percent, which obligates the Group to five end-of-year payments of $26,379.75. Thus, loan payments total $131,898.75, of which $31,898.75 is interest and $100,000 is repayment of principal.

Term loans have three major advantages over publicly placed debt: speed, flexibility, and low administrative costs. Because they are negotiated directly between the lender and the borrower, formal documentation is minimized. The key provisions of the loan can be worked out much more quickly, and with more flexibility, than can those for a public issue, and it is not necessary for a term loan to go through the Securities and Exchange Commission (SEC) registration process. A further advantage of term loans over publicly placed debt has to do with future flexibility: If a bond issue is held by many different bondholders, it is virtually impossible to alter the terms of the agreement, even though new economic conditions may make such changes desirable. With a term loan, the borrower can generally negotiate with the lender to work out modifications to the contract.

The interest rate on a term loan can be either fixed for the life of the loan or variable (floating). If it is fixed, the rate used will be close to the rate on bonds of equivalent maturity for companies of comparable risk. If the rate is variable, it is usually set at a certain number of percentage points over an index rate, such as the prime rate or the T-bill (short-term U.S. Treasury securities) rate. Then, when the index rate goes up or down, so does the rate of interest on the outstanding balance of the term loan.

Bonds

Like a term loan, a bond is a long-term contract under which a borrower agrees to make payments of interest and principal, on specific dates, to the holder of the bond. Although bonds are similar to term loans, a bond issue is generally registered with the SEC, advertised, offered to the public through investment bankers, and actually sold to many different investors. Indeed, thousands of individual and institutional investors may participate when a large firm such as Columbia/HCA Healthcare sells a bond issue, while there is generally only one lender (or very few lenders) in the case of a term loan. Also, it should be noted that a bond issue can be sold to one party (or to just a few). In this case, the issue would be a private placement.

Bonds are generally issued with maturities in the range of 20 to 30 years, but shorter maturities, such as 7 to 10 years, are occasionally used, as are longer maturities. In fact, in 1995, Columbia/HCA Healthcare issued $200 million of noncallable 100-year bonds, following the issuance of 100-year bonds by Disney and Coca-Cola in 1993. These ultra-long-term bonds had not been used by any company since the 1920s.

A bond's interest rate is generally fixed, although in recent years, there has been an increase in the use of various types of floating rate bonds. Also, bonds typically pay only interest over the life of the bond, with the entire amount of principal (or par value) being returned to lenders at maturity.

Mortgage Bonds

With a mortgage bond, the issuer pledges certain real assets as security for the bond. To illustrate, Mid-Texas Healthcare System recently needed $40 million to purchase land and to build a new hospital. Bonds in the amount of $20 million, secured by a mortgage on the property, were issued. If the company defaults on the bonds, the bondholders could foreclose on the hospital and sell it to satisfy their claims.

Mid-Texas could, if it so chose, also issue second mortgage bonds secured by the same $40 million hospital. In the event of bankruptcy and liquidation, the holders of these second mortgage bonds would have a claim against the property only after the first mortgage bondholders had been paid off in full. Thus, second mortgages are sometimes called junior mortgages, or junior liens, because they are junior in priority to claims of senior mortgages, or first mortgage bonds.

The number of mortgage bonds that can be issued by a firm is virtually always limited in the bond indenture (the debt contract) to a specified percentage of the firm's total bondable property, which generally includes all plant and equipment. For example, Mid-Texas can issue first mortgage bonds totaling up to 60 percent of its fixed assets. If fixed assets totaled $500 million, and if the firm had $250 million of first mortgage bonds outstanding, then it could, by the 60 percent of property test, issue another $50 million of bonds.

Debentures

A debenture is an unsecured bond, and as such, has no lien against specific property as security for the obligation. For example, Mid-Texas Healthcare System has $20 million of debentures outstanding. These bonds are not secured by real property but, rather, are backed by the revenue-producing power of the corporation. Debenture holders are, therefore, general creditors whose claims in the event of bankruptcy are protected by property not otherwise pledged. In practice, the use of debentures depends on the nature of the firm's assets and its general credit strength. If a firm's credit position is exceptionally strong, it can issue debentures—it simply does not need to pledge specific assets as collateral for debt. Debentures are also issued by companies with only a small amount of assets suitable as collateral. Finally, companies that have used up their capacity to borrow in the lower-cost mortgage market may be forced to use higher-cost debentures. These companies' debentures will be quite risky, and their interest rates will be correspondingly high.

Subordinated Debentures

The term subordinate means "below," or "inferior." Thus, subordinated debt has a claim on assets in the event of bankruptcy only after senior debt has been paid off. Debentures may be subordinated either to designated notes payable—usually bank loans—or to all other debt. In the event of bankruptcy and liquidation, holders of subordinated debentures cannot be paid until senior debt, as named in the debenture, has been paid. Subordinated debentures are normally quite risky, and hence such debt carries interest rates that are much higher than the rates on top quality debt. To illustrate, Consolidated Pharmacy Distribution, a mail-order prescription drug company, has $10 million in debentures outstanding that are subordinated to the company's accounts payable (trade credit) and notes payable. The debentures have a 10-year maturity and an interest rate of 16.5 percent, over twice as much as the 8 percent rate on its first mortgage bonds.

Municipal Bonds

Municipal bonds are long-term debt obligations issued by states and their political subdivisions, such as counties, cities, port authorities, and so on. Short-term municipal securities are used primarily to meet temporary cash needs, while municipal bonds are usually used to finance capital projects.

The type of municipal bond of specific interest to the healthcare industry is the revenue bond. Here, revenues derived from not-for-profit healthcare facilities are pledged as security for the bond, which is technically issued by a government-sponsored agency, although the agency has no responsibility for meeting promised payments. Most municipal bonds are sold in serial form; that is, a portion of the issue comes due periodically, anywhere from six months after issue to 30 years or more. Municipal bonds are typically issued in denominations of $5,000, or integral multiples of $5,000, and although most municipal bonds are tax-exempt, some are taxable to investors.

In contrast to corporate bonds, municipal bonds are not required to be registered with the SEC. However, prior to bringing municipal debt to market, issuers are required to prepare an official statement that contains relevant financial information about the issuer and the nature of the bond issue. Prior to 1994, issuers were not required to provide periodic financial updates, so it was very difficult for investors to obtain credit information about municipal bonds after initial issue. However, in November 1994, the SEC introduced new rules that require issuers to (1) provide annual financial statements that update the information contained in the official statement, and (2) release information on material events that could affect bonds' values as such events occur. This information is not sent directly to investors but, rather, resides in data banks that can be easily accessed by investment bankers, mutual fund managers, and institutional investors. In effect, by making the information available to investment bankers who handle public trades, any individual who wants to buy or sell a municipal bond will also have access to current information affecting the bond's value.

Whereas the vast majority of federal government and corporate bonds are held by institutions, close to half of the municipal bonds outstanding are held by individual investors. The primary attraction of most municipal bonds, as discussed in Chapter 1, is their exemption from federal and state (in the state of issue) taxes. For example, in August 1996, the rate of return on highly rated 30-year corporate bonds was about 8 percent, while the rate on similar-risk healthcare munis was about 6 percent. To an individual investor in the 40 percent federal-plus-state tax bracket, the muni bond's equivalent taxable yield was $6\%/(1 - 0.40) = 6\%/0.6 = 10.0\%$. It is easy to see why high tax bracket investors are so enthusiastic about municipal bonds!

To illustrate the use of municipal bonds by a healthcare provider, consider the $56 million in municipal bonds issued in May 1996 by the Jacksonville Health Facilities Authority. The Authority is a public body created under Florida's Health Facilities Authorities Act for the sole purpose of issuing health facilities municipal revenue bonds and then loaning the proceeds to the qualifying healthcare provider. For this particular bond issue, the provider is River City Medical Center, a not-for-profit hospital, and the primary purpose of the issue is to raise funds to build and equip a children's hospital facility. The bonds are secured solely by the revenues of River City Medical Center; so the actual issuer, the Jacksonville Health Facilities Authority, has no responsibility whatever regarding payment of interest or principal on the issue. The bonds are rated AAA, not on the basis of the financial strength of River City Medical Center, but because the bonds are insured by the Municipal Bond Investors Assurance (MBIA) Corporation. (Bond ratings and bond insurance, or credit enhancement, will be discussed in more detail later in the chapter.) Table 3–1 shows the maturities and interest rates associated with the issue.

Here are some relevant points about this municipal bond issue:

1. The issue is a serial issue; that is, the $56,000,000 in bonds is composed of 13 series, or individual issues, with maturities ranging from about 2 years to 30 years.

TABLE 3-1

River City Medical Center Municipal Bond Issue: Maturities, Amounts, and
Interest Rates

Maturity*	Amount	Interest Rate
1998	$ 705,000	4.70%
1999	740,000	4.85
2000	785,000	5.00
2001	825,000	5.15
2002	880,000	5.30
2003	925,000	5.40
2004	985,000	5.50
2005	1,050,000	5.60
2006	1,115,000	5.70
2007	1,190,000	5.80
2010	5,590,000	6.20
2015	9,435,000	6.30
2025	31,775,000	6.40
	$56,000,000	

* All serial issues mature on June 1 of the listed year.

2. Interest rates increase across series as the maturities increase. (The relationship between interest rates and maturity is discussed later in the chapter.)

3. The bonds that mature in 2010, 2015, and 2025 have sinking fund provisions (which also will be discussed shortly), whereby the hospital must place a specified dollar amount with a trustee each year to ensure that funds are available to retire the bonds as they become due.

4. Although it is not shown in the table, River City's debt service requirements—that is, the total annual amount of principal and interest that it has to pay on the issue—are relatively constant over time, at about $4,500,000 per year. The purpose of structuring the series in this way is to match the overall maturity of the bonds to the maturity of the asset being financed. The children's hospital has a life of about 30 years. During this time, it will be generating revenues more or less evenly, and its value will decline more or less evenly. Thus, the bond series was structured so that the debt service requirements can be met by the revenues associated with the

children's hospital. At the end of 30 years, the debt will be paid off, and River City probably will be planning for a replacement facility or major renovation that would be funded, at least in part, by a new debt issue.

DEBT CONTRACT PROVISIONS

A firm's managers are most concerned about (1) the interest rate that the firm must pay on its debt issues and (2) any provisions that might restrict the firm's future actions. This section discusses features that could affect either the interest rate or the firm's future flexibility.

Bond Indentures

An indenture is a legal document, which may be several hundred pages long, that spells out the rights of both the bondholders and the issuing corporation. The indenture includes a set of restrictive covenants that cover such points as the conditions under which the issuer can pay off the bonds prior to maturity, the financial condition the company must maintain to issue additional debt, and, for investor-owned firms, any restrictions against the payment of dividends. The purpose of restrictive covenants is to protect bondholders from managerial actions that would negatively affect the creditworthiness of the company and hence have an adverse effect on the value of the bond issue.

The trustee is an official (usually of a bank) who represents the bondholders and makes sure that the terms of the indenture are being carried out. The trustee is responsible for trying to keep the covenants from being violated and for taking appropriate action if a violation does occur. What constitutes "appropriate action" varies with the circumstances. It might be that to insist on immediate compliance would result in bankruptcy and possibly large losses on the bonds. In such a case, the trustee might decide that the bondholders would be better served by giving the company a chance to work out its problems and thus avoid forcing it into bankruptcy.

Call Provisions

A call provision gives the issuer the right to call a bond for redemption prior to maturity; that is, the right to pay off the bondholders in entirety and retire the issue. If it is used, the call provision generally states that the company must pay an amount greater than the initial amount borrowed (par or face value). The additional sum required, called a call premium, is often set equal to one year's interest if the bond is called during the first year, with the premium declining at a constant rate over the life of the issue. Many callable bonds offer a period of call protection. For example, some bonds are not callable until 5 or 10 years after the original issue date. This type of call provision is known as a deferred call.

To illustrate call provisions, consider River City Medical Center's bond issue contained in Table 3–1. All bonds that mature in 2006 and later are subject to call after December 31, 2005. If the call is made in 2006 and 2007, the call premium is 2 percent, or $20 for each $1,000 in face value. The premium drops to 1.5 percent for calls in 2008 and 2009, 1 percent for calls in 2010 and 2011, 0.5 percent for calls in 2012 and 2013, and zero for any calls beyond 2013.

The call privilege is valuable to the issuer but potentially detrimental to bond investors, especially if the bond is issued in a period when interest rates are cyclically high. In general, bonds are called when interest rates have fallen because the issuer usually replaces the old, high-interest issue with a new lower-interest issue. Thus, investors are forced to reinvest the principal returned in a call in new securities at lower rates. The added risk to investors inherent in a call provision causes the interest rate on a new issue of callable bonds to exceed that on a similar issue of noncallable bonds.

Sinking Funds

A sinking fund provides for the systematic retirement of a bond issue. Typically, a sinking fund provision requires the issuer to retire a portion of its bonds each year. Some sinking funds, such as the one on the River City Medical Center bonds, require the issuer to deposit money with the trustee, who invests the funds and then uses the accumulated sum to retire the entire bond issue when it matures. Sometimes the stipulated sinking fund payment is tied to the sales or earnings of the current year, but usually it is a mandatory fixed amount. If it is mandatory, failure to meet the sinking fund payment causes the bond issue to be thrown into default, which could force the issuer into bankruptcy.

In most cases, the issuer is given the right to handle the sinking fund in either of two ways:

1. The issuer may call in for redemption at par value (thus without a premium) a certain percentage of the bonds each year; for example, it might call 2 percent of the total original amount of the issue each year. Bonds are numbered serially, and the ones called for redemption are determined by a lottery.

2. If the bonds are actively traded, which occurs only for large issues by major corporations, the issuer may buy the required amount of bonds on the open market.

The issuer will choose the lowest-cost method. Therefore, if interest rates have risen, which, as you will see in Chapter 5, will cause bond prices to fall, the issuer will buy the bonds in the open market if they are actively traded. Otherwise, the issuer will call the bonds. Note that a call for sinking fund purposes is quite different from a refunding call. A sinking fund call requires no call premium, and only a small percentage of the issue is callable in any one year.

The River City issue contained in Table 3–1 has a sinking fund provision on the series with maturities of 2010, 2015, and 2025. Since municipal bonds are typically not actively traded, the sinking fund provision specifically calls for the funds to be placed in the hands of the trustee, who will ensure that they are used to retire the series when they mature.

Although a sinking fund is designed to protect the bondholders by assuring that the issue is retired in an orderly fashion, it must be recognized that, like a call provision, a sinking fund may at times work to the detriment of bondholders. On balance, however, securities that provide for a sinking fund and continuing redemption are regarded as being safer than bonds without sinking funds, so adding a sinking fund provision to a bond issue will lower the interest rate required on the bond.

BOND RATINGS

Since the early 1900s, bonds have been assigned quality ratings that reflect their probability of going into default, that is, the probability that the issuer will fail to make a promised interest or principal payment. The two major rating agencies are Moody's Investors Service (Moody's) and Standard & Poor's Corporation (S&P), which rate both corporate and municipal bonds. These agencies' rating designations are shown in Table 3–2.

TABLE 3–2

Bond Ratings

Credit Risk	Moody's	Standard & Poor's
Prime	Aaa	AAA
Excellent	Aa	AA
Upper medium	A	A
Lower medium	Baa	BBB
Speculative	Ba	BB
Very speculative	B	B
	Caa	CCC
		CC
Default	Ca	D
	C	

Note: Both Moody's and S&P use modifiers for bond ratings below triple A. S&P uses a plus and minus system; thus, A+ designates the strongest A rated bonds and A– the weakest. Moody's uses a 1,2, or 3 designation, with 1 denoting the strongest and 3 the weakest; thus, within the double A category, Aa1 is the best, Aa2 is average, and Aa3 is the weakest. Triple A bonds have no modifiers in either system.

Bonds with a BBB (using the S&P ratings) and higher rating are called investment grade; they are the lowest-rated bonds that many banks and other institutional investors are permitted by law to hold. Double B and lower bonds are speculative grade, or "junk bonds," with a fairly high probability of going into default; many financial institutions are prohibited from buying them.

Bond Rating Criteria

Although rating assignments are subjective, they are based on both qualitative characteristics, such as quality of management, and quantitative factors, such as measures of a firm's financial strength. Analysts at the rating agencies have consistently stated that no precise formula is used to set a firm's rating—many factors are taken into account, but not in a mathematically precise manner. Statistical studies have borne out this contention. Researchers who have tried to predict bond ratings on the basis of quantitative data have had only limited success, indicating that the agencies do indeed use a good deal of judgment to establish a firm's rating.

Table 3–3 presents a financial glimpse of stand-alone hospitals rated recently by Standard & Poor's. Note that these hospitals are

TABLE 3–3

Standard & Poor's 1993 New Hospital Ratings

Rating	Number of Hospitals	Bed Size	Average		
			Occupancy Rate	Profit Margin	Debt Ratio
AA	6	621	81%	9.3%	26%
AA–	3	554	65	5.3	25
A+	15	494	77	5.7	40
A	19	290	62	5.5	36
A–	32	247	64	5.0	38
BBB+	20	224	58	4.6	41
BBB	19	269	68	2.4	59
BBB–	9	192	68	5.5	38

Source: *Standard & Poor's Corporation CreditWeek Municipal.*

not part of chains nor did they use credit enhancement, as discussed in the next major section. Standard & Poor's indicated that during this time of upheaval in the healthcare industry, other business fundamentals besides financial indicators were considered when assigning credit ratings. Among these factors are location, market position, institutional characteristics, operating efficiency, and attractiveness to managed care plans.

Importance of Bond Ratings

Bond ratings are important both to firms and to investors. First, a bond's rating is an indicator of its default risk, so the rating has a direct, measurable influence on the default risk premium set by investors and hence on the bond's interest rate. (Default risk premiums will be discussed later in the chapter.) Second, most corporate (taxable) bonds are purchased by institutional investors, not by individuals, and many of these institutions are restricted to investment-grade securities. Also, most individual investors who buy municipal bonds are unwilling to take high risks in their bond purchases. Thus, if a firm's bonds fall below BBB, it will have a harder time trying to sell new bonds since the number of potential purchasers is reduced by the low rating. As a result of their higher risk and more restricted market, lower-grade bonds have much higher interest rates than do high-grade bonds. This point is highlighted in Table 3–4, which shows that investors require higher interest rates on both corporate and municipal bonds with lower ratings.

Changes in Ratings

A change in a firm's bond rating will have a significant effect on both its ability to borrow long-term capital and on the cost of that capital. Rating agencies review outstanding bonds on a periodic basis, occasionally upgrading or downgrading a bond as a result of the issuer's changed circumstances. Also, an announcement that a company plans to sell a new debt issue, or to merge with another company and to pay for the acquisition by exchanging bonds for the stock of the acquired company, will trigger rating agency reviews and possible rating changes. If a firm's situation has deteriorated somewhat, but its bonds have not been reviewed and downgraded, it may choose to use a term loan or short-term debt rather than to finance through a public bond issue. This will perhaps postpone a rating agency review until the situation has improved.

TABLE 3–4

Representative Long-Term Interest Rates, May 1996

Rating	Interest Rate	
	Taxable*	Municipal**
U.S. Treasury	7.2%	—
AAA	8.1	6.4%
AA	8.4	6.6
A	8.6	6.8
BBB	9.5	7.9
BB	10.4	8.6
B	11.4	10.5
CCC	13.2	11.2

* The non-Treasury taxable bonds are corporate issues.
** The tax-exempt bonds are municipal healthcare issues.

To illustrate a ratings change, Moody's raised its rating on HCA senior unsecured bonds from Ba to Baa when the Columbia-HCA merger occurred, and thus pushed HCA's debt into the investment-grade category. In the announcement, Moody's stated that the upgrade reflects "the significant improvement in bondholder debt protection resulting from the merger with Columbia Healthcare."

CREDIT ENHANCEMENT

Credit enhancement, or bond insurance, is a relatively recent development for upgrading a municipal bond issue's rating to AAA. The three largest bond insurers are the Municipal Bond Investors Assurance (MBIA) Corporation, AMBAC Indemnity Corporation, and Financial Guaranty Insurance Corporation, a subsidiary of General Electric Capital Corporation. Currently, almost 60 percent of all new healthcare municipal issues carry bond insurance.

Regardless of the inherent credit rating of the issuer, the bond insurance company guarantees that bondholders will receive the promised interest and principal payments. Thus, bond insurance protects investors against default by the issuer. Because the insurer gives its guarantee that payments will be made, the bond carries the credit rating of the insurance company, not the issuer. For example, in our earlier discussion of the bonds issued by the Jacksonville Health Facilities Authority on behalf of River City Medical Center, we noted that the bonds were rated AAA because of MBIA insurance. The hospital itself has an A rating, and hence bonds issued without credit enhancement would be rated A. The guarantee by MBIA resulted in the AAA rating.

Credit enhancement gives the issuer access to the lowest possible interest rate, but not without a cost. Bond insurers typically charge an up-front fee of about 0.2 to 0.5 percent of the total debt service over the life of the bond. Of course, the lower the hospital's inherent credit rating, the higher the cost of bond insurance. About 70 percent of newly issued insured municipal bonds have an underlying credit rating of AA or A. The remainder are still of investment grade, carrying a BBB rating.

Thus far, issuers have defaulted on very few insured bonds. For example, in its 20-year experience, MBIA has had to cover only two defaults: a $20 million hospital issue and a $12 million housing issue. However, many insurance analysts question the ability of bond insurers to cover defaulted payments should a severe recession occur. Their concern is that bond insurers do not have sufficient reserves to cover a large number of defaults. Further, the market as a whole has some reservations about bond insurance because interest rates on AAA insured issues tend to be slightly higher than rates on bonds that carry an uninsured AAA rating.

THE COST OF INVESTMENT CAPITAL

Capital in a free economy is allocated through the price system. The interest rate is the price paid to borrow debt capital; whereas, in the case of equity capital, investors' returns come in the form of dividends and capital gains (or losses). The four most fundamental factors affecting the supply of and demand for investment capital, and hence the cost of money, are (1) production opportunities, (2) time preferences for consumption, (3) risk, and (4) inflation.

To see how these factors operate, visualize the situation facing Kim Greene, a physician/entrepreneur who is planning to found a new home healthcare firm. She does not have all the capital needed to start the firm, so she must go to the debt markets for additional capital. If she estimated that the firm would be highly profitable, she could afford to pay a higher interest rate to potential creditors than if the firm were barely profitable. Obviously, her ability to pay for borrowed capital depends on the prospective firm's own investment opportunities—the higher her expected return on the home healthcare business, the more she could offer to pay potential lenders for use of their savings.

How attractive Ms. Greene's offer would appear to lenders would depend in large part on their time preferences for consumption. For example, one potential lender, Bob Wright, might be thinking of retirement, and he might be willing to loan funds at a relatively low rate because his preference is for future consumption. Another person, John Davis, might have a wife and several young children to clothe and feed, so he might be willing to lend funds out of current income, and hence forego consumption, only if the interest rate is very high. Mr. Davis is said to have a high time preference for consumption and Mr. Wright a low time preference.

The risk inherent in the prospective home healthcare business, and thus in Ms. Greene's ability to repay the loan, would also affect the return investors would require: The higher the perceived risk, the higher the required rate of return. Because of risk aversion, investors would simply be unwilling to lend to high-risk businesses unless the interest rate was higher than on loans to low-risk businesses.

Finally, since the value of money in the future is affected by inflation, the higher the expected rate of inflation, the higher the interest rate demanded by savers. In closing, note that our illustration implies that savers would lend directly to businesses needing capital, but, in most cases, the funds would actually pass through a financial institution, such as a bank, mutual fund company, or insurance company.

INTEREST RATE LEVELS

Debt capital is allocated among borrowers by interest rates: Firms with the most profitable investment opportunities are willing and able to pay the most for capital, so they tend to attract it away from inefficient firms or from those whose products or services are not in demand. Of course, the U.S. economy is not completely free in the sense of being influenced only by market forces. Federal, state, and local governments have agencies that help individuals or groups, as stipulated by Congress, to obtain credit on favorable terms. Among those eligible for government grants or subsidies are not-for-profit healthcare firms. Still, most capital in the U.S. economy is allocated through the price system.

Figure 3–1 shows how supply and demand forces interact to determine interest rates in two capital markets. Markets A and B represent two of the many capital markets in existence. The going interest rate, k_d, is initially 10 percent for the low-risk securities in Market A. (Note that the letter k is commonly used to represent capital costs, or interest rates, and the subscript d stands for debt.) Borrowers whose credit is strong enough to qualify for Market A can obtain funds at a cost of 10 percent. Riskier borrowers must obtain higher-cost funds in Market B. Investors who are more willing to take risks (less risk averse) invest in Market B with the expectation of receiving a 12 percent return, but also with the realization that the investment is riskier than that in Market A. By riskier, we mean that there is a higher probability that borrowers in Market B will default on their loans; that is, not meet the scheduled interest or principal payments.

FIGURE 3–1

Interest Rates as a Function of Supply and Demand

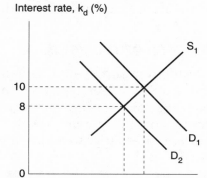

Market A: Low-Risk Securities

Interest rate, k_d (%)

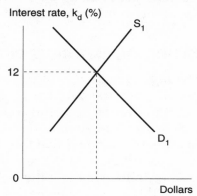

Market B: High-Risk Securities

Interest rate, k_d (%)

If the demand for funds in a market declines, as it typically does during a business recession, the demand curves will shift to the left, as shown in Curve D_2 in Market A. The market-clearing, or equilibrium, interest rate in this example declines to 8 percent. Similarly, you should be able to visualize what would happen if the availability of credit tightened: The supply curve, S_1, would shift to the left, which would raise interest rates and lower the level of borrowing in the economy.

Capital markets are interdependent. For example, if Markets A and B were in equilibrium before the demand shift to D_2 in Market A, investors were willing to accept the higher risk in Market B in exchange for a risk premium of 12% − 10% = 2 percentage points. After the shift to D_2, the risk premium would initially increase to 12% − 8% = 4 percentage points. In all likelihood, this much larger premium would induce some of the lenders in Market A to shift to Market B; this, in turn, would cause the supply curve in Market A to shift to the left (or up) and that in Market B to shift to the right. This transfer of capital between markets would raise the interest rate in Market A and lower it in Market B, thus bringing the risk premium back closer to the original level, two percentage points.

There are many capital markets in the United States. There are markets for short-term loans (called money markets) and long-term loans and equity (called capital markets). These markets are further broken down into markets for specific types of securities; and within each category, there are regional markets as well as different types of submarkets. Regardless of the market, the cost of funds is a function of the supply-and-demand conditions in that market.

SETTING REQUIRED RATES OF RETURN ON DEBT CAPITAL

Although prevailing interest rates result from supply-and-demand conditions in the debt markets, the supply of debt capital at any given interest rate depends on several factors. For any individual debt issue, the most important determinant of the interest rate is its risk. Chapter 2 noted that the riskiness of a security to an investor is the contribution of the security to the riskiness of a well-diversified portfolio. Although the security's market beta is the best measure of this risk, debt investors often think of risk in other terms. In this section, we discuss how interest rates, at least conceptually, can be decomposed into components.

In general, the interest rate on a debt security, which is also its required rate of return, k_d, is composed of a real risk-free rate of interest, k^*, plus premiums that reflect expected inflation, the riskiness of the security, and the security's marketability (or liquidity). This relationship can be expressed as follows:

$$\text{Required rate of return} = k_d = k^* + IP + DRP + LP + PRP$$

Note, however, that $k^* + IP = k_{RF}$, so another form of the interest rate equation is

$$k_d = k_{RF} + DRP + LP + PRP$$

Here

k_d = the required rate of interest on a given debt security.

k^* = the real risk-free rate of interest; k^* is pronounced "k-star," and it is the rate that would exist on a riskless debt security if zero inflation were expected.

k_{RF} = the nominal risk-free rate of interest. This is the interest rate on a security such as a U.S. Treasury bill (a federal short-term security), which is very liquid and free of most risks. Note that k_{RF} includes a premium for expected inflation, so $k_{RF} = k^* + IP$.

    IP = inflation premium. IP is equal to the average expected inflation rate over the life of the security.

  DRP = default risk premium. This premium reflects the possibility that the issuer will not pay interest or principal on a security at the stated time and in the stated amount.

    LP = liquidity premium. This is a premium charged by lenders to reflect the fact that some securities cannot be converted to cash on short notice at a "fair market" price.

  PRP = price risk premium. As shown in Chapter 5, longer-term bonds are exposed to a significant risk of price declines if interest rates rise, and a price risk premium is charged by lenders to reflect this risk.

The following sections discuss the components whose sum makes up the required rate of return on a debt security in more detail.

The Real Risk-Free Rate of Interest (k*)

The real risk-free rate of interest, k^*, is the interest rate that would exist on a riskless security if no inflation were expected, and it may be thought of as the rate of interest that would exist on short-term U.S. Treasury securities in an inflation-free world. The real risk-free rate is not static; it changes over time depending on economic conditions, especially on (1) the rate of return corporations and other borrowers can expect to earn on productive assets and (2) people's time preferences for current versus future consumption. It is difficult to measure k^* precisely, but most experts think it has fluctuated in the range of 2 to 4 percent in the United States in recent years.

The Nominal Risk-Free Rate of Interest (k_{RF})

The nominal risk-free rate, k_{RF}, is the real risk-free rate plus a premium for expected inflation: $k_{RF} = k^* + IP$. In the strictest sense, the risk-free rate is the interest rate on a totally risk-free security—one that has no risk of default, no liquidity risk, and no risk of loss if inflation increases (no price risk). In the United States, the closest thing to a truly risk-free security is a short-term Treasury security, a T-bill.

Treasury bonds, which are longer-term government securities, are free of default and liquidity risks, but T-bonds are exposed to some risk due to changes in the level of interest rates. In general, analysts use the T-bill rate to approximate the short-term risk-free rate and the T-bond rate to approximate the long-term risk-free rate.

Inflation Premium (IP)

Inflation has a major impact on interest rates because it erodes the purchasing power of the dollar and lowers the real rate of return on investments. To illustrate, suppose you save $1,000 and invest it in a Treasury security that matures in one year and pays 5 percent interest. At the end of the year, you will receive $1,050—your original $1,000 plus $50 of interest. Now suppose the rate of inflation during the year is 10 percent, and it affects all items equally. If beer had cost $1.00 per bottle at the beginning of the year, it would cost $1.10 at the end of the year. Therefore, your $1,000 would have bought $1,000/$1 = 1,000 bottles at the beginning of the year but only $1,050/$1.10 = 955 bottles at the end. Thus, in real terms, you would be worse off: You would receive $50 of interest, but it would not be sufficient to offset inflation. You would thus be better off buying 1,000 bottles of beer (or some other storable asset such as land, timber, apartment buildings, wheat, or gold) than buying the Treasury security.

Investors are well aware of the impact of inflation, so when they lend money, they build an inflation premium (IP) equal to the expected inflation rate over the life of the security into the required rate of return. Therefore, if the real risk-free rate of interest were $k^* = 3\%$, and if inflation were expected to be 4 percent (and hence IP = 4%) during the next year, then the required rate of interest on 1-year T-bills would be 7 percent.

It is important to note that the rate of inflation built into interest rates is the rate of inflation expected in the future, not the rate experienced in the past. Thus, the latest reported figures might show an annual inflation rate of 3 percent, but that is for a past period. If people on the average expect a 6 percent inflation rate in the future, then 6 percent would be built into the current rate of interest. Note also that the inflation rate reflected in the interest rate on any security is the average rate of inflation expected over the security's life. Thus, the inflation premium built into a 1-year bond is the expected inflation rate for the next year, but the inflation premium built into a 30-year bond is the average rate of inflation expected over the next 30 years.

Expectations for future inflation are closely related to, although not perfectly correlated with, rates experienced in the recent past. Therefore, if the inflation rate reported for last month increased, people would tend to raise their expectations for future inflation, and this change in expectations would cause an increase in interest rates.

Default Risk Premium (DRP)

The risk that a borrower will default on a loan also affects the market interest rate on a security: The greater the default risk, the higher the interest rate lenders charge. Treasury securities have no default risk; thus, they carry the lowest interest rates on taxable securities in the United States. For corporate and municipal bonds, the higher the bond's rating, the lower its default risk, the lower its default risk premium, and consequently, the lower its required interest rate.

Liquidity Premium (LP)

A highly liquid asset is one that can be sold quickly at a predictable "fair market" price and thus can be converted to a known amount of cash on short notice. Active markets, which provide liquidity, exist for government bonds and for the stocks and bonds of larger corporations. Real estate, as well as securities issued by small companies, including healthcare organizations that issue municipal bonds, are illiquid—they can be sold to raise cash, but not quickly and not at a predictable price. If a security is not liquid, investors will add a liquidity premium (LP) when they establish the market rate on the security. It is very difficult to measure liquidity premiums with precision, but a differential of at least two percentage points is thought to exist between the least liquid and the most liquid financial assets of similar default risk and maturity.

Price Risk Premium (PRP)

U.S. Treasury securities are free of default risk in the sense that one can be virtually certain that the federal government will pay interest on its bonds and will also repay the principal amount when the bonds mature. Therefore, the default risk premium on Treasury securities is essentially zero. Further, active markets exist for Treasury securities, so their liquidity premiums are also close to zero. Thus, as a first approximation, the rate of interest on a Treasury bond should be the risk-free rate, k_{RF}, which is equal to the real risk-free rate, k^*, plus an inflation premium, IP.

However, an adjustment is needed for long-term Treasury bonds. The market prices of long-term bonds decline sharply whenever interest rates rise, and since interest rates can and do rise, all long-term bonds, even Treasury bonds, have an element of risk called price risk. For example, if you bought a 30-year Treasury bond in 1972 for $1,000 when the long-term interest rate was 7 percent, and held it until 1981, when T-bond rates were about 14.5 percent, the value of your bond would have declined to about $514. That would represent a loss of almost half your money, and it demonstrates that long-term bonds, even U.S. Treasury bonds, are not riskless.

As a general rule, the bonds of any organization, from the U.S. government to Beverly Enterprises, have more price risk the longer the maturity of the bond. Therefore, a price risk premium (PRP), which is higher the longer the years to maturity, must be included in the required interest rate. The effect of price risk premiums is to raise interest rates on long-term bonds relative to those on short-term bonds. This premium, like the others, is extremely difficult to measure, but (1) it seems to vary over time, rising when interest rates are more volatile and uncertain and falling when they are more stable, and (2) in recent years, the price risk premium on 30-year T-bonds appears to have generally been in the range of one to two percentage points.

Although long-term bonds are heavily exposed to price risk, short-term bonds are heavily exposed to reinvestment rate risk. When short-term bonds mature and the funds are reinvested, or "rolled over," a decline in interest rates would result in reinvestment at a lower rate and hence would lead to a decline in interest income. To illustrate, suppose you had $100,000 invested in one-year Treasury securities, and you lived on the income. In 1981, short-term rates were about 15 percent, so your annual income would have been about $15,000. However, your income would have declined to about $9,000 by 1983 and to about $5,000 by 1996. Had you invested your money in long-term bonds, your income (but not the value of the principal) would have been stable. Thus, although "investing short" preserves one's principal, the interest income provided by short-term bonds varies from year to year, depending on reinvestment rates.

Note that long-term bonds also have some reinvestment rate risk. To actually earn the stated interest rate on a long-term bond, the interest payments must be reinvested as they are received in other securities that pay the bond's stated rate. If interest rates fall, the interest payments would be reinvested at a lower rate; thus, the realized return would be less than the stated rate. However, the reinvestment rate risk on a long-term bond is less than on a short-term bond because only the interest payments (rather than interest plus principal) must be reinvested over time.

In closing, note that in early 1996 the U.S. Treasury announced that it would soon begin to issue long-term bonds that are indexed to inflation. Although the details of the new bonds have not been finalized, one possible approach would be to link both the face value of the bonds and interest payments to inflation. Thus, if inflation were 5 percent in the first year of issue, the face value of a $1,000 bond would be increased to $1,050 and interest payments would increase proportionally. At maturity, the bonds would repay an amount greater than the original investment that would depend on realized inflation over the life of the issue. Because interest rate movements are primarily caused by inflation, these indexed bonds will be free of almost all risk. Thus, when such bonds are issued, their interest rate will be the real, risk-free rate.

A Healthcare Example

To understand better how an interest rate is developed using the above factors, consider Kim Greene's plan to found a new home healthcare business. She has asked a local bank to grant a 10-year, $100,000 loan to help get the business started. Here is the bank's assessment of the loan and the interest rate that they would charge if the loan is made.

$$k_d = k^* + IP + DRP + LP + PRP$$
$$= 2\% + 4\% + 5\% + 2\% + 1\% = 14\%$$

where

k^* = the real risk-free rate of interest = 2%.

IP = inflation premium = expected annual rate of inflation over the next 10 years = 4%.

DRP = default risk premium = the premium for providing debt capital to a relatively risky start-up business = 5%.

LP = liquidity premium = the premium for granting a loan that would be difficult to sell to another lender = 2%.

PRP = price risk premium = the premium for taking price risk on a 10-year loan = 1%.

THE TERM STRUCTURE OF INTEREST RATES

At certain times, such as in 1996, short-term interest rates are lower than long-term rates; whereas, at other times, such as in 1980, short-term rates are higher than long-term rates. The relationship between long- and short-term rates, which is called the term structure of interest rates, is important to healthcare managers, who must decide whether to borrow by issuing long- or short-term debt, and to investors, who must decide whether to buy long- or short-term debt. Thus, it is important to understand (1) how long- and short-term interest rates are related to each other and (2) what causes shifts in their relative positions.

To begin, one can look up in a source such as *The Wall Street Journal* or the *Federal Reserve Bulletin* the interest rates on bonds of various maturities at a given point in time. For example, the tabular section of Figure 3–2 presents interest rates for Treasury issues of different maturities on two dates. The set of data for a given date, when plotted on a graph, is called a yield curve. As can be seen in the figure, the yield curve changes both in position and in shape over time. Had the yield curve during January of 1982 been drawn, it would have been essentially horizontal, for long-term and short-term bonds at that time had about the same rate of interest.

Figure 3–2 shows yield curves for U.S. Treasury securities, but yield curves can be constructed for corporate bonds or for municipal (tax-exempt) bonds. For example, yield curves could be developed for Columbia/HCA Healthcare Corporation, for the not-for-profit River City Medical Center in Jacksonville, or for any other company that borrows money over a range of maturities. Had these yield curves been constructed and plotted on Figure 3–2, the yield curves for Columbia/HCA would have been above those for Treasury securities on the same date because the corporate yields would include default risk premiums, but they would have had the

FIGURE 3-2

U.S. Treasury Bond Interest Rates on Two Dates

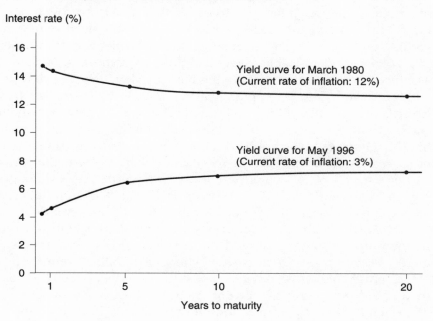

same general shape as the Treasury curves. Conversely, the curves for River City Medical Center would probably have plotted below the Treasury curves because the tax exemption benefit generally outweighs the default risk premium. In each case, the riskier the corporation—that is, the lower its bonds are rated—the higher its yield curve.

Historically, long-term rates have been above short-term rates in most years, so usually the yield curve has been upward sloping. An upward-sloping curve would be expected if (1) inflation is expected to increase in the future, or (2) the inflation premium is relatively constant across all maturities, in which case the price risk premium will push long-term rates above short-term rates. Since an upward-sloping yield curve is most prevalent, people often call this shape a normal yield curve. Conversely, a yield curve that slopes downward is called an inverted, or abnormal, yield curve. Thus, in Figure 3–2, the yield curve for March 1980 was inverted, but the one for May 1996 was normal.

INTEREST RATES AND BUSINESS DECISIONS

The yield curve for May 1996, shown in Figure 3–2, indicates how much the U.S. government had to pay at that time to borrow money for 1 year, 5 years, 10 years, and so on. A taxable healthcare firm would have had to pay somewhat more, while a not-for-profit provider would probably have had to pay somewhat less, but assume for the moment that we are back in May 1996 and that the yield curve in Figure 3–2 applies to all companies. Now suppose that River City Medical Center has decided (1) to build a new outpatient clinic with a 20-year life, which will cost $10 million and (2) to raise the $10 million by selling debt. If it borrowed in 1996 on a short-term basis—say, for one year—its interest cost for that year would be only 4.6 percent, or $460,000; whereas, if it used long-term (20-year) financing, its cost would be 7.1 percent, or $710,000. Therefore, at first glance, it would seem that River City should use short-term debt.

However, if the hospital uses short-term debt, it will have to renew the loan every year, and the rate charged on each renewal loan will reflect the then-current short-term rate. Interest rates could return to their March 1980 levels, so by 1999 or 2000 the hospital could be paying 14 percent, or $1,400,000, per year. On the other hand, if River City used long-term financing in 1996, its interest costs would remain constant at $710,000 per year, so an increase in interest rates in the economy would not hurt it.

Does this suggest that firms should always avoid short-term debt? Not necessarily. If inflation remains low for the remainder of the 1990s, so will interest rates. If River City had borrowed on a long-term basis for 7.1 percent in May 1996, it would be at a major disadvantage if its debt were locked in at that rate while its competitors that used short-term debt that cost 4.6 percent in May 1996 were able to continually renew that debt at a low rate. On the other hand, federal deficits might drive inflation and interest rates up to new record levels. In that case, all borrowers would wish they had borrowed on a long-term basis in 1996.

Financing decisions would be easy if managers could develop accurate forecasts of future interest rates. Unfortunately, predicting future interest rates with consistent accuracy is somewhere between difficult and impossible—people who make a living by selling interest rate forecasts say it is difficult, but many others say it is impossible.

Even though it is difficult, if not impossible, to predict future interest rate levels, it is easy to predict that interest rates will fluctuate—they always have and they always will. This being the case, sound financial policy for healthcare businesses calls for using a mix of long- and short-term debt, as well as equity (or fund capital), in such a manner that the firm can survive in all but the most severe, and hence unlikely, interest rate environments. Furthermore, the optimal financing policy depends in an important way on maturities of the firm's assets. In general, to reduce risk, managers try to match the maturities of securities with the maturities of the assets being financed. The issue of debt maturities will be revisited in Chapter 10, which discusses capital structure and debt-maturity decisions.

EQUITY FINANCING

The second major type of financing is equity financing. Equity, or ownership, capital comes in several forms. According to accounting classification, for-profit corporations issue two forms of equity: common stock and preferred stock. However, unlike common stock, preferred stock generally does not carry voting rights. Furthermore, preferred stock has a fixed claim against a firm's earnings rather than a claim against residual earnings. For these reasons, from a financial perspective, preferred stock is more of a debt security than an equity security. Since preferred stock is not widely used in the healthcare industry, this book will focus on common stock.

Most for-profit firms have only one type of common stock, but in some instances several types of common stock, called classified stock, are used to meet the special needs of the company. Generally, when special classifications of stock are used, one type is designated Class A, another Class B, and so on. Small, new companies seeking to obtain funds from outside sources frequently use different types of common stock. For example, when Bay Area Genetic Research, Inc., went public in 1996, its Class A stock was sold to the public and paid a dividend but carried no voting rights for five years. Its Class B stock was retained by the organizers of the company and carried full voting rights for five years, but dividends could not be paid on the Class B stock until the company had established its earning power by building up retained earnings to a designated level. The firm's use of classified stock allowed the public to take a position in a conservatively financed growth company without sacrificing income, while the founders retained absolute control during the crucial early stages of the firm's development. At the same time, outside investors were protected against excessive withdrawals of funds by the original owners. As is often the case in such situations, the Class B stock was also called founders' shares.

Note that "Class A," "Class B," and so on, have no standard meanings. Most firms have no classified shares, but a firm that does could designate its Class B shares as founders' shares and its Class A shares as those sold to the public, while another could reverse these designations. Other firms could use the A and B designations for entirely different purposes.

Investor-owned firms have two sources of equity financing: earnings retentions and new stock sales. (All net income that is not paid out as dividends is automatically retained by the firm and added to the firm's equity base.) Not-for-profit firms can, and do, retain earnings, but they do not have access to the equity markets; that is, they cannot sell stock to raise equity capital. Not-for-profit firms can, however, raise equity capital through government grants and charitable contributions. The equity capital in not-for-profit firms is often called fund capital, but it serves the same purpose as common stock in for-profit firms.

Individuals, as well as firms, are motivated to contribute to healthcare organizations for a variety of reasons, including concern for the well-being of others, the recognition that often accompanies large contributions, and tax deductibility. Since only contributions to not-for-profit firms are tax deductible, this source of funding is, for all practical purposes, not available to investor-owned healthcare entities.

SETTING REQUIRED RATES OF RETURN ON COMMON STOCK

As discussed in Chapter 2, the relevant riskiness of a stock to a well-diversified investor is its market risk, and the appropriate measure of market risk is the stock's market beta. Stock betas will be covered in more detail in Chapter 6, but for now recognize that many investment advisory firms, such as Merrill Lynch and Value Line, compute and publish stock betas for thousands of publicly traded companies. The key question here is this: What is the relationship between risk as measured by beta and return? That is, what rate of return will investors require on a stock to compensate them for assuming a given amount of risk as measured by its market beta coefficient? To begin our discussion, here are the relevant terms:

$E(R)$ = expected rate of return on a given stock.

k_s = required rate of return on a given stock. Note that if $E(R)$ is less than k_s, you would not purchase this stock, or you would sell it if you owned it. If $E(R)$ were greater than k_s, you would want to buy the stock. You would be indifferent if $E(R) = k_s$.

k_{RF} = risk-free rate of return. In this context, it is generally measured by the return on long-term U.S. Treasury bonds.

b = market beta coefficient of the stock. The beta of an average stock is $b_A = 1.0$.

k_M = required rate of return on a portfolio consisting of all stocks, which is the market portfolio. k_M is also the required rate of return on an average ($b_A = 1.0$) stock.

RP_M = market risk premium = $(k_M - k_{RF})$. This is the additional return over the risk-free rate required to compensate an investor for assuming average ($b_A = 1.0$) risk.

RP_s = risk premium on the stock in question = $(k_M - k_{RF})b$. The stock's risk premium is less than, equal to, or greater than the premium on an average stock, depending on whether its beta is less than, equal to, or greater than 1.0. If $b = b_A = 1.0$, then $RP_s = RP_M$.

The market risk premium, RP_M, depends on the degree of aversion that investors in the aggregate have to risk. Assume T-bonds currently yield $k_{RF} = 8\%$ and an average-risk stock (with $b_A = 1.0$) has a required rate of return of $k_M = 12\%$. Under these conditions, the market risk premium is 4 percentage points.

$$RP_M = k_M - k_{RF} = 12\% - 8\% = 4 \text{ percentage points}$$

It follows that if one stock were twice as risky as another, its risk premium would be twice as high, and, conversely, if its risk were only half as much, its risk premium would be half as large. Furthermore, a stock's riskiness is measured by its market beta coefficient. Therefore, if the market risk premium, RP_M, and the stock's risk as measured by its market beta coefficient, b, are known, the stock's risk premium is found as the product $(RP_M)b$. For example, if b = 0.5 for Northwest Home Healthcare, Inc. (NHH) and RP_M = 4%, then RP_s is 2 percentage points.

$$\text{Risk Premium for NHH} = RP_{s(NHH)} = (RP_M)b$$
$$= (4\%)(0.5) = 2.0\%$$

To summarize, given estimates of k_{RF}, k_M, and b, the required rate of return on any stock can be estimated. For example, the required rate of return on NHH's stock is 10 percent.

$$k_{s(NHH)} = k_{RF} + (k_M - k_{RF})b$$
$$= 8\% + (12\% - 8\%)(0.5)$$
$$= 8\% + (4\%)0.5 = 10\%$$

This equation is called the Security Market Line (SML). It is an extremely important financial tool because it provides the link between risk and required returns, at least within a market risk framework. Without this link, one could talk in great detail about risk, but it would not be possible to quantify how investors should "price" risk into their investment decisions. The Security Market Line (SML) is the "bottom line," or "useful end," of a widely used equilibrium risk/return model called the Capital Asset Pricing Model (CAPM).

If some other stock, say, Boston Biotechnologies (BB), were riskier than Northwest Home Healthcare and had b = 2.0, then its required rate of return would be 16 percent.

$$k_{s(BB)} = 8\% + (4\%)2.0 = 16\%$$

An average stock, with b = 1.0, would have a required return of 12 percent, the same as the market return.

$$k_{s(A)} = 8\% + (4\%)1.0 = 12\% = k_M$$

The SML is often expressed in graph form, as in Figure 3–3, which shows the SML when k_{RF} = 8% and k_M = 12%. Note the following points:

1. Required rates of return are shown on the vertical axis, while risk as measured by market beta is shown on the horizontal axis.

2. Riskless securities have b = 0; therefore, k_{RF} appears as the vertical axis intercept in Figure 3–3.

FIGURE 3–3

Security Market Line

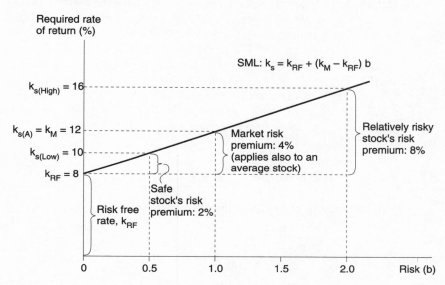

3. The slope of the SML reflects the degree of risk aversion in the economy; the greater the average investor's aversion to risk, (a) the steeper the slope of the line, (b) the greater the risk premium for any stock, and (c) the higher the required rate of return on all stocks.

4. The values for k_s worked out above for stocks with b = 0.5, b = 1.0, and b = 2.0 agree with the values shown on the graph.

Both the plot of the SML and a company's position on the X axis change over time due to changes in interest rates, investors' risk aversion, and individual company's betas. Thus, the SML, as well as a company's risk, must be evaluated on the basis of current information.

The SML is a key element of the risk/return relationship when market risk is the relevant risk in financial decision making. Thus, you will use the SML again both in Chapter 5, to value financial assets, and in Chapter 6, to develop a firm's opportunity cost of capital.

————

Here is Dr. Brooks's explanation of how interest rates are set on a particular loan and why rates fluctuate over time:

Basically, investors set interest rates on a debt security to earn a return that (1) compensates them for the time value of money, (2) protects them against inflation, and (3) compensates them for the risks inherent in the investment. To accomplish this, they charge a base rate called the real, risk-free rate, then add premiums to this rate that reflect expected inflation and the riskiness of the investment. The higher the risk and inflation expectations, the higher the interest rate. Interest rates for the debt of Barnett University Hospital vary over time for several reasons, the most important being changes in inflation expectations. In the early 1980s, inflation was running in double digits, so interest rates were high. By 1996, inflation was down to about 3 percent, so interest rates were relatively low.

SELF-ASSESSMENT EXERCISES

3–1   a. Briefly describe the following types of debt:
      (1) Term loan
      (2) Bond
      (3) Mortgage bond
      (4) Senior debt; junior debt
      (5) Debenture
      (6) Subordinated debenture
      (7) Municipal bond
    b. Briefly explain the following debt features:
      (1) Indenture
      (2) Restrictive covenant
      (3) Trustee
      (4) Call provision
      (5) Sinking fund

3–2   a. What are the two major bond rating agencies? What do bond ratings measure? How do investors interpret bond ratings? (That is, what is the difference between an A-rated bond and a B-rated bond?)
    b. Why are bond ratings important to investors? Why are the ratings important to firms that issue bonds?
    c. What is credit enhancement?

3–3   a. The four fundamental factors that affect the supply of and demand for investment capital, and hence the cost of money, are (1) productive opportunities, (2) time preferences for consumption, (3) risk, and (4) inflation. Explain how each of these factors affects the cost of money.

b. Investors' required rate of return (or interest rate demanded) on a debt security, k_d, can be expressed by the following equation.

$$k_d = k^* + IP + DRP + LP + PRP$$

Define each term of the equation, and explain how it affects the required rate of return.

3–4 a. What is a yield curve? Is the yield curve static, or does it change over time? What is the difference between a normal yield curve and an inverted yield curve?

b. What impact does the yield curve have on debt financing decisions?

3–5 a. Write out the equation for the Security Market Line (SML). Describe each term in the equation. Why is the SML such a valuable tool in financial management?

b. Suppose Value Line reports that Beverly Enterprises, a for-profit nursing home chain, has a beta coefficient of 1.25. Assume further that the risk-free rate (the current interest rate on long-term Treasury bonds) is 7.4 percent, and the required rate of return on the market (or an average stock) is 12.4 percent.

(1) What is the market risk premium?

(2) What is the required rate of return on Beverly's stock?

(3) Assume inflation expectations increase, and the risk-free rate increases to 8.5 percent. What is Beverly's required rate of return under these conditions? (Assume that the market risk premium does not change.)

(4) Finally; return to the original conditions, but now assume that Beverly's market risk decreases so that its beta coefficient falls to 1.10. Now what is the required rate of return on Beverly's stock?

SELECTED REFERENCES

Aderholdt, John M., and Charles R. Pardue. "A Guide to Taxable Debt Financing Alternatives." *Healthcare Financial Management,* July 1989, pp. 58–66.

Aderholdt, John M., and Robert H. Rasmussen. "Using Derivatives to Hedge Against the Unexpected." *Healthcare Financial Management,* February 1996, pp. 62–69.

Carlile, Larry L., and Bruce M. Serchuk. "The Coming Changes in Tax-Exempt Health Care Finance." *Journal of Health Care Finance,* Fall 1995, pp. 1–42.

Cleverley, William O., and Paul C. Nutt. "The Decision Process Used for Bond Rating—and Its Implications." *Health Services Research,* December 1984, pp. 615–37.

"A Creditor's Perspective on the Hospital Industry." *Topics in Health Care Financing,* Summer 1993, pp. 12–20.

Culler, Steven D. "Assessing Hospital Credit Risk: A Banker's View." *Topics in Health Care Financing,* Summer, 1993, pp. 35–43.

Demby, Hillary J. "Overcoming Financial Challenges with Bond Insurance." *Healthcare Financial Management,* March 1995, pp. 48–49.

Dunn, Kenneth C., Geoffrey B. Shields, and Joanne B. Stern. "The Dynamics of Leveraged Buy-Outs, Conversions, and Corporate Reorganizations of Not-For-Profit Healthcare Institutions." *Topics in Health Care Financing,* Spring 1991, pp. 5–20.

Elrod, James L., Jr. "Can Municipal Bond Futures Contracts Minimize Financial Risk?" *Healthcare Financial Management,* April 1986, pp. 40–44.

Flaherty, Mary Pat. "Planned Giving Programs as a Source of Financing: Creating a 'Win-Win' Situation for a Healthcare Organization and Its Donors." *Topics in Health Care Financing,* Spring 1991, pp. 70–81.

Harris, John P., and Jeannette B. Price. "Finding Money Under Your Nose Using New Capital Techniques." *Healthcare Financial Management,* July 1988, pp. 24–30.

Kaplan, Robert S., and Gabriel Urwitz. "Statistical Models of Bond Ratings: A Methodological Inquiry." *Journal of Business,* April 1979, pp. 231–61.

Kaufman, Kenneth, and Mark L. Hall. *The Capital Management of Health Care Organizations.* Ann Arbor, MI: Health Administration Press, 1990.

LeBuhn, James. "Primary Market Derivatives: Satisfying Investor Appetites." *Journal of Health Care Finance,* Winter 1994, pp. 11–21.

Mullner, Ross, Dale Matthews, Joseph D. Kubal, and Stephen Andes. "Debt Financing: An Alternative for Hospital Construction Funding." *Healthcare Financial Management,* April 1983, pp. 18–24.

Nemes, Judith. "Dealing with the Authorities." *Modern Healthcare,* October 14, 1991, pp. 22–29.

Odegard, Bradley M. "Tax-Exempt Financing Under the Tax Reform Act of 1986." *Topics in Health Care Financing,* Summer 1988, pp. 35–45.

Shields, Geoffrey B., and George C. McKann. "Raising Healthcare Capital Through the Public Equity Markets." *Topics in Health Care Financing,* Fall 1991, pp. 21–36.

Sims, William B. "Financing Strategies for Long-Term Care Facilities." *Healthcare Financial Management*, March 1984, pp. 42–54.

Sterns, Jay B. "Emerging Trends in Health Care Finance." *Journal of Health Care Finance*, Winter 1994, pp. 1–10.

Sykes, C. Scott, Jr. "The Role of Equity Financing in Today's Healthcare Environment." *Topics in Health Care Financing*, Fall 1991, pp. 1–4.

Wallace, Cindy. "Not-For-Profits Competing for Capital by Selling Stock in Alternative Ventures." *Modern Healthcare*, August 16, 1985, pp. 32–38.

West, David A. "Debt Financing in the 1980s: Is the Risk for Non-Profit Hospitals Too Great?" *Healthcare Financial Management*, April 1983, pp. 56–62.

Woodward, Mark A. "Interest Rate Swaps: Financial Tool of the '90s." *Healthcare Financial Management*, November 1993, pp. 56–64.

4

Discounted Cash Flow (DCF) Analysis

*R*obert MacGregor, the Northwest regional manager of ElderCare, Inc., a long-term care company, had a great idea. His mother needed to be placed in a nursing home in her hometown of Harper, Oregon, but there just weren't any beds available at the town's only existing facility. So, he took on the task of developing a plan to be presented to the firm's board of directors to build a new facility in Harper. The project would cost $10 million, but he expected that it would generate annual operating cash inflows of about $1 million.

Robert's plan for the board presentation was to review the overall concept, present the contractor's bid, discuss the expected annual revenues and operating costs, and then sell the project to the board on the basis of the company recovering its investment in about 10 years. That is, the expected cash inflows of $1 million per year over a 10-year period would total $10 million, the cost of the project. As Robert put it, all cash flows generated after 10 years would be "pure gravy" to the company.

However, before Robert finalized his board presentation, he wanted to get some input from Ellen Richards, a local banker. They had worked closely on another project, and Robert valued her financial know-how and judgment as to how best to sell his idea. Keep Robert's presentation plan in mind as you read the chapter, and see if you can come up with a better approach for his sales pitch. At the end of the chapter, you will find out how Ellen reacted to Robert's plan.

INTRODUCTION

The values of most assets—including securities such as stocks and bonds, real assets such as lithotripters and hospital wings, and even entire firms—stem solely from the future cash flows that the asset is expected to generate. The process of valuing future cash flows, which is called discounted cash flow analysis, or time value of money analysis, is vital to most business decisions because such decisions almost always involve future cash flows. In fact, of all the techniques used in financial decision making, none is more important than discounted cash flow analysis.

Although most readers of this book will not actually have to perform time value of money calculations, the best way to understand the concept is to understand the underlying mathematics. The math isn't difficult, and financial calculators are available for under $30 that can do the hard part for you. If you want to get the most out of this chapter, buy or borrow a financial calculator and follow along as the examples are presented. In that way, you will gain an excellent appreciation for why time value is important and how it will be applied to healthcare financial analysis and decision making. (Financial calculators are distinguished from other calculators in that they can perform time value of money analyses, including bond valuation and NPV/IRR analyses.)

TIME LINES

One of the most important tools in discounted cash flow analysis is the time line. Time lines make it easier to visualize when the cash flows in a particular financial analysis are expected to occur. To illustrate the time line concept, consider the following time line, which shows five periods.

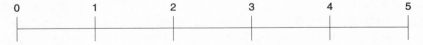

Time 0 is today; Time 1 is one period from today, or the end of Period 1; Time 2 is two periods from today, or the end of Period 2; and so on. Thus, the values on top of the tick marks represent the end of each time period. Off the time line, time periods are usually designated as t = 0, t = 1, and so on, where the letter t stands for time. Often, the periods are years; but other time intervals, such as semiannual periods, quarters, months, or even days, are also used. If the time periods were years, the interval from 0 to 1 would be Year 1, and t = 1 would represent both the end of Year 1 and the beginning of Year 2.

Cash flows are shown on a time line directly below the tick mark that matches the flow's actual time of occurrence, and interest rates are shown directly above the time line between tick marks. Unknown cash flows, which you are trying to find in the analysis, often are indicated by question marks.

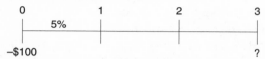

Here, the interest rate for each of the three periods is 5 percent; a single amount, or lump sum, cash outflow of $100 is made at t = 0; and the t = 3 value is unknown. We know the $100 is an outflow to the individual or firm doing the analysis because it is shown as a negative cash flow; that is, it has a minus sign. (Negative cash flows, or outflows, are sometimes designated by parentheses rather than minus signs.)

Now consider the following situation, where an unknown lump sum cash outflow must be made today to receive $100 at t = 2.

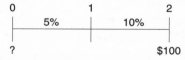

The interest rate is 5 percent during the first period, but 10 percent during the second period. Generally, the interest rate is constant over all periods, in which case it is indicated only in the first period to avoid cluttering the time line.

Times lines are useful when first learning discounted cash flow analysis, but even experienced financial analysts approach complex problems by first creating a time line of cash flows. The time line may be an actual line, as illustrated in this chapter, or it may be a series of columns (or sometimes rows) on a spreadsheet. Time lines will be used throughout the book to help you get into the habit of creating your own time lines when conducting analyses that involve future cash flows.

FUTURE VALUE OF A SINGLE CASH FLOW (COMPOUNDING)

A dollar in hand today is worth more than a dollar to be received in the future because current consumption is more valuable than future consumption. (Or as we noted in Chapter 1, a Big Mac today is better than a Big Mac tomorrow.) Also, if you have a dollar now, you can put it a savings account (or some other investment), earn a return, and end up with more than a dollar in the future. The process of going from today's values, called present values, to values in the future is called compounding. In this chapter, the discussion of compounding will begin with single cash flows (lump sums), and then, after the basic concepts are covered, the discussion will turn to multiple cash flows.

To illustrate compounding, suppose Green Valley Community Hospital had $100 in excess cash that it deposited in a bank account that paid 5 percent interest each year. How much would the hospital have at the end of one year? To begin, here are the terms that will be used:

PV = $100 = present value, or beginning amount, of the account.

i = 5% = interest rate the bank pays on the account per year. The interest is based on the balance at the beginning of each year, and it is paid at the end of the year. Expressed as a decimal, $i = 0.05$.

Interest = dollars of interest earned during the year = Beginning amount multiplied by i.

FV_n = future value, or ending amount, of the account at the end of n years. Whereas PV is the value now, FV_n is the value n years into the future, after the interest earned has been added to the account. Thus, FV_1 is the value of the account at $t = 1$, or after one year.

In our example, $n = 1$, so FV_n can be calculated as follows:

$$FV_n = FV_1 = PV + \text{Interest}$$
$$= PV + PV(i)$$
$$= PV(1 + i)$$

Thus, the future value at the end of one year, FV_1, equals the present value multiplied by 1.0 plus the interest rate.

These concepts can now be used to find how much Green Valley's $100 will be worth at the end of one year if it is invested in an account that pays 5 percent interest.

$$FV_1 = PV(1 + i) = \$100(1 + 0.05) = \$100(1.05) = \$105$$

What would be the value of the $100 if the hospital left its money in the account for five years? Here is a time line set up to show the amount at the end of each year:

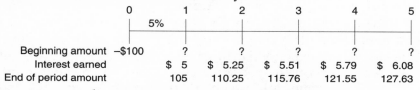

Here are the relevant points about the time line:

1. The account is opened with a $100 deposit—this is shown as an outflow at t = 0.
2. The hospital earns $100(0.05) = $5 of interest during the first year, so the amount at t = 1 is $100 + $5 = $105.
3. The account starts the second year with $105, earns $5.25 on the now larger amount, and ends the second year with $110.25. The second year's interest, $5.25, is higher than the first year's interest, $5, because the hospital earned $5(0.05) = $0.25 interest on the first year's interest.
4. This process continues, and because the beginning balance is higher in each succeeding year, the annual interest income increases.
5. The total interest earned, $27.63, is reflected in the account's final balance at t = 5, $127.63.

Note that the t = 2 value, $110.25, is equal to

$$
\begin{aligned}
FV_2 &= FV_1(1 + i) \\
&= PV(1 + i)(1 + i) \\
&= PV(1 + i)^2 \\
&= \$100(1.05)^2 = \$110.25
\end{aligned}
$$

Continuing, the balance at t = 3 is

$$
\begin{aligned}
FV_3 &= FV_2(1 + i) \\
&= PV(1 + i)^3 \\
&= \$100(1.05)^3 = \$115.76
\end{aligned}
$$

and

$$FV_5 = \$100(1.05)^5 = \$127.63$$

In general, the future value of a lump sum at the end of n years can be found by applying this equation:

$$FV_n = PV(1 + i)^n$$

Future values, as well as most other discounted cash flow problems, can be solved in three ways:

1. *Use a regular calculator.* One can simply use a regular calculator, either by multiplying the beginning value by $(1 + i)$ n times or by using the exponential function to raise $(1 + i)$ to the nth power. For this problem, you would enter $1 + i = 1.05$ and multiply it by itself four times, or else enter 1.05, then press the y^x (exponential) function key, then enter 5. In either case, you would get 1.2763 (if you set your calculator to display four decimal places) as the answer, which you would then multiply by $100 to get the final answer, $127.63.

2. *Use a financial calculator.* Financial calculators have been programmed to solve many types of discounted cash flow problems. The necessary equations are programmed directly into the calculator, and the data are entered into the equations using the time value of money input keys pictured below.

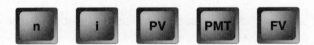

On some financial calculators, these keys are actually buttons on the face of the calculator; on others they are shown on the display after accessing the time value of money menu. Also, most calculators now use upper case n and i, and hence the keys show N and I, and other calculators use yet other symbols on their time value of money keys such as INT/YR for interest rate.

Note that there are five calculator keys that correspond to the five time value of money variables that are commonly used:

n (or N or some other symbol) = number of periods (years in our example).

i (or I or some other symbol) = interest rate per period.

PV = present value.

PMT = payment. This key is used only if the cash flows involve a series of equal payments (an annuity).

FV = future value.

This chapter deals with situations that involve only four of the variables at any one time—three of the variables will be known, and the calculator will solve for the fourth (unknown) variable. In Chapter 5, in the bond valuation section, all five of the variables will be used in the analysis.

To find the future value of $100 after five years at 5 percent interest using a financial calculator, just enter PV = 100, i = 5, and n = 5, and then press the FV key, and the answer 127.63 (rounded to two decimal places) will appear. Many financial calculators require that cash flows be designated as either inflows or outflows (shown as positive or negative values). Applying this logic to our illustration, Green Valley deposits, or puts in, the initial amount (which is an outflow to the hospital) and receives, or takes out, the ending amount (which is an inflow to the hospital). If your calculator requires that you follow this sign convention, the PV would be entered as –100.

Note also that some calculators require you to press a "Compute" key before pressing the FV key. Finally, note that financial calculators permit you to specify the number of decimal places that are displayed, even though 12 or more significant digits are actually used in the calculations. Most analysts generally display two places for answers in dollars or percentages, and four places for decimal answers, but the final answer should be rounded to reflect the accuracy of the input values; it makes no sense to say that the expected rate of return on a particular investment is 14.63827 percent when the cash flows are highly uncertain. The nature of the analysis dictates how many decimal places should be displayed.

3. *Use a computer.* Computers, along with spreadsheet programs such as Excel, Lotus 1-2-3, and QuattroPro, can also be used to solve discounted cash flow problems. Spreadsheet programs contain a set of preprogrammed time value functions, and spreadsheet users can create their own formulas to perform tasks that have not been preprogrammed. The discounted cash flow formulas that are provided are part of a series of functions called @func-

tions (pronounced "at functions"). Like any formula, @functions consist of a number of arithmetic calculations combined into one statement. By using @functions, spreadsheet users can save the time and tedium of building formulas from scratch. We will not discuss spreadsheet solutions in this chapter, but Appendix B contains spreadsheet applications, including discounted cash flow applications for this chapter.

The most efficient way to solve most time value of money problems is to use a financial calculator or a spreadsheet. However, financial analysts must understand the basic mathematics behind the calculations so they can set up complex problems before solving them. In addition, healthcare managers need to understand the underlying logic in order to comprehend stock and bond valuation, lease decisions, capital investment decisions, and other topics important to healthcare financial analysis and decision making.

PRESENT VALUE OF A SINGLE CASH FLOW (DISCOUNTING)

Suppose Green Valley Community Hospital has been offered the chance to purchase from a local broker a low-risk security that will pay $127.63 at the end of five years. The local bank is currently offering 5 percent interest on a five-year certificate of deposit (CD), and the hospital's managers regard the security being offered as being as safe as the bank CD. The 5 percent interest rate available on the bank CD is the hospital's opportunity cost rate, or the rate of return it could earn on alternative investments of similar risk. (Opportunity costs will be discussed in detail in the next section.) How much would the hospital be willing to pay for this security that promises to return $127.63 after five years?

From the future value example presented in the previous section, we saw that an initial amount of $100 invested at 5 percent per year would be worth $127.63 at the end of five years. Thus, Green Valley should be indifferent to the choice between $100 today and $127.63 at the end of five years. The $100 is defined as the present value, or PV, of $127.63 due in five years when the opportunity cost rate is 5 percent. If the price of the security is anything less than $100, the hospital should buy it; if the price is greater than $100, the hospital should turn it down. If the price is exactly $100, the hospital could buy it or turn it down because that is the security's "fair value."

In general, the present value of a cash flow due n years in the future is the amount which, if it were on hand today, would grow to equal the future amount when invested at the opportunity cost rate. Since $100 would grow to $127.63 in five years at a 5 percent interest rate, $100 is the present value of $127.63 due five years in the future when the opportunity cost rate is 5 percent.

Finding present values is called discounting, and it is simply the reverse of compounding—if you know the PV, you compound it to find the FV; if you know the FV, you discount it to find the PV. What follows is the solution to Green Valley's discounting problem.

Time Line

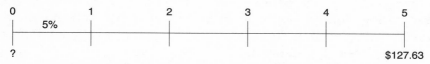

To develop the discounting equation, simply solve the compounding equation for the PV.

$$\text{Compounding: } FV_n = PV(1 + i)^n$$

$$\text{Discounting : } PV = \frac{FV_n}{(1+i)^n}$$

Regular Calculator Solution

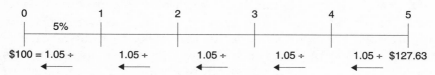

Here, divide $127.63 by 1.05 five times in succession to obtain the present value, $100.

Financial Calculator Solution

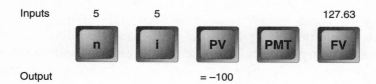

OPPORTUNITY COSTS

The opportunity cost concept plays a very important role in discounted cash flow analysis and hence in healthcare financial analysis and decision making. To illustrate, suppose you found the winning Florida lottery ticket and now have $1 million to invest. Should you assign a cost to these funds? At first blush, it might appear that this money has zero cost to you since its acquisition was purely a matter of good luck. However, as soon as you think about what to do with the $1 million, you have to think in terms of the opportunity costs involved. By using the funds to invest in one alternative, say buying the stock of Columbia/HCA Healthcare, you must forego the opportunity to make some other investment, say buying Treasury bonds. Thus, there is an opportunity cost associated with the $1 million investment even though your lottery winnings were, for all practical purposes, "free."

Since one investment decision automatically negates all other possible investments with the same funds, the cash inflows from any investment must be discounted at a rate that reflects the return that could be earned on foregone opportunities, regardless of the source of the funds. But the number of foregone opportunities is virtually infinite, so which one should be chosen to set the opportunity cost rate?

The opportunity cost rate to be applied in discounted cash flow analysis is the rate that could be earned on alternative investments of similar risk. It would not be logical to assign a very low opportunity cost rate to a series of very risky cash flows, or vice versa. This concept is one of the cornerstones of financial analysis and decision making, so it is worth repeating. *The opportunity cost rate (discount rate) to apply to investment cash flows is the rate that could be earned on alternative investments of similar risk, regardless of the source of the investment funds.*

Generally, opportunity cost rates are obtained by looking at rates that could be earned (at least expectationally) on securities such as stocks and bonds because they are more easily measured than rates of return on real assets such as hospital beds, MRI machines, lithotripters, and the like. For example, assume Green Valley Community Hospital was considering building a nursing home. The first step in the analysis would be to forecast the cost of the facility and the cash flows that it would likely produce. Then, these cash flows would have to be discounted at some opportunity cost rate. Would the hospital's opportunity cost rate be (1) the expected rate of return on Treasury bonds; (2) the expected rate of return on the stock of Beverly Enterprises, which owns some 850 nursing homes; or (3) the expected rate of return on pork belly futures? (Pork belly futures are very risky investments that involve commodity contracts for delivery at some time in the future.) The answer is the expected rate of return on Beverly Enterprises because that is the rate of return that could be earned on alternative investments of similar risk. Treasury securities are low-risk investments, so they would understate the opportunity cost rate in owning a nursing home. Conversely, pork belly futures are very high risk investments, so that rate of return is probably too high to apply to a nursing home investment.

Note that owning a single nursing home is riskier than owning a chain that has geographical diversification, so the true opportunity cost is probably somewhat higher than the return expected on Beverly Enterprises' stock. Also, it would be much easier for Green Valley to sell stock that it owned than it would be to sell a nursing home, so the nursing home investment should have yet an additional premium to account for its lack of liquidity. Finally, note that the source of the funds used for the nursing home investment is not relevant to the analysis. Green Valley may obtain the needed funds by issuing tax-exempt debt or by soliciting contributions, or it may even have excess cash accumulated from retained earnings. The discount rate applied to the nursing home cash flows depends on the riskiness of those cash flows, not on the source of the investment funds.

The bottom line here is that some discount rate has to be applied to discount future cash flows. The proper rate is the rate that best reflects the riskiness inherent in the future cash flows, and this rate is normally established by looking at the expected returns available on securities of similar risk. (Chapter 8 presents a detailed discussion on how the riskiness of a cash flow stream can be assessed.)

SOLVING FOR INTEREST RATE AND TIME

It should be clear that compounding and discounting are reciprocal processes and that we have been dealing with one equation in two different forms. Further, we have been working with four time value of money variables: PV, FV, i, and n. If you know the values of three of the four variables, you (normally with the help of your financial calculator or spreadsheet) can find the value of the fourth. Thus far, you have known the interest rate, i, the number of years, n, and either the PV or the FV. In some situations, though, you will need to solve for either interest rate, i, or time, n.

Solving for Interest Rate, i

Suppose Green Valley can buy a bank CD for $78.35 that will return $100 after five years. Here, we know PV, FV, and n, but we do not know i, the interest rate that the bank is paying. These types of situations are solved as follows, and the answer is 5.0 percent.

Time Line

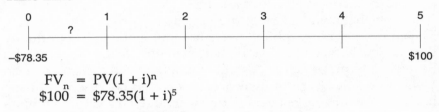

$$FV_n = PV(1 + i)^n$$
$$\$100 = \$78.35(1 + i)^5$$

Financial Calculator Solution

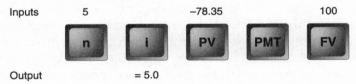

Solving for Time, n

Suppose the bank told Green Valley's managers that a CD pays 5 percent interest each year, that it costs $78.35, and that at maturity the hospital would receive $100. How long must the hospital keep its money invested in the CD? Here, we know PV, FV, and i, but we do not know n, the number of periods. Here is how to solve this type of problem, and the answer is 5 years.

Time Line

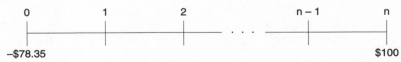

$$FV_n = PV(1 + i)^n$$
$$\$100 = \$78.35(1.05)^n$$

Financial Calculator Solution

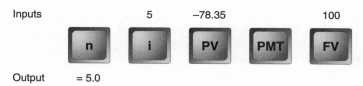

Inputs   5   −78.35   100

n   i   PV   PMT   FV

Output   = 5.0

ANNUITIES

An annuity is a series of equal payments at fixed intervals for a specified number of periods. Annuity payments, which are given the symbol PMT, can occur at the beginning or end of each period. If the payments occur at the end of each period, as they typically do, the annuity is an ordinary, or deferred, annuity. If payments are made at the beginning of each period, the annuity is an annuity due. Since ordinary annuities are far more common in actual situations, the term *annuity* without additional description usually refers to payments that occur at the end of each period.

Future Value of Ordinary Annuities

A series of equal payments at the end of each period constitutes an ordinary annuity. If Green Valley Community Hospital were to deposit $100 at the end of each year for three years in a bank account that paid 5 percent interest per year, how much would the hospital accumulate at the end of three years?

Time Line

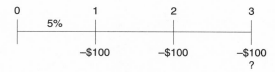

```
0          1          2          3
|    5%    |          |          |
|          |          |          |
        −$100      −$100      −$100
                                 ?
```

Note that the future value of an annuity is always defined as occurring at the end of the last period, so the future value of an ordinary annuity coincides with the annuity's final payment.

Regular Calculator Solution

One approach to the problem is to compound each cash flow to t = 3 and then sum the individual future values.

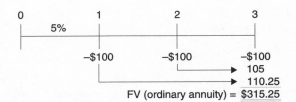

Financial Calculator Solution

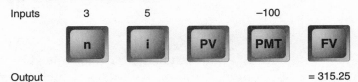

Output   = 315.25

In effect, a financial calculator performs the tasks on the time line above. Note that in annuity problems, the PMT key is used in conjunction with either the PV or FV key, along with the n and i keys.

Future Value of Annuities Due

Had the three $100 payments in the previous example been made at the beginning of each year, the annuity would have been an annuity due. Each payment would be shifted to the left one year, so each payment would be compounded for one extra year. In an annuity due, the future value occurs one period after the final payment.

Time Line

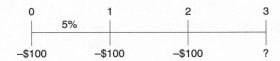

Regular Calculator Solution

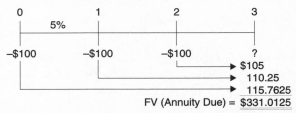

In an annuity due, as compared with an ordinary annuity, all of the cash flows are compounded for one additional period; hence, the future value of an annuity due is greater than the future value of a similar ordinary annuity by $(1 + i)$. Thus, the future value of an annuity due also can be found as follows:

$$\text{FV (Annuity due)} = \text{FV (Ordinary annuity)} \times (1 + i)$$
$$= \$315.25(1.05) = \$331.01$$

Financial Calculator Solution

Most financial calculators have a switch or key marked DUE or BEGIN (or some variation of these words) that permits you to change the setting from end-of-period payments (ordinary annuity) to beginning-of-period payments (annuity due). When this mode is activated, the display will normally show a word or symbol to signify that the calculator is in the annuity-due mode. Thus, to deal with annuities due, press the beginning-of-period switch or key and proceed as before.

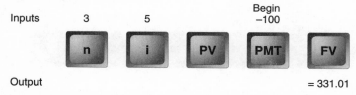

Since most problems will deal with end-of-period cash flows, don't forget to switch your calculator back to the end-of-period mode.

Present Value of Ordinary Annuities

Suppose Green Valley were offered the following alternatives by a potential contributor: (1) a three-year annuity with payments of $100 at the end of each year or (2) a lump sum payment today. If the hospital accepts the annuity, it would deposit the payments in a bank account that pays 5 percent interest per year. Similarly, the lump sum payment would be deposited into the same account. (Thus, the hospital's opportunity cost rate is 5 percent.) How large must the lump sum payment today be to make it equivalent to the annuity?

Time Line

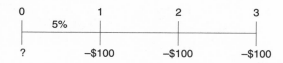

Note that the present value of an annuity is always defined as occurring at the beginning of the first period, so the present value of an ordinary annuity occurs one period before the annuity's first payment.

Regular Calculator Solution

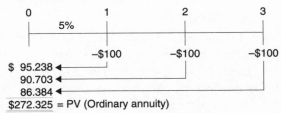

Financial Calculator Solution

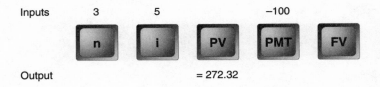

One especially important application of the annuity concept relates to loans with constant payments, such as term loans to businesses, mortgage loans, and auto loans. With such loans, the loan amount is the present value of an ordinary annuity, and the loan payments constitute the annuity stream. Term loans will be discussed in more depth in a later section on amortization.

Present Value of Annuities Due

Since its payments come in faster, an annuity due is more valuable than an ordinary annuity. Note that the present value of an annuity due coincides with the first payment.

Time Line

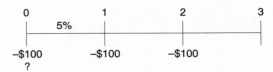

Regular Calculator Solution

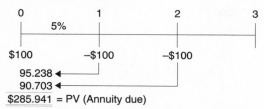

The present value of an annuity due can be thought of as the present value of an ordinary annuity that is compounded for one period, so it also can be can found as follows:

$$\text{PV (Annuity due)} = \text{PV (Ordinary annuity)} \times (1 + i)$$
$$= \$272.32(1.05) = \$285.94$$

Financial Calculator Solution

Activate the beginning-of-period mode, and then the following:

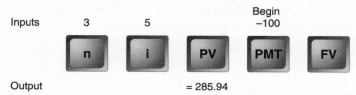

Again, since most problems will deal with end-of-period cash flows, don't forget to switch your calculator back to the end-of-period mode.

UNEVEN CASH FLOW STREAMS

The definition of an annuity includes the words *constant amount*—annuities involve payments that are the same in every period. Although some financial decisions, such as bond valuation (discussed in the next chapter), do involve constant payments, most decisions involve uneven, or nonconstant, cash flows. For example, common stocks typically pay an increasing stream of dividends over time; and capital projects, such as the operation of an MRI, do not normally generate constant operating cash flows.

In general, the term payment (PMT) is reserved for annuity situations, where the time line amounts are constant, while the term cash flow (CF) when applied to more than one flow denotes uneven amounts. Financial calculators are set up to follow this convention, so if you are using one and dealing with uneven cash flows, you need to use the CF, not the PMT, function.

Present Value

The present value of an uneven cash flow stream is simply the sum of the present values of the individual cash flows. For example, suppose Green Valley's managers are trying to find the present value of the following cash flow stream associated with a new project, and the opportunity cost rate is 6 percent.

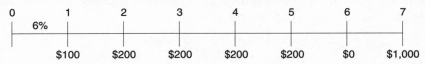

Regular Calculator Solution

One approach is to simply find the present value of each individual cash flow using a regular calculator and then sum these values to find the present value of the stream, $1,413.24.

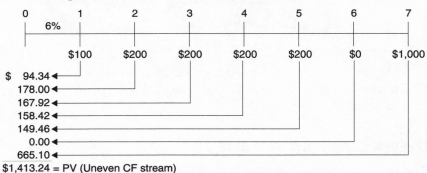

The present value can also be found by treating the cash flows in t = 2 through t = 5 as an ordinary annuity.

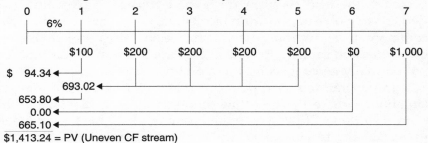

Here, the annuity present value occurs at t = 1 (one period before the first payment), so it had to be discounted for one more year to get the t = 0 value. Alternatively, the annuity payments could be treated as an annuity due, in which case the PV, $734.60, would have to be discounted two years at 6 percent to get the t = 0 value. The end result is the same.

The present value of a cash flow stream can always be found by summing the present values of the individual cash flows. However, cash flow regularities within the stream may allow the use of shortcuts, such as shown above. Also, in some situations, you may want to find the value of a cash flow stream at some point in time other than t = 0. In that situation, proceed as above, but compound and discount the individual cash flows to some other point on the time line, say t = 2.

Financial Calculator Solution

Problems involving uneven cash flows can be solved in one step with most financial calculators. The procedure is to (1) input the individual cash flows, in chronological order, into the calculator's cash flow registers, usually designated as CF_0 and CF_j (CF_1, CF_2, CF_3, and so on) or just CF_j (CF_0, CF_1, CF_2, CF_3, and so on); (2) enter the discount rate; and (3) push the NPV key. For this illustration, enter 0, 100, 200, 200, 200, 200, 0, and 1000 in that order into the calculator's cash flow registers, enter i = 6, and then push NPV to obtain the answer, 1,413.19. (A rounding difference occurs here.)

Three points should be noted. First, when dealing with the cash flow registers, the term *NPV* rather than PV is used to represent present value. The N in NPV stands for the word net, so NPV is the abbreviation for net present value. Net present value simply means the sum of the present values of a stream of both positive and negative cash flows (inflows and outflows); in effect, the inflows and outflows are "netted out" on a present value basis. The Green Valley example has no negative cash flows; but if it did, we would simply input them into the cash flow registers as negative numbers.

Second, note that annuity payments can be entered into the cash flow registers more efficiently on most calculators by using the n_j (or N_j) key. This key allows you to specify the number of times that a constant payment occurs within the uneven cash flow stream. (On some calculators, you are prompted to enter the number of times the cash flow occurs.) In this illustration, you would enter $CF_0 = 0$, $CF_1 = 100$, $CF_2 = 200$, $n_j = 4$, $CF_3 = 0$, and $CF_4 = 1000$. Enter $i = 6$, press the NPV key, and 1,413.19 appears in the display.

Finally, note that amounts entered into a calculator's cash flow registers remain in those registers until they are cleared. Thus, if you had previously worked an analysis with eight cash flows and then moved to an analysis with only four cash flows, the calculator would assume that the final four cash flows from the first analysis belonged to the second analysis. Be sure to clear the cash flow registers before starting a new analysis!

Future Value

The future value of an uneven cash flow stream (sometimes called the terminal value) is found by compounding each payment to the end of the stream and then summing the individual future values.

Regular Calculator Solution

The FV of each individual cash flow can be found using a regular calculator, and then these values can be summed to find the future value of the stream, $2,124.92.

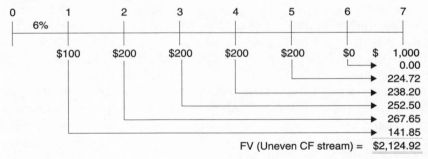

FV (Uneven CF stream) = $2,124.92

Financial Calculator Solution

Some financial calculators have a net future value (NFV) key, which, after the cash flows have been entered into the cash flow registers, can be used to obtain the future value of an uneven cash flow stream. However, most healthcare financial decisions involve the present value of an asset's cash flow stream rather than its future value because the present value represents today's value, which decision makers can compare to the cost of the asset.

Solving for Interest Rate, i

Although it is relatively easy to solve for i when the cash flows are lump sums or annuities, it is more difficult to solve for i when the present or future value is given and the cash flows are uneven. One can use a trial-and-error technique, in which various values of i are chosen until the correct one is found. Alternatively, a financial calculator's internal rate of return (IRR) function can be used when the present value is known. The use of the IRR function will be presented in Chapter 7 in conjunction with capital investment profitability measures.

SEMIANNUAL AND OTHER NONANNUAL COMPOUNDING PERIODS

All of the examples thus far have assumed that interest is compounded once a year, or annually. This is called annual compounding. Suppose, however, that Green Valley Community Hospital puts $100 into a bank account that pays 6 percent annual interest compounded semiannually. How much would the hospital accumulate at the end of one year, two years, or some other period? Semiannual compounding means that interest is paid each six months, so interest is earned more often than under annual compounding.

To illustrate semiannual compounding, assume that the $100 is placed into the account for three years. The following situation occurs under annual compounding.

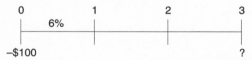

$$FV = PV(1 + i)^n = \$100(1.06)^3 = \$119.10$$

Now consider what happens under semiannual compounding. In this situation, $n = 2(3) = 6$ semiannual periods and $i = 6/2 = 3\%$ per semiannual period. Here is the solution.

Time Line

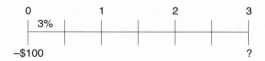

$$FV_n = PV(1 + i)^n = \$100(1.03)^6$$

Regular Calculator Solution

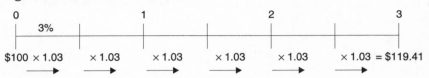

Financial Calculator Solution

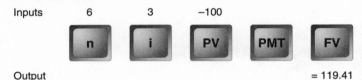

We see that the $100 deposit grows to $119.41 under semiannual compounding but only to $119.10 under annual compounding. This result occurs because interest on interest is being earned more frequently.

Semiannual and other compounding periods can also be used for discounting, and for both lump sum cash flows and annuities. First, consider the case of an ordinary annuity of $100 per year for three years discounted at 8 percent compounded annually.

Time Line

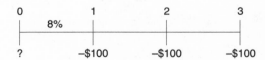

Financial Calculator Solution

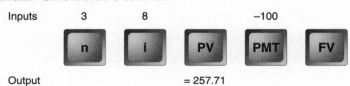

Now suppose the annuity calls for payments of $50 every six months for three years, and the interest rate is 8 percent compounded semiannually.

Time Line

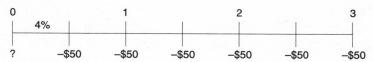

```
0              1              2              3
|   4%   |     |      |      |      |      |
?      -$50  -$50   -$50   -$50   -$50   -$50
```

Financial Calculator Solution

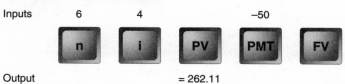

```
Inputs      6        4                      -50
          [ n ]   [ i ]    [ PV ]  [ PMT ]  [ FV ]

Output                              = 262.11
```

The semiannual payments come in a little earlier, so the $50 semi-annual annuity is a little more valuable than the $100 annual annuity. Note, though, that an annuity with annual payments but semiannual compounding cannot be treated in the same way. The discount rate period must match the annuity period, so if there are annual payments, then an annual discount rate (as calculated in the next section) must be used.

EFFECTIVE ANNUAL RATES

Throughout the economy, different compounding periods are used for different types of investments. For example, bank accounts often compound interest monthly or daily, most bonds pay interest semiannually, and stocks generally pay quarterly dividends. (Some banks and savings and loans even pay interest compounded continuously. Since continuous compounding is rarely used in health-care financial analysis and decision making, it will not be covered in this book.) If investments having different compounding periods are to be properly compared, their returns must be put on a common basis. The interest rates that are typically provided by banks and other institutions are stated (or nominal) rates, which do not reflect the impact of compounding more frequently than once a year. The rate that does reflect the impact of intra-year compounding is called the effective annual rate.

We found earlier that the future value of $100 after three years under semiannual compounding at a 6 percent stated rate is $119.41. The effective annual rate is that rate that produces the same ending (future) value under annual compounding. Thus, in the example, the effective annual rate is the rate that would produce an account value of $119.41 at t = 3 under annual compounding. The solution is 6.09 percent.

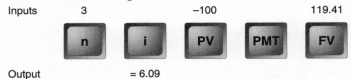

Inputs   3   −100   119.41

Output   = 6.09

Thus, if one bank offered to pay 6 percent interest with semiannual compounding on its savings accounts, while another offered 6.09 percent with annual compounding, they would both be paying the same effective annual rate, and hence the ending amount in each account would be the same.

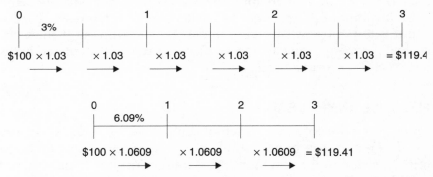

Given the nominal rate and number of compounding periods per year, the effective annual rate can be determined by using the following equation:

$$\text{Effective annual rate} = \left(1 + \frac{i_{\text{Stated}}}{m}\right)^m - 1.0$$

Here i_{Stated} is the stated (nominal) interest rate and m is the number of compounding periods per year. For example, the effective annual rate when the stated rate is 6 percent and semiannual compounding occurs is 6.09 percent.

$$\text{Effective annual rate} = \left(1 + \frac{0.06}{2}\right)^2 - 1.0$$
$$= (1.03)^2 - 1.0$$
$$= 1.0609 - 1.0 = 0.0609 = 6.09\%$$

Note that most financial calculators are programmed to calculate the EAR or, given the EAR, to calculate the stated rate. This process is called interest rate conversion. On most calculators, simply enter the stated rate and the number of compounding periods per year and then press the EFF% key to find the EAR.

Semiannual compounding, or, for that matter, any compounding that occurs more than once a year, can be handled in two ways. First, the n and i inputs can be expressed as periodic variables rather than annual variables. In the example, use n = 6 periods rather than n = 3 years and i = 3% per period rather than i = 6% per year. Second, find the effective annual rate and then use this rate as an annual rate over the number of years. In the example, use i = 6.09% and n = 3 years.

For another illustration of effective annual rates, consider the interest rate charged on credit cards. Many banks charge 1.5 percent per month, and, in their advertising, state that the annual percentage rate (APR) is 18.0 percent. However, the true cost rate to credit card users is the effective annual rate of 19.6 percent.

$$\text{Effective annual rate} = (1.015)^{12} - 1.0 = 0.196 = 19.6\%$$

The different types of interest rates will be reviewed in the last section of the chapter.

AMORTIZATION SCHEDULES

One important application of discounted cash flow analysis involves loans that are to be paid off in equal installments over time, such as automobile loans, home mortgage loans, and most healthcare business debt other than very short-term loans and long-term bonds. If a loan is to be repaid in equal periodic amounts (monthly, quarterly, or annually), it is said to be an amortized loan, and the payment schedule for such a loan is called an amortization schedule. (The word *amortize* comes from the Latin *mors*, meaning death, so an amortized loan is one that is killed off over time.)

To illustrate, suppose ElderCare borrows $100,000 from First BankCorp for kitchen renovations in one of its nursing homes. The loan terms call for repayment in three equal payments at the end of each of the next three years. First BankCorp is to receive 6 percent interest on the loan balance that is outstanding at the beginning of each year. The first task is to determine the amount that

ElderCare must repay each year, or the annual payment. To find this amount, recognize that the $100,000 loan represents the present value of an annuity of PMT dollars per year for three years, discounted at 6 percent.

Time Line

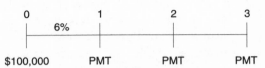

Financial Calculator Solution

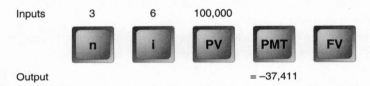

Therefore, if ElderCare pays First BankCorp $37,411 at the end of each of the next three years, the percentage cost to ElderCare, and the rate of return to First BankCorp, will be 6 percent.

Each payment consists partly of interest and partly of a repayment of principal. This breakdown is given in the amortization schedule shown in Table 4-1. The interest component is largest in the first year, and it declines as the outstanding balance of the loan is reduced

TABLE 4-1

Loan Amortization Schedule, 6% Rate

Year	Beginning Amount	Payment	Repayment of Interest*	Remaining Principal**	Balance
(1)	(2)	(3)	(4)	(5)	(6)
1	$100,000	$ 37,411	$ 6,000	$ 31,411	$68,589
2	68,589	37,411	4,115	33,296	35,293
3	35,293	37,411	2,118	35,293	0
		$112,233	$12,233	$100,000	

* Interest is calculated by multiplying the loan balance at the beginning of the year by the interest rate. Therefore, interest in Year 1 is $100,000(0.06) = $6,000; in Year 2 it is $68,589(0.06) = $4,115; and in Year 3 it is $35,293(0.06) = $2,118.
** Repayment of principal is equal to the payment of $37,411 minus the interest charge for each year. For example, in Year 1, the principal repayment is $37,411 − $6,000 = $31,411.

over time. For tax purposes, each year a taxable business borrower reports as a deductible cost the interest payments in Column 4, while the lender reports these same amounts as taxable income.

Financial calculators are programmed to calculate amortization tables—you just key in the inputs and then press one button to get each entry in the amortization table.

A REVIEW OF INTEREST RATE TYPES

This chapter discussed three different interest rate types: stated, or nominal, rate; periodic rate; and effective annual rate. To correctly perform discounted cash flow analysis when making healthcare financial decisions, it is essential that you understand the differences between the three and how each one is used in actual situations. Thus, to end the chapter, we review some of the finer points concerning interest rate types.

Stated, or Nominal, Rate

The stated, or nominal, rate is the rate that is typically stated in financial contracts. Convention in the stock, bond, mortgage, commercial loan, consumer loan, and other markets calls for terms to be expressed in stated rates. So if you talk with a banker, broker, or mortgage lender about rates, the stated rate, which is an annual rate, will normally be quoted. However, to be meaningful, the stated rate must be accompanied by the number of compounding periods per year. For example, a bank account might offer 5 percent interest compounded quarterly, a money market mutual fund might offer a 4 percent rate with interest paid monthly, or a term loan to a business might have terms of 12 percent, compounded monthly. You should never use the stated rate for calculations (that is, never use i_{Stated} on a time line or in your calculator) unless compounding occurs once a year, in which case the stated rate is also the periodic rate and the effective annual rate.

Periodic Rate

The periodic rate is the rate charged by a lender or paid by a borrower per period. It can be a rate per year (in which case the stated rate equals the periodic rate), per six-month period, per quarter, per month, per day, or per any other time interval. For example, a bank might charge 1.5 percent per month on its credit card loans, or a finance company might charge 3 percent per quarter on consumer loans. Note that Periodic rate = i_{Stated}/m, which implies that i_{Stated} = (Periodic rate)(m), where m is the number of compounding periods per year. To illustrate, the finance company loan calls for 3 percent per quarter, so:

$$i_{Stated} = \text{(Periodic rate)(m)} = (3\%)(4) = 12\%,$$

and

$$\text{Periodic rate} = i_{Stated}/m = 12\%/4 = 3\% \text{ per quarter.}$$

When compounding occurs more frequently than once a year, the periodic rate, rather than the stated rate, must be used in calculations. (In some situations, the effective annual rate could also be used, but never the stated rate.) To illustrate the use of the periodic rate with a lump-sum calculation, consider a $1,000 loan at 12 percent, compounded quarterly, that must be paid back after two years.

Time Line

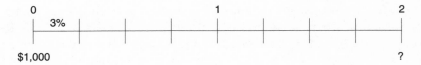

Here, we have quarterly compounding, so we must apply the quarterly periodic rate to find the future value of the loan.

Financial Calculator Solution

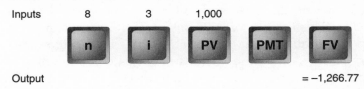

The periodic rate can be used with annuity payments when the number of payments per year corresponds to the number of compounding periods per year. To illustrate use of the periodic rate with an annuity, assume that you make eight quarterly payments of $100 into an account that pays 12 percent, compounded quarterly. What would you accumulate after two years?

Time Line

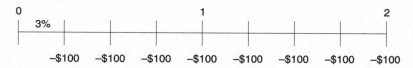

Here, we have quarterly payments and compounding, so we can apply the quarterly periodic rate to find the future value of the annuity.

Financial Calculator Solution

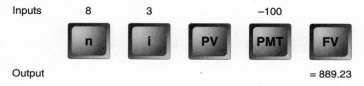

Effective Annual Rate

The effective annual rate is the rate which, under annual compounding (m = 1), would produce the same results as a given nominal rate with m greater than 1. The effective annual rate (EAR) is found as follows:

$$EAR = \left(1 + \frac{i_{Stated}}{m}\right)^m - 1.0$$

In the EAR equation, i_{Stated}/m is the periodic rate and m is the number of periods per year. For example, suppose you could use either the 1 percent per month credit card loan or the 3 percent per quarter consumer loan to make a purchase. Which one should you choose? To answer this question, the cost rate of each alternative must be expressed as an EAR.

Credit card loan: EAR = $(1 + 0.01)^{12} - 1.0$
$= (1.01)^{12} - 1.0 = 1.126825 - 1.0$
$= 0.126825 = 12.6825\%$

Consumer loan: EAR = $(1 + 0.03)^4 - 1.0$
$= (1.03)^4 - 1.0 = 1.125509 - 1.0$
$= 0.125509 = 12.5509\%$

Thus, the consumer loan is slightly less costly than the credit card loan. This result should have been intuitive to you because both loans have the same 12 percent stated rate, but you would have to make monthly payments on the credit card, while under the consumer loan terms you only would have to make quarterly payments. In making monthly payments, you would be paying the loan back faster and hence have money available for a shorter time.

The EAR is also used when the interest rate compounding period occurs more often than the period between payments or cash flows. For example, if payments occur semiannually but interest is compounded quarterly, the EAR must be used. Here, the EAR is really an "effective semiannual rate" calculated as $(1 + i_{Stated}/4)^2 - 1.0$, which is then applied to the semiannual payment stream. To illustrate, assume that you make four semiannual payments of $100 into an account that pays 12 percent, compounded quarterly. What would you accumulate after two years?

Time Line

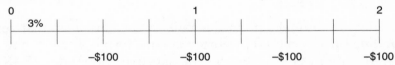

Now, you must calculate the *semiannual* EAR, because, although the compounding is quarterly, the payments occur semiannually.

$$\text{Semiannual EAR} = (1 + 0.03)^2 - 1.0$$
$$= (1.03)^2 - 1.0 = 1.0609 - 1.0$$
$$= 0.0609 = 6.09\%$$

Financial Calculator Solution

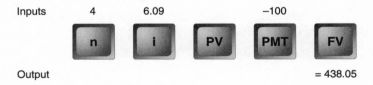

Note that the number of periods, n, must equal the number of payments when using the annuity formulas (and financial calculator PMT key). If the value for n that you are using in a calculation does not match the number of payments, something is wrong!

Although Ellen liked Robert's general approach to the presentation, she was bothered by the calculation of the 10-year "payback period." She recognized that money has time value, so a dollar expected to be received 10 years from now cannot be treated the same as a dollar that will be received today. Indeed, a dollar to be received 10 years from now is worth much less than a dollar received today.

Ellen was confident that at least a few of the board members understood discounted cash flow concepts, so she was convinced Robert would not be able to sell the project to the board using his current approach. To help her friend out, she gave Robert some hints about how he could include the time value of money in his presentation and hence head off any criticism from board members who would recognize the flaw in his logic. Specifically, she suggested that Robert put all of the cash flows from the proposed nursing home on a time line, discount the flows to t = 0, and then sum the present values to get a feel for the inherent profitability of the project. (As you will see in Chapter 7, this is exactly how proposed projects are evaluated financially.)

Armed with a rational way of presenting the project, Robert made one of the best proposals the board had ever seen. Of course, Robert's reputation (and career potential) was enhanced by the presentation, but more importantly, his mother's hometown got the new nursing home that it sorely needed.

SELF-ASSESSMENT EXERCISES

4–1   Consider a six-year, 8 percent savings certificate that costs $1,000.

    a. If interest is compounded annually, what will be the value of the certificate when it matures?

    b. Now assume the interest on the savings certificate is compounded semiannually. What is the value of the certificate at maturity under semiannual compounding?

4–2   a. A friend promises to pay you $600 two years from now if you loan him $500 today. What annual interest rate is your friend offering?

b. You are offered an investment opportunity with the "guarantee" that your investment will double in five years. Assuming annual compounding, what annual rate of return would this investment provide?

4-3   You decide to begin saving today toward the purchase of new carpeting for your home in five years. Each year, you plan to put $1,000 in a savings account paying 6 percent interest compounded annually.

a. If the payments are made at the end of each year, how much will you accumulate after five years?

b. What would be the ending amount if the payments were made at the beginning of each year?

c. What would be the ending amount if $500 payments were made at the end of each six-month period for five years and the account paid 6 percent compounded semiannually?

4-4   a. What is the present value of $1,000 to be received at the end of eight years? Assume an interest rate of 7 percent.

b. How much would you be willing to pay today for an investment that would return $800 at the end of each of the next six years? Assume a discount rate of 5 percent.

c. What is an opportunity cost rate? What role does the opportunity cost concept play in discounted cash flow analysis?

4-5   a. What is the present (t = 0) value of the following cash flows if the discount rate is 12 percent?

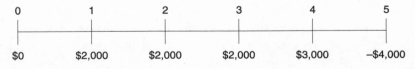

b. What is the effective annual percentage rate (EAR) of 12 percent compounded monthly?

SELECTED REFERENCES

For a better appreciation of the capabilities of financial calculators, see your calculator's owner's manual. For example, Hewlett-Packard. *HP-17B Business Calculator Owner's Manual*, January 1988.

For more information on spreadsheet @functions, see Gasteiger, Daniel. *The Lotus Guide to @Functions*. Cambridge, MA: Lotus Publishing, 1988.

5

CHAPTER

Financial Asset Valuation

George Takamoto, the Medical Director of Monterey Peninsula Health Alternatives, a California HMO, has been bothered by a delicate family situation. George's sister-in-law, a broker with Merrill Lynch, has been insisting that George buy a large block of Merck stock for his self-funded retirement plan. Her rationale for "pushing" the stock was the strong buy recommendation put out by Merrill's New York-based drug industry analyst. The analyst's recommendation, in turn, was based on fundamental analysis performed by his staff that indicated the stock was undervalued by the market.

George's first concern regarding his sister-in-law's recommendation was that he did not understand fundamental analysis. After reading up a bit on the topic at the local library, George discovered that fundamental analysis is the process of valuing a firm's stock on the basis of its future prospects and hence its ability to maintain or increase its dividend payments. (He also found out that technical analysis involves analyzing past stock price movements for certain patterns that indicate whether a stock should be bought or sold.) Although fundamental analysis made sense, he still was not convinced that he should take his sister-in-law's advice.

*After you read this chapter, you will have a better feel for how finan-
cial assets (stocks and bonds) are valued and how investors make choices
as to what types of securities to buy and from which companies. As you
read through the chapter, think about George's problem and what you
would do if you were in his shoes. At the close of the chapter, you will
learn his decision.*

INTRODUCTION

This chapter discusses financial asset valuation, with emphasis on
the valuation of stocks and bonds. The discussion applies the risk,
required return, and discounted cash flow concepts developed in
Chapters 2, 3, and 4. Your reaction at this point might be this: Why
should I have to worry about stock and bond valuation when
what I really want to learn is healthcare financial analysis and
decision making? There are many reasons why financial asset valuation concepts are important to healthcare decision making. Here
are just a few:

1. The lifeblood of any business is capital. In fact, one of the
   most common reasons for small business failures is insufficient capital. Therefore, it is vital that healthcare managers understand how investors make capital allocation
   decisions.
2. For investor-owned firms, stock price maximization is an
   important goal, if not the most important; so healthcare
   managers of for-profit firms must know how investors
   value the firm's securities to understand how managerial
   actions affect stock price.
3. For healthcare managers to make financially sound capital
   investment (plant and equipment) decisions, it is necessary to estimate the business's cost of capital. As demonstrated in Chapter 6, stock and bond valuation is a necessary skill in this process, whether the business is for-profit
   or not-for-profit.
4. Capital assets are valued in the same general way as
   financial assets. Thus, financial asset valuation provides
   healthcare managers with an excellent foundation to learn
   capital asset valuation techniques, the heart of capital

investment decision making within firms. The concepts presented here are crucial to a good understanding of Chapters 7 and 8.

5. One decision that many healthcare managers must face is the appropriate mix of debt and equity financing. An understanding of stock and bond valuation is critical to this decision, so the concepts presented in this chapter will be used again in Chapter 10.

THE GENERAL VALUATION MODEL

In almost all situations, individuals and institutions buy financial assets (securities) for one reason: to receive the cash flows that the security is expected to produce. Since the values of financial assets stem from streams of expected cash flows, all such assets are valued by the same four-step process:

1. *Estimate the expected cash flow stream.* This involves estimating both the expected cash flow in each period and the riskiness of the cash flows. For some types of securities, such as Treasury securities, the estimation process is quite easy—the interest and principal repayment stream is known with some certainty. For other types of securities, such as the stock of a biotechnology start-up company that is not yet paying dividends, the estimation process can be very difficult.

2. *Set the required rate of return.* The required rate of return on the cash flow stream is established on the basis of the stream's riskiness and the returns available on alternative investments of similar risk. Again, in some situations, it will be fairly easy to assess the riskiness of the estimated cash flow stream; in other situations, it may be quite difficult. Once the riskiness is assessed, the opportunity cost principle is applied. By investing in one security, the funds are no longer available to purchase alternative securities of similar risk. This opportunity loss sets the required rate of return on the security being valued.

3. *Discount the expected cash flows.* Each cash flow is now discounted at the security's required rate of return.

4. *Sum the present values.* The final step is to sum the present values of the individual cash flows to find the value of the security.

The following time line formalizes the valuation process.

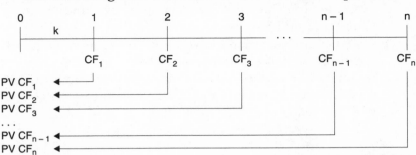

Here, CF_t is the expected cash flow at each Period t, k is the required rate of return (opportunity cost rate) on the security, and n is the number of periods for which cash flows are expected. The periods can be months, quarters, semiannual periods, or years, depending on the frequency of the cash flows expected from the security.

Note that the general valuation model can be applied to both financial assets, such as stocks and bonds, and capital (or real) assets, such as land, buildings, equipment, and even whole businesses. Each of the asset types requires a somewhat different application of the general valuation model, but the basic approach remains the same. This chapter deals with the valuation of two basic business securities: stocks and bonds. Chapters 7, 8, and 9 will discuss real asset valuation.

DEBT VALUATION

The discussion of security valuation begins with debt valuation. Bonds are used as the illustration, but the procedures discussed are applicable to a wide variety of debt securities. As a starter, here is a review of some basic definitions essential to the bond valuation process.

1. *Par value.* The par value is the stated face value of the bond; it is often set at $1,000 or $5,000. The par value generally represents the amount of money the firm borrows per bond and promises to repay at some future date.

2. *Maturity date.* Bonds generally have a specified maturity date on which the par value will be repaid. For example, Premier

Health Systems, a for-profit managed care company, issued $50 million worth of $1,000 par value bonds on January 1, 1996. The bonds will mature on December 31, 2010, so they had a 15-year maturity at the time they were issued. Note that the effective maturity of a bond declines each year it is outstanding. Thus, on January 1, 1997, Premier's bonds will have a 14-year maturity; on January 1, 1998, the bonds will have a 13-year maturity, and so on.

3. *Coupon rate.* A bond requires the issuer to pay a specific amount of interest each year (or, more typically, every six months). The rate of interest is called the coupon interest rate, or just the coupon rate. For example, Premier's bonds have a 10 percent coupon rate, so each $1,000 bond pays 0.10($1,000) = $100 in interest each year. The dollar amount of annual interest, in this case $100, is called the coupon payment. (The term coupon goes back to the time when bonds were bearer bonds. Bearer bonds had small coupons attached, one for each interest payment. To collect each interest payment, bondholders would tear, or "clip," the coupon from the bond and send it to the issuer, or take it to a bank, where it would be exchanged for the dollar payment. Today, however, almost all bonds are registered bonds, and interest payments are automatically sent by the issuer to the registered owner.)

4. *New issues versus outstanding bonds.* A bond's value is determined by the dollar amount of its coupon payments—the higher the amount, other things held constant, the higher the bond's value. At the time a bond is issued, its coupon rate is generally set at a level that will cause the bond to sell at its par value. In other words, the coupon rate is set at the interest rate that investors require on bonds of that risk. A bond that has just been issued is called a new issue. Once the bond has been on the market for a while, about a month, it is classified as an outstanding bond, or a seasoned issue. New issues sell close to par, but since a bond's coupon payments are generally fixed over the life of the bond, when economic conditions, and hence interest rates, change, a seasoned bond will sell for more or less than its par value.

5. *Debt service requirements.* Firms that issue bonds are concerned with their total debt service requirements, which include both interest expense and repayment of principal. For Premier, the debt service requirement is 0.10($50 million) = $5 million per year until maturity. In 2010, the firm's debt service requirement will be $5 million in interest plus $50 million in principal repayment, for a total of $55 million. In Premier's case, only interest is paid until maturity, so the entire principal amount must be repaid at that time. Many issues are structured so that the debt service requirements are more or less constant over time. In this situation, the issuer pays back a portion of the principal each year over the life of the bond.

 6. *Required rate of return,* k_d. Investors set required rates of return on bonds on the basis of the bond's risk (the riskiness of the expected cash flow stream) and the expected returns available on alternative investments of similar risk. A conceptual model for setting a bond's required rate of return was presented in Chapter 3.

The Basic Bond Valuation Model

A bond calls for the payment of a specific amount of interest for a certain number of years and for the repayment of par on the bond's maturity date, and its value is found as the present value of this cash flow stream. If we assume that the bond's coupon payments are made annually (in fact, almost all bonds have semiannual coupon payments), the cash flow stream looks like this:

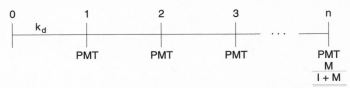

Here

 PMT = dollars of interest paid each year = Coupon rate × Par value.

 M = par, or maturity, value.

 n = number of years until maturity. n declines each year after the bond is issued.

Here are the cash flows from Premier's bonds on a time line:

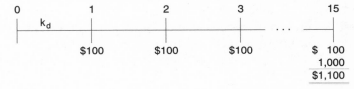

If the bonds were issued with a coupon rate set at the current interest rate for other bonds of similar risk (10 percent), and if investors actually required a rate of return on the issue of 10 percent, the value of the bond at time of issue would be $1,000.

Present value of a 15-year, $100 payment
   annuity when discounted at 10 percent = $ 760.61
Present value of a $1,000 lump sum when
   discounted 15 years at 10 percent   =   239.39
Value of bond   = $1,000.00

The value of the bond can also be found using most financial calculators:

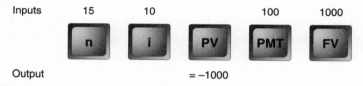

With a financial calculator, input n = 15, i = 10, PMT = 100, and FV = 1,000, and then press the PV key to get the answer, –1,000. Here, the coupon payments and par value are treated as inflows to the investor, so the bond's value is displayed as a negative number. Also, note that in bond valuation, all five of a calculator's time value of money keys are used since bonds involve both an annuity stream (payment) and a lump sum.

If k_d remained constant at 10 percent over time, what would be the value of the bond one year after it was issued? Now, the term to maturity is only 14 years (n = 14), but the bond's value remains at $1,000:

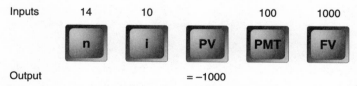

Now suppose that interest rates in the economy fell immediately after Premier issued the bonds, and, as a result, k_d decreased from 10 percent to 5 percent. The coupon rate and par value are fixed by contract, so they remain unaffected by changes in the level of interest rates, but now the opportunity cost rate (required rate of return) is 5 percent rather than 10 percent. At the end of the first year, with 14 years remaining, the value of the bond would be $1,494.93.

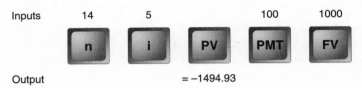

The mathematics of the bond value increase should be clear (a lower discount rate leads to a higher present value), but what is the logic behind it? The fact that k_d has fallen to 5 percent means that if you had $1,000 to invest, you could buy new bonds such as Premier's (every day some 10 to 20 companies sell new bonds), except that these new bonds would only pay $50 in interest each year. Naturally, you would favor interest payments of $100 over interest payments of $50, so you would be willing to pay more than $1,000 for Premier's bonds. All investors would recognize this and, as a result, the Premier bonds would be bid up in price to $1,494.93, at which point they would provide the same rate of return as new bonds of similar risk, 5 percent.

Assuming that interest rates stay constant at 5 percent over the next 14 years, what would happen to the value of a Premier bond? It would fall gradually from $1,494.93 at present to $1,000 at maturity, when the company would redeem each bond for $1,000. To illustrate, calculate the value of the bond one year later, when it has 13 years remaining to maturity.

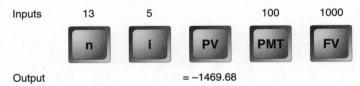

The value of the bond with 13 years to maturity is $1,469.68.

Notice that if you purchased the bond at a price of $1,494.93, and then sold it one year later with interest rates still at 5 percent, you would have a capital loss of $25.25. Your rate of return on the bond over the year consists of an interest, or current, yield plus a capital gains (or loss in this case) yield.

$$\text{Interest yield} = \$100/\$1{,}494.93 = 0.0669 \quad = \quad 6.69\%$$
$$\text{Capital gains yield} = -\$25.25/\$1{,}494.93 = -0.0169 = \underline{-1.69}$$
$$\text{Total yield} = \$74.75/\$1{,}494.93 = 0.0500 \quad = \quad \underline{5.00\%}$$

Had interest rates risen from 10 to 15 percent immediately after the bonds were issued rather than fallen, the value of each bond would have declined to $713.78 at the end of the first year. If interest rates then held constant at 15 percent, the bond would have a value of $720.84 at the end of the second year. So the total yield to investors would have been

$$\text{Interest yield} = \$100/\$713.78 = 0.1401 \quad = 14.01\%$$
$$\text{Capital gains yield} = \$7.06/\$713.78 = 0.0099 \quad = \underline{\ 0.99}$$
$$\text{Total yield} = \$107.06/\$713.78 = 0.1500 = \underline{15.00\%}$$

Figure 5–1 graphs the values of the Premier bond over time, assuming that interest rates (1) remain constant at 10 percent, (2) immediately fall to 5 percent and then remain constant at that level, and (3) immediately rise to 15 percent and remain constant at that level. Of course, interest rates do not remain constant nor does a bond's term to maturity. Also, occasionally a bond's credit quality (risk) changes over time. Thus, a bond's value fluctuates as interest rates, term to maturity, and credit quality change. Figure 5–1 illustrates the following important points about changes in interest rates:

1. Whenever the going rate of interest, k_d, is equal to the coupon rate, a bond will sell at its par value.
2. When interest rates fall after a bond is issued, the bond's value rises above its par value, and the bond is said to sell at a premium.
3. When interest rates rise after a bond is issued, the bond's value falls below its par value, and the bond is said to sell at a discount.
4. Bond prices and interest rates are inversely related. Increasing rates lead to falling prices, and decreasing rates lead to increasing prices.
5. The price of a bond will always approach its par value as its maturity date approaches, provided the issuing firm does not default on the bond.

FIGURE 5–1

Bond Values over Time

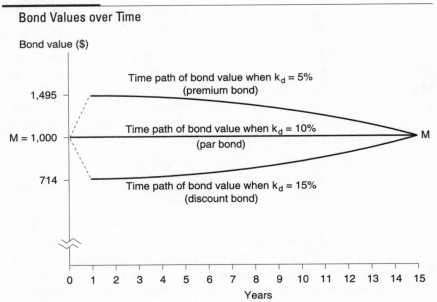

Yield to Maturity on a Bond

Up to this point, the illustration has treated the bond's required rate of return, k_d, as known, and then the value of the bond was calculated. In reality, investors' required rates of return on securities are not observable, but bond prices are listed in local newspapers and *The Wall Street Journal* or quoted by securities' brokers. Suppose the Premier bond had 14 years remaining to maturity, and the bond was selling at a price of $1,200. What rate of interest, or yield to maturity (YTM), would you earn if you bought the bond at this price and held it to maturity? To find the answer, use your financial calculator as follows:

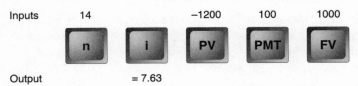

The yield to maturity, 7.63 percent in this example, is identical to the total rate of return discussed in the previous section. In other words, the YTM is the promised rate of return on the bond if it is bought at the current price and held to maturity. The YTM is also the expected rate of return on the bond if it cannot be called (redeemed prior to maturity) and if there is zero probability that the firm will default on the bond payments. The YTM for a bond that sells at par consists entirely of an interest yield, but if the bond sells at a discount or premium, the YTM consists of the interest yield plus a positive or negative capital gains yield.

Bond Values with Semiannual Compounding

Although some bonds pay interest annually, most actually pay interest semiannually, or every six months. To apply the valuation concepts to semiannual bonds, the bond valuation procedures must be modified as follows:

1. Divide the annual interest payment, PMT, by 2 to determine the dollar amount paid each six months.
2. Multiply the number of years to maturity, n, by 2 to determine the number of semiannual interest periods.
3. Divide the annual required rate of return, k_d, by 2 to determine the semiannual required rate of return.

These changes result in the following model for valuing a bond that pays semiannual interest:

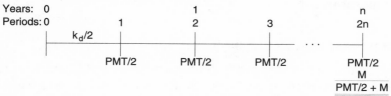

To illustrate the use of the semiannual bond valuation model, assume that the Premier bonds pay $50 every six months rather than $100 at the end of each year. Thus, each interest payment is only half as large, but there are twice as many of them. When the going rate of interest is 5 percent (2.5 percent on a semiannual basis), the value of Premier's bonds with 14 years left to maturity is $1,499.12:

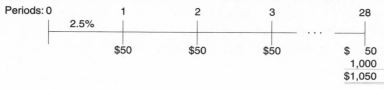

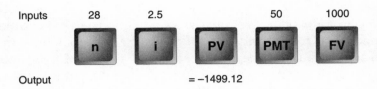

Similarly, if the bond were actually selling for $1,400 with 14 years to maturity, its YTM would be 5.80 percent.

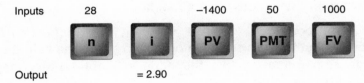

Note that the solution value for i, 2.90 percent, is the semiannual YTM, so it is necessary to multiply it by 2 to get the annual, or stated YTM. Of course, the effective annual YTM on the bond is somewhat greater than the stated 5.80 percent. However, it is convention in the bond markets to quote all rates on a stated basis; so the procedures outlined in this section are correct when bonds, which almost all have semiannual coupons, are being compared. However, when the returns on securities with different payment periods are being compared, all returns should be expressed on an effective annual rate basis.

Interest Rate Risk on a Bond

As we know, interest rates fluctuate over time, and fluctuating rates create two types of interest rate risk for bondholders: price risk and reinvestment rate risk. (These topics were introduced in Chapter 3.) To further develop these concepts, suppose you bought some 10 percent Premier bonds when they were issued at a price of $1,000. If interest rates rose, the value of your bonds would fall. Thus, bond investors are exposed to the risk of loss of value from changing interest rates, which is called price risk. An investor's exposure to price risk depends on the maturity of the bonds. This point can be easily demonstrated by showing how the value of a 1-year bond with a 10 percent coupon rate fluctuates with changes in interest rates, and then comparing these changes with those on a 14-year bond.

Figure 5–2 shows the values of 1-year and 14-year bonds at several different market interest rates. Notice how much more sensitive the value of the long-term bond is to changes in interest rates. For bonds with similar coupons, the longer the maturity of the bond, the greater its price changes in response to a given change in interest rates. Thus, even if the default risk on two bonds is the same, the one with the longer maturity is exposed to more price risk.

Although a 1-year bond exposes the buyer to less price risk than a 14-year bond, the 1-year bond carries with it more reinvestment rate risk, at least if your holding period, or investment horizon, is greater than one year. For example, assume your daughter is now eight years old, and you are saving for her first year's college tuition. If you invest in a 10-year bond, the interest payments you will receive over your 10-year investment horizon are known with some certainty. However, if you invest in a 1-year bond, you will have to reinvest the principal at the end of the first year. If interest rates fall, the interest earned in the second year will be less than that earned during the first year. If interest rates continue to fall over your 10-

FIGURE 5–2

Price Risk

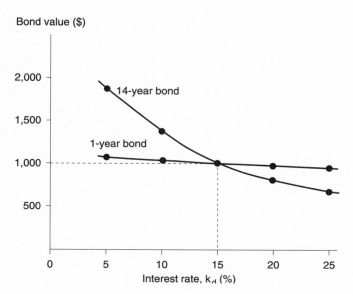

year investment horizon, the amount saved for your daughter's college tuition will be much less if you invested in successive 1-year bonds than if you initially had bought a 10-year bond.

Thus, bond investors face both price risk and reinvestment rate risk as a result of interest rate fluctuations over time. Which risk is most meaningful to a particular investor depends on the circumstances; but, in general, interest rate risk, including both price and reinvestment rate risk, is reduced by matching the maturity of the bond with the anticipated investment horizon. Thus, if you planned to provide for your daughter's college education by investing in bonds, and the funds would be needed in 10 years, your interest rate risk would be minimized by buying a 10-year bond because it would match your investment horizon. Similarly, when firms issue bonds to finance capital investments, the lowest risk maturity is that which matches the maturity of the assets being financed.

STOCK VALUATION

Common stock represents the ownership of a corporation, but to most investors a share of common stock is simply a piece of paper entitling the owner to the following cash flows:

1. Stock entitles the bearer to dividends, but only if (a) the company has earnings to support dividends, and (b) management chooses to pay dividends rather than retain the earnings for reinvestment within the firm. Whereas a bond contains a promise to pay interest, common stock provides no such promise (in a legal sense) to pay dividends—if you own a stock, you may expect a dividend, but your expectations may not in fact be met. To illustrate, Beverly Enterprises' dividend grew from $0.08 a share in 1979 to $0.20 a share in 1987, and investors were expecting this growth to continue. However, problems in the nursing home industry caused the firm to lower its dividend to $0.05 in 1988 and to omit it entirely in 1989. As of today, Beverly has not yet reinstituted its common stock dividend.

2. Stock can be sold at some future date, hopefully at a price greater than the purchase price. If the stock is actually sold at a price above its purchase price, the investor will receive a capital gain. Generally, at the time people buy common stocks, they expect to receive capital gains; otherwise, they would not buy stocks.

However, after the fact, one can end up with capital losses rather than capital gains. Beverly Enterprises' stock price dropped from $20 in 1986 to $5 in 1988. The capital gains purchasers expected in 1986 turned out to be actual capital losses if they sold the stock in 1988.

Definitions Used in Stock Valuation

Here are the terms used in valuing common stock:

D_0 = last dividend actually paid on the stock, which is typically assumed to have occurred yesterday, regardless of when the last dividend payment was actually made. Since D_0 is a historical cash flow, it is known with certainty.

$E(D_t)$ = dividend the stockholder expects to receive at the end of Year t. $E(D_1)$ is the first dividend expected, and it is generally assumed that it will be paid at the end of one year; $E(D_2)$ is the dividend expected at the end of two years; and so forth. $E(D_1)$ represents the first cash flow a new purchaser of the stock will receive. Note that all future dividends are expected values, so the estimate of $E(D_t)$ may differ among investors. Also, note that stocks generally pay dividends quarterly, so in theory stocks should be valued on the basis of quarterly cash flows. However, most analysts work on an annual basis because the data generally are not precise enough to warrant the refinement of a quarterly valuation model.

P_0 = actual market price of the stock today, which is known and identical to all investors.

$E(P_t)$ = expected price of the stock at the end of each Year t. $E(P_0)$ is the value of the stock today as seen by a particular investor based on his or her estimate of the stock's expected dividend stream and riskiness, $E(P_1)$ is the price expected at the end of one year, and so on. Whereas P_0 is fixed and is identical for all investors, $E(P_0)$ will differ among investors depending on their assessments of the stock's dividend stream and its riskiness. $E(P_0)$, an investor's estimate of the stock value today, could be above or below P_0, the current stock price, but an investor would buy the stock only if his or her estimate of $E(P_0)$ were equal to or greater than P_0.

$E(g_t)$ = expected dividend growth rate in Year t. Different investors may use different $E(g_t)$s to value a firm's stock.

k_s = required rate of return on the stock, considering both its riskiness and the returns available on other investments. In Chapter 3, we discussed how the Security Market Line (SML) of the Capital Asset Pricing Model can be used to estimate k_s. Note, however, that different investors will use different estimates of the stock's market risk (different beta coefficients), as well as different values for other inputs to the SML, so different investors will set different required rates of return on the same stock.

$E(R)$ = expected rate of return, or the return which an investor who buys the stock expects to receive. $E(R)$ could be above or below k_s, but one would buy the stock only if $E(R)$ were equal to or greater than k_s.

$E(D_1)/P_0$ = expected dividend yield on the stock during the first year of ownership. If the stock is expected to pay a dividend of $1 during the next 12 months, and if its current price is $10, then the expected dividend yield is $1/$10 = 0.10 = 10%.

$(E(P_1) - P_0)/P_0$ = expected capital gains yield on the stock during the first year of ownership. If the stock sells for $10 today, and if it is expected to rise to $10.50 at the end of the first year, the expected capital gain is $E(P_1) - P_0 = \$10.50 - \$10.00 = \$0.50$, and the expected capital gains yield is $0.50/$10 = 0.050 = 5.0%.

Expected Dividends as the Basis for Stock Values

In the earlier discussion of bond valuation, the value of a bond was found as the present value of interest payments over the life of the bond plus the present value of the bond's maturity (or par) value. Stock prices are likewise determined as the present value of a stream of cash flows, and the basic stock valuation model is similar to the bond valuation model. What are the cash flows that stocks provide to their holders? First, think of yourself as an investor who buys a stock with the intention of holding it (in your family) forever. In this case, all that you (and your heirs) will receive is a stream of dividends, and the value of the stock today is calculated as the present value (PV) of an infinite stream of dividends.

$E(P_0)$ = PV of infinite stream of expected future dividends

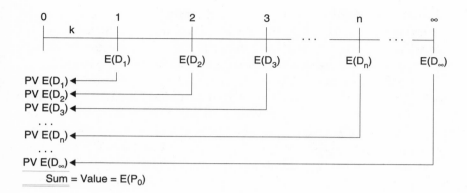

What about the more typical case, in which you expect to hold the stock for a finite period and then sell it—what would be the value of the stock in this case? The value of the stock is again the present value of the expected dividend stream. To see this, recognize that for any individual investor, expected cash flows consist of expected dividends plus the expected sale price of the stock. However, the sale price the current investor receives will depend on the dividends some future investor expects to receive. Therefore, for all present and future investors in total, expected cash flows must be based on expected future dividends. To put it another way, unless a business is liquidated or sold to another concern, the cash flows it provides to its stockholders consist only of a stream of dividends; therefore, the value of a share of its stock must be the present value of that expected dividend stream.

The validity of this concept can also be confirmed by asking the following question: Suppose you buy a stock and expect to hold it for one year. You will receive dividends during the year plus the value $E(P_1)$ when you sell out at the end of the year, but what will determine the value of $E(P_1)$? The answer is that it will be determined as the present value of the dividends during Year 2 plus the stock price at the end of that year, which in turn will be determined as the present value of another set of future dividends and an even more distant stock price. This process can be continued ad infinitum, and the ultimate result is that the value of a stock is the present value of its expected dividend stream, regardless of the holding period of the investor performing the analysis. (Occasionally, stock shares could have additional value, such as the value of a controlling interest when an investor buys 51 percent of a company's outstanding stock. However, in most situations, the sole value inherent in stock ownership stems from the cash flows expected to be passed from the company to its shareholders.)

Investors periodically lose sight of the long-run nature of stocks as investments and forget that in order to sell a stock at a profit, one must find a buyer who will pay the higher price. If you analyzed a stock's value on the basis of expected future dividends, concluded that the stock's market price exceeded a reasonable value, and then bought the stock anyway, you would be following the "bigger fool" theory of investment: You may be a fool to buy the stock at its excessive price, but you believe that when you get ready to sell it, you can find someone who is an even bigger fool. The bigger fool theory was widely followed in the summer of 1987, just before the stock market lost over one-third of its value.

The concept of the value of a stock being the present value of the expected dividend stream holds for all situations: Dividends can be rising, falling, or constant, or they can even fluctuate more-or-less randomly. Thus, stocks can always be valued by projecting the expected dividend stream and then finding the present value of that stream. It is not even necessary to project the stream for more than, say, 50 years. Because of the time value of money, dividends beyond that point contribute an insignificant amount to a stock's value today. Needless to say, it is generally not possible to have much confidence in the values of expected dividends projected over a 50-year period, so stock valuation must be viewed as something of an approximation.

Constant Growth

Often, the projected stream of dividends follows a systematic pattern, in which case it is possible to develop a simplified (that is, easier to evaluate) version of the general stock valuation model. This section discusses the most common simplifying assumption, constant growth.

Although the dividends of only a few firms actually grow at a constant rate, the assumption of constant growth is often made because it makes the forecasting of individual dividends over a long time period unnecessary. For a constant growth company, $E(g_{t-1}) = E(g) = E(g_{t+1})$, and so on, so the dividend growth rate is constant for all years. Under this assumption, the dividend in any future Year t may be forecast as $E(D_t) = D_0[1 + E(g)]^t$, where D_0 is the last dividend paid (and hence is known with certainty) and $E(g)$ is the constant expected rate of growth. Alternatively, each year's dividend is $E(g)$ percent greater than the previous dividend, so $E(D_t) = E(D_{t-1})[1 + E(g)]$. For example, if Minnesota Health Systems, Inc., (MHS) just paid a dividend of $1.82 (that is, $D_0 = 1.82), and if investors expect a 10 percent constant growth rate, the estimated dividend one year hence will be $E(D_1) = $1.82(1.10) = 2.00; $E(D_2)$ will be $$1.82(1.10)^2 = 2.20; and the estimated dividend five years hence will be

$$E(D_5) = D_0[1 + E(g)]^5 = \$1.82(1.10)^5 = \$2.93$$

Using this method of estimating future dividends, it is certainly possible to determine the expected future cash flow stream (the dividends), calculate the present value of, say, the first 50 dividends, and then sum these present values to find the value of MHS's stock—the value of any stock is equal to the present value of its expected future dividend stream.

However, if $E(g)$ is assumed to be constant, a stock can be valued using a simplified model, where k_s is the required rate of return on the stock.

$$E(P_0) = \frac{D_0\left[1 + E(g)\right]}{k_s - E(g)} = \frac{E(D_1)}{k_s - E(g)}$$

If $D_0 = 1.82, $E(g) = 10\%$, and $k_s = 16\%$ for Minnesota Health Systems, the value of its stock would be $33.33.

$$E(P_0) = \frac{\$1.82(1.10)}{0.16 - 0.10} = \frac{\$2.00}{0.06} = \$33.33$$

Note that a necessary condition for the derivation of the constant growth model is that the required rate of return on the stock is greater than its constant dividend growth rate; that is, k_s is greater than $E(g)$. If the equation is used when k_s is not greater than $E(g)$, the results will be meaningless. However, to qualify as a constant growth stock, dividends must be expected to grow at the constant growth rate forever (or at least for 50 years). Although stocks can have $E(g_t)$ greater than k_s for short periods, $E(g_t)$ cannot exceed k_s for a prolonged period, and hence $E(g)$, the constant growth rate, cannot exceed k_s. Note also that the constant growth model can be applied to any situation where the cash flows are growing at a constant rate; its usefulness is not restricted to stock valuation.

How does an investor determine k_s, his or her required rate of return on a particular stock? One way is to use the Security Market Line (SML) of the Capital Asset Pricing Model that was discussed in Chapter 3. Assume that MHS's market beta, as reported by a financial advisory service, is 1.5. Furthermore, assume that the interest rate on long-term Treasury bonds (the risk-free rate) is 7 percent, and the required rate of return on the market (on an average-risk stock) is 13 percent. Then, according the SML, the required rate of return on MHS's stock is 16.0 percent.

$$k_{s(MHS)} = k_{RF} + (k_M - k_{RF})b_{MHS}$$
$$= 7\% + (13\% - 7\%)(1.5)$$
$$= 7\% + (6\%)1.5 = 16\%$$

Here, k_{RF} is the risk-free rate, k_M is the required rate of return on the market (or the required rate of return on a $b = 1.0$ stock), and b_{MHS} is Minnesota Health System's market beta.

Growth in dividends occurs primarily as a result of growth in earnings per share (EPS). Earnings growth, in turn, results from a number of factors, including the inflation rate and the amount of earnings the company retains and reinvests. Regarding inflation, if output (in units) is stable, and if both sales prices and input costs increase at the inflation rate, EPS also will grow at the inflation rate. EPS will also grow as a result of the reinvestment, or plowback, of earnings. If the firm's earnings are not all paid out as dividends (that is, if some fraction of earnings is retained), the dollars of investment behind each share will rise over time, which should lead to growth in productive assets and hence growth in earnings and dividends.

When using the constant growth model, the most critical input is $E(g)$, the expected constant growth rate in dividends. Investors can make their own $E(g)$ estimates on the basis of historical dividend growth, but $E(g)$ estimates are also available from brokerage and investment advisory firms. Chapter 6 contains more information on estimating dividend growth rates.

Expected Rate of Return on a Constant Growth Stock

The constant growth model to value stocks can be solved for k_s, the required rate of return, to find a stock's expected rate of return, $E(R)$. (The k_s value is a required rate of return, but when we transform the model, we are finding an expected rate of return.) Obviously, the transformation requires that the required rate of return equal the expected rate of return, or $k_s = E(R)$. This equality holds if the stock is in equilibrium, a condition that will be discussed later in the chapter.

$$\begin{matrix} \text{Expected} & \text{Expected} & \text{Expected growth} \\ \text{rate of} & = \text{dividend} + & \text{rate, or capital} \\ \text{return} & \text{yield} & \text{gains yield} \end{matrix}$$

$$E(R) \;=\; \frac{E(D_1)}{P_0} \;+\; E(g)$$

Thus, if you buy a stock for a price $P_0 = \$33.33$, and if you expect the stock to pay a dividend $E(D_1) = \$2.00$ one year from now and to grow at a constant rate $E(g) = 10\%$ in the future, your expected rate of return is 16.0 percent:

$$E(R) = \frac{\$2.00}{\$33.33} + 10.0\% = 6.0\% + 10.0\% = 16.0\%$$

In this form, we see that $E(R)$ is the expected total return on the stock and that it consists of an expected dividend yield, $E(D_1)/P_0 = 6.0\%$, plus an expected growth rate or capital gains yield, $E(g) = 10\%$.

Suppose this analysis had been conducted on January 1, 1997, so $P_0 = \$33.33$ is Minnesota Health System's January 1, 1997, stock price and $E(D_1) = \$2.00$ is the dividend expected at the end of 1997. What is the value of $E(P_1)$, the company's stock price at the end of 1997 (or the beginning of 1998)? We would again apply the constant growth model, but this time we would use the 1998 dividend, $E(D_2) = E(D_1)[1 + E(g)] = \$2.00(1.10) = \$2.20$.

$$E(P_1) = \frac{E(D_2)}{k_s - E(g)} = \frac{\$2.20}{0.06} = \$36.67$$

Now notice that $E(P_1) = \$36.67$ is 10 percent greater than $P_0 = \$33.33$: $\$33.33(1.10) = \$36.67$. Thus, we would expect to make a capital gain of \$36.67 − \$33.33 = \$3.34 during 1997 and hence a capital gains yield of 10 percent:

$$\text{Capital gains yield} = \frac{\text{Capital gain}}{\text{Beginning price}} = \frac{\$3.34}{\$33.33} = 0.100 = 10.0$$

If the analysis were extended, in each future year the expected capital gains yield would always equal E(g) because the stock price would grow at the 10 percent constant dividend growth rate. The expected dividend yield in 1998 (Year 2) could be found as follows:

$$\text{Dividend yield} = \frac{E(D_2)}{E(P_1)} = \frac{\$2.20}{\$36.67} = 0.060 = 6.0\%$$

The dividend yield for 1999 (Year 3) could also be calculated, and again it would be 6 percent. Thus, for a constant dividend growth stock, the following conditions must hold:

1. The dividend is expected to grow forever (or at least for a long time) at a constant rate, E(g).
2. The stock price is expected to grow at this same rate.
3. The expected dividend yield is a constant.
4. The expected capital gains yield is also a constant, and it is equal to E(g).
5. The expected total rate of return in any Year t is equal to the expected dividend yield plus the expected growth rate (expected capital gains yield): $E(R_t) = E(D_{t+1})/E(P_t) + E(g)$. (Note that this equality holds also for nonconstant growth stocks.)

The term *expected* should be clarified: It means expected in a statistical sense. Thus, if Minnesota Health System's dividend growth rate is expected to remain constant at 10 percent, this means that the growth rate in each year can be represented by a probability distribution with an expected value of 10 percent, not that the growth rate is literally expected to be exactly 10 percent in each future year. In this sense, the constant growth assumption is reasonable for many large, mature companies.

Nonconstant Growth

What happens when a company does not meet the constant growth assumption? For example, what if Minnesota Health System's dividend was expected to grow at 30 percent for three years and then to settle down to a constant growth rate of 10 percent? In this situation, the constant growth model does not apply, so some other technique must be used to value the stock. Although nonconstant stock valuation models are not that complicated, they are beyond the scope of a book on healthcare financial management. Suffice it to note that the value of MHS's stock would be $53.86 under the nonconstant growth assumption, which is significantly higher than the $33.33 value of the stock assuming 10 percent constant growth. Dividend growth of 30 percent for three years followed by 10 percent constant growth creates a more valuable expected dividend stream than straight constant growth at 10 percent.

SECURITY MARKET EQUILIBRIUM

Investors will want to buy a security if its expected rate of return exceeds its required rate of return or, put another way, when its value exceeds its current price. Conversely, investors will want to sell a security when its required rate of return exceeds its expected rate of return or when its current price exceeds its value. When more investors want to buy a security than to sell it, its price is bid up; and when more investors want to sell a security than to buy it, its price falls. In equilibrium, these two conditions must hold:

1. The expected rate of return on a security must equal its required rate of return to the marginal investor. This means that no investor owning the stock believes that its expected rate of return is less than its required rate of return, and no investor who does not own the stock believes that its expected rate of return is greater than its required rate of return.

2. The market price of a security must equal its value to the marginal investor.

If these conditions do not hold, trading will occur until they do. Of course, security prices are not constant. A security's price can swing wildly as new information becomes available to the market that changes investors' expectations concerning the security's cash flow stream or risk or when the general level of returns (interest rates) changes. But evidence suggests that security prices, especially those of the U.S. Treasury and of large companies that are actively traded, adjust rapidly to disequilibrium situations. Thus, most people believe that the bonds of the U.S. Treasury and the bonds and stocks of major corporations are generally in equilibrium. The key to the rapid movement of security prices towards equilibrium is market efficiency, which is discussed in the next section.

INFORMATIONAL EFFICIENCY

A securities market, say the market for long-term U.S. Treasury bonds, is informationally efficient if (1) all information relevant to the values of the securities traded can be obtained easily and at low cost, and (2) the market contains many buyers and sellers who act rationally on this information. If these conditions hold, current market prices will contain all information of possible relevance; hence, future price movements will be based solely on new information as it becomes known.

The Efficient Markets Hypothesis (EMH), which has three forms, formalizes the theory of informational efficiency:

1. The weak form of the EMH holds that all information contained in past price movements is fully reflected in current market prices. Therefore, information about recent trends in a security's price, or a bond's yield, is of no value in choosing which security will "outperform" the market. Here, the term *outperform* means that the security will provide a return in excess of that required by its riskiness.

2. The semistrong form of the EMH holds that current market prices reflect all publicly available information. Therefore, it makes no sense to spend hours and hours analyzing economic data and financial reports because whatever information you might find, whether it be good or bad, has already been absorbed by the market and is embedded in current prices.

3. The strong form of the EMH holds that current market prices reflect all relevant information, whether publicly available or privately held. If this form holds, then even investors with "inside information," such as corporate officers, would find it impossible to earn abnormal returns (returns in excess of that justified by the riskiness of the investment), even when they invest in the securities of their own companies.

The EMH is a hypothesis, not a proven fact. However, hundreds of empirical tests have been conducted to try to prove (or disprove) the EMH, and the results are relatively consistent. Most tests support the weak and semistrong forms of the EMH for well-developed markets such as the U.S. markets for large firms' stocks and bonds, and for Treasury securities. Supporters of these forms of the EMH note that there are some 100,000 or so full-time, highly trained, professional analysts and traders operating in these markets. Furthermore, most of the analysts and traders work for companies such as Citibank, Fidelity Investments, Merrill Lynch, Prudential Insurance, and the like, which have billions of dollars available to take advantage of undervalued securities. Finally, as a result of disclosure requirements and electronic information networks, new information about widely followed securities is almost instantaneously available. With immediate information, and many analysts processing the information and passing it to traders who have the funds to act on it, security prices in major markets adjust almost immediately as new developments occur; hence, it is very difficult, if not impossible, to "beat the market."

If markets were not efficient, the better managers of stock and bond mutual funds and pension plans would be able to consistently outperform the broad averages over long periods of time. In fact, very few managers can consistently better the broad averages, and, during most years, mutual fund managers, on average, underperform the market. Of course, in any year, a large percentage of mutual fund managers will outperform the market, and a large percentage will underperform the market. This is known with certainty. But, for an investor to beat the market by investing in mutual funds, he or she must identify the successful managers beforehand, and this seems very difficult, if not impossible, to do.

In spite of the evidence, many theorists, and even more Wall Streeters, believe that "pockets of inefficiency" do exist. In some cases, entire markets may be inefficient. For example, the markets for the securities issued by small companies may be inefficient because there are neither enough analysts ferreting out information on these companies nor sufficient numbers of investors trading these securities. Also, many people even believe that individual securities traded in efficient markets are occasionally priced inefficiently, or that investor emotions can drive prices too high during raging bull markets or too low during whimpering bear markets.

Still, most theorists believe, for the most part, that the prices of securities traded in the major U.S. securities markets reflect all publicly available information. Virtually no one, however, believes that strong-form efficiency holds. Studies of legal purchases and sales by people with inside information indicate that insiders can make abnormal profits by trading on that information. It is even more apparent that insiders can make abnormal profits if they trade illegally on specific information that has not been disclosed to the public, such as a takeover bid, a research and development breakthrough, and the like.

The EMH has important implications for investment decisions. Since security prices do appear to generally reflect all public information, most actively followed and traded securities are in equilibrium and fairly valued. This does not mean that new information could not cause a security's price to soar or to plummet, but it does mean that stocks and bonds, in general, are neither undervalued or overvalued. Therefore, an investor with no inside information can only expect to earn a return on an investment that compensates him or her for the amount of risk assumed. Also, since the EMH applies to bond markets, bond prices and hence interest rates, reflect all current public information. Thus, it is impossible to consistently forecast future interest rates—interest rates change in response to new information, and this information could either lower or raise rates.

Finally, note that managers may have information about their own firms that is unknown to the general public. This condition is called asymmetric information, and it can have a profound effect on managerial decisions. For example, suppose a drug manufacturer has made a breakthrough in AIDS research, but it doesn't want to announce the development until it completes the final series of tests. The firm might want to delay any new securities offerings because securities could probably be sold under more favorable terms once the announcement is made. This scenario does not mean that markets are inefficient but, rather, that markets are not strong-form efficient. Managers can and should act on inside information for the benefit of their firms, but inside information cannot legally be used for personal benefit.

THE RISK/RETURN TRADE-OFF

Most financial decisions involve alternative courses of action. For example, should a hospital invest its excess funds in Treasury bonds yielding 7 percent or in Continental Airlines bonds yielding 12 percent? Should a group practice buy a replacement piece of equipment now or wait until next year? Should a joint venture outpatient diagnostic center purchase a small, limited-use magnetic resonance imaging (MRI) system or a large, and more expensive, multipurpose system? In general, the alternative courses of action will have different expected rates of return, and one might be tempted to automatically accept the alternative with the higher expected return. However, this approach to financial decision making would be incorrect. In efficient markets, those alternatives that offer higher returns will also entail higher risk. The correct question to ask when making financial decisions, then, is not which alternative has the higher expected rate of return but, rather, which alternative has the higher return after adjusting for risk. In other words, which alternative has the higher return over and above the return commensurate with that alternative's riskiness?

To illustrate the risk/return trade-off, suppose Columbia/HCA Healthcare's stock has an expected rate of return of 14 percent, while its bonds yield 9 percent. Does this mean that investors should flock to buy the company's stock and ignore the bonds? Of course not—the higher expected rate of return on the stock merely reflects the fact that the stock is riskier than the bonds. Those investors who are not willing to assume much risk will buy Columbia's bonds, while those that are less risk averse will buy the stock. From the perspective of Columbia's managers and other stakeholders, financing with stock is less risky than using debt, so the firm is willing to pay the higher cost of equity to limit the firm's risk exposure.

The moral of this story is simple. There are three key questions involved in every financial decision: (1) What is the expected return? (2) What is the risk? (3) How does the return compare with that required to asume the assessed level of risk? For decisions that involve the major capital (stock and bond) markets, expected returns will usually be just sufficient to compensate for the risk incurred—no more, no less. To obtain higher rates of return, investors will have to assume more risk. Thus, be wary when you receive an unsolicited call promising a low-risk, high-return investment opportunity. Except in extremely rare instances (and I have never seen one), such claims are pure fabrications. (After all, if the deal is that good, it would be fully subscribed by professional investors in private transactions, not mass marketed to the general public.)

In spite of the efficiency of major securities markets, the markets for products and services (that is, markets for real assets such as MRI systems) are usually not efficient; hence, returns are not necessarily related to risk. Thus, hospitals, group practices, and other healthcare businesses can make real asset investments and achieve returns in excess of those required by the riskiness of the investment. Furthermore, the market for innovation (the market for ideas) is not efficient; hence, people like Bill Gates, the founder of Microsoft, can become billionaires at a relatively young age. However, when excess returns are found in the product, service, or idea markets, new entrants quickly join the innovators, and competition over time will usually force rates of return down to efficient market levels. The result is that later entrants can expect returns that are just commensurate with the risks involved.

George Takamoto, after wrestling with the decision regarding a large purchase of Merck stock, finally made up his mind. What tipped the balance was a discussion of market efficiency that he read in his daughter's finance text. "After all," said George, "what makes the Merrill analyst smarter than the rest of the market? If everyone else thought that Merck was undervalued, they would have already bought the stock, and the buy orders would have pushed the price up to the point where it was fairly valued."

In the end, George disregarded his sister-in-law's advice. But in the process of dealing with the situation, he learned a great deal about financial asset valuation. These insights later proved useful to him in understanding how the HMO's cost of capital is developed, as well as in understanding how capital investments are valued by businesses.

SELF-ASSESSMENT EXERCISES

5–1   a. How are all financial assets valued?

   b. What is price risk?

   c. What is reinvestment rate risk?

5–2   a. Twin Oaks Health Center has a bond issue outstanding with a coupon rate of 7 percent and four years remaining until maturity. The par value of the bond is $1,000, and the bond pays interest annually. Determine the current value of the bond if present market conditions justify a 14 percent required rate of return.

   b. Now suppose Twin Oaks' four-year bond had semiannual coupons. Now what would be its current value? (Assume a 14 percent stated required rate of return, or 7 percent per semiannual period, but note that this procedure results in an effective annual required rate of return of about 14.5 percent.)

   c. Now assume that Twin Oaks' bond had a semiannual coupon but 20 years remaining to maturity. What is the current value under these conditions? (Again assume a 14 percent stated required rate of return, although the actual required rate of return would probably be greater than 14 percent because of increased price risk to investors due to the longer maturity.)

5–3   Tidewater Home Healthcare, Inc., has a bond issue outstanding with eight years remaining to maturity, a coupon rate of 10 percent with interest paid semiannually, and a par value of $1,000. If the current market price of the bond is $1,251.22, what is its yield to maturity (YTM)?

5–4   a. Better Life Nursing Home, Inc., has maintained a dividend payment of $4 per share for many years. The same dollar amount is expected to be paid in future years. If investors require a 12 percent rate of return on investments of similar risk, determine the value of the company's stock.

b. Your stockbroker is trying to get you to buy the stock of HealthSouth, a regional HMO. The stock has a current market price of $25; its last dividend ($D_0$) was $2.00; and the company's earnings and dividends are expected to increase at a constant growth rate of 10 percent. Your required rate of return on this stock is 20 percent. From a strict valuation standpoint, should you buy the stock?

c. Lucas Drugs' last dividend was $1.50. Its current equilibrium stock price is $15.75, and its expected dividend growth rate is a constant 5 percent. If the stockholders' required rate of return is 15 percent, what is the expected dividend yield and expected capital gains yield for the coming year?

5–5   a. Precision Surgical Company, a medical equipment manufacturer, has been hard hit by increased competition. Analysts predict that earnings (and dividends) will decline at a rate of 5 percent annually into the foreseeable future. If the company's last dividend (D_0) was $2.00, and investors require a rate of return of 15 percent, what will be the company's stock price in three years?

b. What is the value of the stock of a firm that is never expected to pay a dividend?

SELECTED REFERENCES

There are no references that pertain exclusively to the valuation of stocks and bonds issued by healthcare companies. For two seminal works on valuation, see:

Durand, David. "Growth Stocks and the St. Petersburg Paradox." *Journal of Finance*, September 1957, pp. 348–63.

Williams, John Burr. *The Theory of Investment Value*. Cambridge, MA: Harvard University Press, 1938.

For a more in-depth treatment of financial asset valuation, see Brigham, Eugene F. and Louis C. Gapenski. *Financial Management: Theory and Practice*. Fort Worth, TX: Dryden Press, 1997.

6

CHAPTER

The Cost of Capital

Sister Mary Margaret of St. Sebastian's Hospital was perplexed. Deep down in her heart she knew that the mission of the not-for-profit hospital was to provide healthcare services to the community, with special emphasis on helping those without the financial resources to seek treatment elsewhere. But the hospital's board of trustees had just turned down a project she had proposed to construct a neonatal care unit that would benefit many of the hospital's indigent patients. The primary objection of the board was that the project's expected profitability did not meet St. Sebastian's minimum acceptable profitability (hurdle rate) for capital investments.

As part of its capital investment analysis process, St. Sebastian's financial staff estimates the cost of the hospital's debt capital, as well as the cost of its fund capital, and then combines these costs to form the hospital's overall cost of capital. Projects with projected returns less than the hospital's cost of capital are financially unattractive, and the board rarely gives the go-ahead to such projects.

It was not at all clear to Sister Mary Margaret why the hospital should worry about its cost of capital. Furthermore, the whole process was somewhat of a mystery. Especially puzzling was the need to attach a cost to St.

Sebastian's fund capital. No contributor requires an explicit return for fur-
nishing this capital, so why couldn't it be considered free? To get a better feel
for the cost of capital concept, Sister Mary Margaret decided to enroll in an
evening healthcare finance course taught at a local university. As you will
learn at the end of this chapter, her efforts were well rewarded.

INTRODUCTION

The cost of capital is an extremely important concept in healthcare
financial management. All firms, whether investor-owned or not-
for-profit, have to raise funds to buy the assets required to meet
their business objectives. Hospitals, nursing homes, clinics, group
practices, and so on, all need assets to provide services. The funds
to acquire these assets come in many shapes and forms, including
contributions, profit retention, equity sales to stockholders, and
debt capital supplied by creditors such as banks, bondholders,
lessors, and suppliers. Most of the capital raised by businesses has
a cost, which is either explicit, such as the interest payments on
debt, or implicit, such as the opportunity cost associated with equity (fund) capital. Since many business decisions require the cost of
capital as an input, it is necessary for all healthcare managers to
understand the cost of capital concept. Furthermore, healthcare
managers of small organizations, without financial staffs, need to
be able to estimate the cost of capital for their own businesses.

The goal of the cost of capital estimation process is to estimate
the firm's overall cost of capital, which is then used as the hurdle
rate to evaluate capital investment opportunities. For example,
assume St. Sebastian's hospital has a cost of capital of 10 percent. If
a new investment, say, an MRI, is expected to return at least 10 percent, then it is financially attractive to the hospital. If the MRI is
expected to return less than 10 percent, accepting it will have an
adverse effect on the hospital's financial soundness.

In establishing a firm's cost of capital, the first step is to identify the specific sources of capital to be included in the estimate.
Once the capital components have been identified, the next step is
to estimate the cost of each component. Finally, the component
costs are combined in a weighted average to estimate the firm's
overall cost of capital.

Capital Components

Capital, as the term is used here, refers to the entire right-hand side of the balance sheet because the liabilities and equity (fund capital) listed here represent the sources of funds used to acquire the assets shown on the left-hand side. Which sources of capital should be included in the cost of capital estimate? The cost of capital is used primarily in capital investment decision making; hence, it should focus on those capital sources that are typically used to finance long-term (fixed) assets. For most firms, long-term assets are funded with long-term (permanent) capital; so, clearly, a firm's cost of capital estimate should include the costs of long-term debt and equity.

What about short-term interest-bearing debt, often notes payable to banks? If a firm uses notes-payable financing only as temporary financing to support seasonal or cyclical cash needs, it should not be included in the cost of capital estimate. However, if a business uses short-term debt as part of its permanent financing mix, such debt should be included in the firm's cost of capital estimate. As discussed in Chapter 10, the use of short-term debt to finance permanent assets is highly risky, and it is not common under normal conditions. Therefore, short-term debt will be excluded from the cost of capital discussion presented here.

Finally, should short-term, non-interest-bearing liabilities such as payables and accruals be included in the cost of capital estimate? In general, the answer is no because such liabilities are not used to finance capital assets.

Debt Tax Benefits

In developing the component costs, the issue of debt tax benefits arises for investor-owned companies. In Chapter 10, you will see that the use of debt financing creates a tax benefit to the issuer because interest expense is tax deductible, while the dividends paid to stockholders have no impact on the paying firm's taxes. When conducting capital investment analyses, the tax benefit associated with debt financing can be incorporated either in the cash flows of the project being analyzed or in the firm's cost of capital. Since it is generally easier to incorporate the tax benefit of debt financing in the cost of capital, this approach will be used throughout the book. Thus, the tax benefits to investor-owned firms associated with debt financing will be recognized in the component cost of debt estimate, resulting in an after-tax cost of debt. For not-for-profit firms, the benefits arising from the issuance of tax-exempt debt will be incorporated directly by estimating a relatively low cost of debt.

Capital Pass-Through Payments

Capital pass-through payments are separate payments made by some third-party payers to compensate healthcare providers for capital costs. Such payments were especially important under Medicare reimbursement to hospitals. When used by payers, capital pass-through payments typically are made for depreciation expense, interest expense, and lease and rental payments. These benefits, when they occur, must be recognized in any financial analysis. To accomplish this, the interest pass-through benefit is typically incorporated in the cost of capital estimate. However, capital pass-through payments are being phased out by most third-party payers, including Medicare; hence, their impact on financial decision making is diminishing over time. Because capital pass-through payments are becoming a rarity, they will not be considered here, nor will they be considered in Chapter 7 in the discussion of project cash flows.

Historical versus Marginal Costs

Two very different sets of component costs can be measured: historical, or embedded, costs, which reflect the cost of funds raised in the past, and new, or marginal, costs, which measure the cost of funds to be raised in the future. Historical costs are important in many ways. For example, third-party payers who reimburse on a cost basis are interested in embedded costs. However, our primary purpose in developing a firm's overall cost of capital is to use it in making capital investment decisions, which involve future asset acquisitions and future capital financing. Thus, for our purposes here, the relevant costs are the marginal costs of new funds to be raised in the future (normally during some planning period—say, a year), not the embedded cost of funds raised in the past.

COST OF DEBT

It is unlikely that a firm's managers will know at the start of a planning period the exact types and amounts of debt that will be issued in the future; the type of debt actually used will depend on the specific assets to be financed and on market conditions as they develop over time. Even so, a firm's managers do know what types of debt are typically used by the firm. For example, St. Sebastian's Hospital typically uses bank debt to raise short-term funds to finance temporary needs, and it uses 30-year tax-exempt bonds to raise long-term debt capital. Since St. Sebastian's does not use short-term debt to finance long-term assets, its managers include only long-term debt in their cost of capital estimate, and they assume that this debt will consist solely of 30-year tax-exempt bonds. (If the hospital typically issued serial bonds with different maturities, an average debt cost across all maturities could be used as the cost of debt estimate.)

Suppose St. Sebastian's managers are developing the hospital's cost of capital estimate for the coming year. How should they estimate the hospital's component cost of debt? Most managers would begin by discussing the current interest rate environment with their firms' investment bankers, the institutions that help companies bring their security issues to market. For example, the municipal bond department at Frederick C. Rouse & Company, St. Sebastian's investment banker, estimated that a new 30-year tax-exempt healthcare issue with the same risk as St. Sebastian's would require semiannual interest payments of $30 ($60 annually) per bond to sell at a $1,000 par value. Thus, municipal bond investors currently require a $60/$1,000 = 6.0% return on their investment in the hospital's bonds.

In reality, the cost of the issue to St. Sebastian's would be higher than 6 percent because the hospital must incur costs to sell the bonds. Such costs, which are called issuance, or flotation, costs, consist of accounting costs, legal fees, printing costs, and the fees paid to governmental bond agencies and investment bankers. However, flotation costs on debt issues are typically small, so their impact on the cost of debt estimate is often inconsequential, especially when one considers the uncertainty inherent in the entire cost of capital estimation process. Therefore, it is common practice to ignore flotation costs when estimating the component cost of debt. St. Sebastian's managers follow this practice, so they would estimate the component cost of debt as 6 percent.

$$\text{Tax-exempt component cost of debt} = k_d = 6.0\%$$

If St. Sebastian's currently outstanding debt were actively traded, the current yield to maturity on this debt also could be used to estimate the cost of new debt. For example, St. Sebastian's has a tax-exempt debt issue outstanding that has 20 years (40 semiannual periods) to maturity, a 7 percent coupon, and currently sells in the secondary market for $1,115.57. The yield to maturity on this issue is 6 percent.

Inputs	40		−1115.57	35	1000
	n	i	PV	PMT	FV
Output		= 3.00			

$$\text{YTM} = k_d = 2(3.00\%) = 6.00\%$$

Using the yield to maturity on an outstanding issue to estimate the cost of new debt provides a good estimate for k_d when the remaining life of the old issue approximates the anticipated maturity of the new issue. If this is not the case, then yield curve differentials might cause the estimate to be biased. For example, if the yield curve were upward sloping (interest rates were higher on longer-maturity issues), the yield to maturity on an outstanding 15-year bond would underestimate the cost of a new 30-year issue.

A taxable healthcare organization would use the techniques just described to estimate its before-tax cost of debt. However, the tax benefits of interest payments must then be incorporated into the estimate. To illustrate, consider Puget Sound Health Systems, Inc., an investor-owned company that operates five acute care hospitals in Washington and Oregon. The company's investment bankers indicate that a new 30-year taxable bond issue would require a yield of 10.0 percent. Since the firm's federal-plus-state tax rate is 40 percent, its component cost of debt estimate is also 6 percent.

$$\begin{aligned}
\text{Taxable component cost of debt} &= k_d(1 - T) \\
&= 10.0\%(1 - 0.40) \\
&= 10.0\%(0.60) = 6.0\%
\end{aligned}$$

Note that the component cost of debt to an investor-owned firm is reduced by the (1 − T) term. As discussed previously, reducing Puget Sound's component cost of debt from 10 percent to 6 percent incorporates the benefit associated with interest payment tax deductibility into the debt estimate.

In general, the effective cost of debt is roughly comparable between investor-owned and not-for-profit firms of similar risk. Investor-owned firms have the benefit of tax deductibility of interest payments, while not-for-profit firms have the benefit of being able to issue lower-cost tax-exempt debt.

COST OF EQUITY

Equity capital is raised by investor-owned firms by selling new common stock and by retaining earnings for use by the firm rather than paying them out as dividends to shareholders. Not-for-profit firms raise equity capital through contributions and government grants and by generating an excess of revenues over expenses, none of which can be paid out as dividends. The following sections describe how to estimate the cost of equity capital, both to investor-owned and not-for-profit firms.

The two sources of equity capital to investor-owned firms—retained earnings and new common stock sales—have slightly different costs. The difference arises because flotation costs (issuance expenses) must be incurred on new common stock sales, while the retention of earnings does not require such costs. Although issuance costs are larger for stock issues than for debt issues, the cost differential is rarely material, so many firms elect not to distinguish between the costs of these two equity sources. Thus, the example presented here will assign a single cost to equity capital that will be called the cost of equity, rather than assign separate costs to retained earnings and new common stock sales.

The cost of debt is based on the return that investors require on debt securities. The cost of equity to investor-owned firms can be defined similarly: It is the rate of return that investors require on the firm's common stock. At first glance, it might appear that retained earnings are a costless source of capital to investor-owned firms. After all, dividend payments must be paid on new shares of stock that are issued, but no such payments are required on funds that are obtained by retaining earnings because no additional shares are issued. The reason why a cost of capital must be assigned to retained earnings involves the opportunity cost principle. An investor-owned firm's net income literally belongs to its common stockholders. Employees are compensated by wages, suppliers are compensated by cash payments for supplies, bondholders are compensated by interest payments, governments are compensated by tax payments, and so on. The residual earnings of a firm, its net income, belong to the stockholders and serve to "pay the rent" on stockholder-supplied capital.

Management can either pay out earnings in the form of dividends or retain earnings for reinvestment in the business. If part of the earnings are retained, an opportunity cost is incurred: Stockholders could have received these earnings as dividends and then invested this money in stock, bonds, real estate, commodity futures, and so on. Thus, the firm should earn on its retained earnings at least as much as its stockholders themselves could earn on alternative investments of similar risk. If the firm cannot earn as much as the stockholders can in similar risk investments, the firm's net income should be paid out as dividends rather than retained for reinvestment within the firm. What rate of return can stockholders expect to earn on other investments of equivalent risk? The answer is k_s, the required rate of return on the firm's equity. Investors can earn this return either by buying more shares of the firm in question or by buying the stock of similar firms.

To illustrate this opportunity-cost concept, consider Puget Sound Health Systems, Inc. In 1996, it earned $22 million in net income. If Puget Sound paid all $22 million out to its stockholders as dividends, they would have that cash in hand to invest in securities, including buying more stock of Puget Sound itself. The firm's stockholders would earn a return on these dividend investments. By not paying dividends, Puget Sound is depriving its stockholders of that opportunity. Since Puget Sound is denying its stockholders the chance to earn a return on dividend payments, it has the obligation to earn a return on its retentions. If Puget Sound retains net income without earning at least as much as its stockholders could earn on investments of similar risk, its stock price would fall and it would have difficulty raising new equity capital in the future.

Whereas debt is a contractual obligation with an easily esti-mated cost, it is not nearly as easy to estimate k_s, the firm's cost of equity. Two primary methods are used to estimate k_s: the Capital Asset Pricing Model (CAPM) and the Discounted Cash Flow (DCF) model. These methods should not be regarded as mutually exclu-sive, for neither approach dominates the estimation process. In practice, both approaches should be used to estimate k_s, and then the final value should be chosen on the basis of the analyst's confi-dence in the data at hand.

Capital Asset Pricing Model (CAPM) Approach

The Capital Asset Pricing Model (CAPM), which was introduced in Chapter 3, is a widely accepted corporate finance model that spec-ifies the equilibrium risk/return relationship on risky assets, espe-cially common stocks. Basically, the model assumes that investors consider only one risk factor when setting required rates of returns: the volatility of returns on the stock compared with the volatility of returns on a well-diversified portfolio called the market portfolio, or just the market. The measure of risk in the CAPM is the firm's beta, or beta coefficient, which measures the volatility of the stock's returns relative to the returns on the market. The market, which is a large collection of stocks such as the S&P 500 index, has a beta of 1.0. A stock with a beta of 2.0 has twice the volatility of returns as the market, while a stock with a beta of 0.5 has only half the volatil-ity of returns as the market. Since return volatility is a measure of risk, a low beta stock, defined as having a beta less than 1.0, is less risky than the market; while a high beta stock, defined as having a beta larger than 1.0, is more risky than the market.

Within the CAPM, the equation which relates risk to return is called the Security Market Line (SML).

$$k_s = \text{Risk-free rate} + \text{Risk premium}$$
$$= k_{RF} + (k_M - k_{RF})b$$

Here,

k_{RF} = risk-free rate, the required rate of return on riskless securities.

b = beta coefficient of the stock in question.

$(k_M - k_{RF})$ = market risk premium; the premium above the risk-free rate that investors require to buy a stock with average risk.

$(k_M - k_{RF})b$ = stock risk premium, the premium above the risk-free rate that investors require to buy the stock in question.

Given estimates of (1) the risk-free rate, k_{RF}, (2) the beta of the firm's stock, b, and (3) the required rate of return on the market, k_M, a healthcare manager can estimate the required rate of return on his or her firm's stock (or, for that matter, any stock). This estimate, in turn, can be used as the estimate for the firm's cost of equity.

Estimating the Risk-Free Rate

The starting point for the CAPM cost of equity estimate is k_{RF}, the risk-free rate. Unfortunately, there is no security in the United States that is truly riskless; hence, it is impossible to observe the risk-free rate. Treasury securities are essentially free of default risk, but long-term T-bonds will suffer capital losses if interest rates rise (price risk), and a portfolio invested in short-term T-bills will provide a volatile earnings stream because the rate paid on T-bills varies over time (reinvestment rate risk).

Since it is impossible in practice to find a truly riskless rate, what rate should be used in the CAPM? The preference of most finance professionals is to use the rate on long-term Treasury bonds. Here is the rationale:

1. Capital market rates include a real, riskless rate (generally thought to vary from 2 to 4 percent) plus a premium for inflation that reflects the expected inflation rate over the life of the security, be it 30 days or 30 years. The expected rate of inflation is likely to be relatively high during booms and relatively low during recessions. Therefore, during booms, T-bill rates tend to be high to reflect the high current inflation rate; whereas, in recessions, T-bill rates are generally low. T-bond rates, on the other hand, reflect expected inflation rates over a long period, so they are far less volatile than T-bill rates.

2. Common stocks are generally viewed as long-term investments, and although a particular stockholder may not have a long investment horizon, the majority of stockholders do invest on a long-term basis. Therefore, it is reasonable to think that stock returns embody long-term inflation expectations similar to those embodied in bonds rather than the short-term inflation expecta-

tions embodied in bills, so the cost of equity should be more highly correlated with T-bond rates than with T-bill rates.

3. Treasury bill rates are subject to more random disturbances than are Treasury bond rates. For example, bills are used by the Federal Reserve System (the Fed) to control the money supply, and bills are also used by foreign governments, firms, and individuals as a temporary safe haven for money. Thus, if the Fed decides to stimulate the economy, it drives down the bill rate, and the same thing happens if trouble erupts somewhere in the world and money flows into U.S. dollars seeking a temporary haven. T-bond rates are also influenced by Fed actions and by international money flows but not to the same extent as T-bill rates. This is another reason why T-bill rates are more volatile than T-bond rates and, most experts agree, more volatile than the cost of equity.

In view of the preceding points, it is generally accepted that common equity costs are more logically related to Treasury bond rates than to T-bill rates. Thus, the rate on T-bonds is used most often as the base rate, or k_{RF}, in a CAPM cost-of-equity analysis. T-bond rates can be found in *The Wall Street Journal*, the *Federal Reserve Bulletin*, or even in most local papers. Since the yield curve is relatively flat on the long end (interest rates on 15-year bonds are usually close to those on 30-year bonds), it is common for analysts to use the yield on 20-year T-bonds as the proxy for the risk-free rate.

Estimating the Required Rate of Return on the Market

The required rate of return on the market, k_M, and its derivative, the market risk premium, $RP_M = k_M - k_{RF}$, can be estimated on the basis of (1) historical returns or (2) forecasted returns.

Historical Risk Premiums

Many sources of historical risk premium data are available. One of the most commonly used, which examines market data over long periods of time to find the average annual rates of return on stocks, T-bills, T-bonds, and a set of high-grade corporate bonds, is published annually by Ibbotson Associates. (See *Stocks, Bonds, Bills and Inflation: 1996 Yearbook.* Chicago: Ibbotson Associates, 1996.) To illustrate, Table 6–1 summarizes some results from the 1996 Yearbook, which covers the period 1926 to 1995.

TABLE 6-1

Selected Historical Returns Data, 1926–1995

	Mean	Standard Deviation
Total Return Data:		
Common stocks	12.5%	20.4%
Long-term corporate bonds	6.0	8.7
Long-term Treasury bonds	5.5	9.2
Treasury bills	3.8	3.3
Inflation rate	3.2	4.6
Risk Premium Data:		
Common stocks over T-bills	8.8%	Not reported
Common stocks over T-bonds	7.4	Not reported
T-bonds over T-bills	1.4	Not reported

Source: Ibbotson Associates, *1996 Yearbook.*

Note that common stocks provided the highest average return over the 70-year period, while Treasury bills gave the lowest. T-bills barely covered inflation over the period, but common stocks provided a substantial real (inflation-adjusted) return. However, the superior returns on stock investments had its cost: Stocks were by far the riskiest of the investments listed as judged by standard deviation (which measures dispersion about the mean), and they would also rank as riskiest within a market-risk framework (that is, have the highest beta). To further illustrate the risk differentials, the range on annual returns on stocks was from –43.3 to 54.0 percent, while the range on T-bills was only 0.0 to 14.7 percent. The study provides strong empirical support for the efficient market principle discussed in Chapter 5; namely, higher returns can be obtained only by bearing greater risk.

The study also reported the risk premiums, or differences, among the returns on the various securities. For example, Ibbotson Associates found the average risk premium of stocks over T-bonds to be 7.4 percentage points. Thus, 7.4 percent could be used as RP_M = $k_M - k_{RF}$ in a CAPM cost of equity estimate. However, like the returns, historical risk premiums have large standard deviations, so one must use them with caution. Also, the choice of the beginning and ending years can have a major impact on value calculated. Ibbotson Associates used the longest period available to them, but had their data begun some years earlier or later, or ended earlier, their results would have been significantly affected. Indeed, in many years their data would indicate negative risk premiums, which would lead to the conclusion that Treasury securities have a higher required rate of return than common stocks, which in turn is contrary to both financial theory and common sense. All this suggests that historical risk premiums should be used with caution. As one businessman muttered after listening to a professor give a lecture on the CAPM, "Beware of academics bearing gifts!"

Forecasted Market Returns

The historical approach to risk premiums used by Ibbotson Associates assumes that investors expect future results, on average, to equal past results. However, as noted above, historical risk premiums vary greatly depending on the period selected; and, in any event, investors today probably expect results in the future to be different from those achieved during the Great Depression of the 1930s, during the World War II years of the 1940s, and during the peaceful boom years of the 1950s, all of which are included (and given equal weight with more recent results) in the Ibbotson Associates data. The questionable assumption that future expectations are equal to past realizations, together with the sometimes nonsensical results obtained in historical risk premium studies, has resulted in the second approach: forecasted market returns.

Financial services companies such as Merrill Lynch publish, on a regular basis, a forecast for the expected rate of return on the market. (In reality, these forecasts are for the expected rate of return on some market index, such as the S&P 500 or New York Stock Exchange index.) Since the market is generally in equilibrium, the expected rate of return equals investors' required rate of return, so such estimates can be used for k_M in CAPM cost of equity estimates.

Two potential problems arise when using k_M estimates from investment companies such as Merrill Lynch. First, what is really needed is investors' expectations, not those of security analysts. However, this is probably not a major problem since investors form their own expectations on the basis of professional analysts' forecasts.

The second problem is that there are a number of investment companies besides Merrill Lynch, and, at any given time, their forecasts of expected market returns are generally somewhat different. However, these estimates rarely differ from one another by more than ±0.3 percentage points. Therefore, a single firm's forecast may be considered a "reasonable" proxy for the expectations of investors. Note, though, that forecasted market returns are not stable: They vary over time. Therefore, when using investment company forecasts for k_M in a CAPM cost-of-equity estimate, it is essential to use current forecasts.

Estimating Beta

The last parameter needed for a CAPM cost of equity estimate is the stock's beta coefficient. Recall from Chapter 3 that a stock's beta is a measure of its volatility relative to that of an average stock, and that betas are generally estimated from the stock's market characteristic line, that is, estimated by running a linear regression between past returns on the stock in question and past returns on some market index.

Unfortunately, betas show how risky a stock was in the past; whereas, investors are interested in future risk. It may be that a given company appeared to be quite safe in the past but that things have changed, and its future risk is judged to be higher than its past risk, or vice versa. The hospital industry presents a good example. Prior to 1983, when the industry operated on a cost-plus basis, investor-owned hospitals were among the bluest of the blue chips, with betas well below 1.0. However, when prospective payment began, the industry became much riskier, and hospital betas climbed above 1.0.

Also, there are many firms that calculate and publish betas, and these firms use somewhat different data sets for a given firm (different time periods for returns and different market return proxies) and calculate their betas using slightly different methodologies. Unfortunately, there is no consensus in this regard, so different sources report different betas for the same firm. Where does this leave healthcare managers regarding the proper beta? The choice is a matter of judgment and data availability, for there is no "right" beta. With luck, the betas derived from different sources will, for a given company, be close together. If they are not, then one's confidence in the CAPM cost of capital estimate will be diminished. Of course, analysts who use betas still have the problem that betas measure a firm's past risk, but what is relevant to cost of capital estimates is current and future risk.

Table 6–2 contains the betas of the stocks of some representative investor-owned healthcare firms as provided by Value Line. Value Line uses the New York Stock Exchange Composite Index as its proxy for the market, along with 260 weekly observations of market and firm historical returns. On the basis of this very limited selection, it appears that healthcare firms carry above-average market risk for stockholders. Drug producers carry the lowest risk, with betas of 1.05, while HMOs and high-technology firms carry very high risk, with betas over 1.50. It is interesting to note that the market risk of many of the stocks listed in Table 6–2 increased over the past few years, some substantially. (Pacificare's beta increased from 1.00 to 1.55.) Apparently, the ongoing structural changes in the industry have made investments in most healthcare stocks more risky.

TABLE 6–2

Beta Coefficients for Selected Healthcare Companies

Company	Primary Line of Business	Beta
Alza	Drug delivery systems	1.60
Baxter International	Medical supplies	1.15
Beverly Enterprises	Nursing homes	1.35
Bristol-Myers Squibb	Pharmaceuticals	1.05
Chiron	Biotechnology	1.60
Community Psychiatric Centers	Psychiatric hospitals	1.35
Lincoln National	Diversified insurance	1.05
Manor Care	Nursing homes	1.15
National Medical Enterprises	Diversified hospitals	1.30
Omnicare	Clinical supplies	1.15
PacifiCare Systems	HMO	1.55
Puget Sound Health Systems	Acute care hospitals	1.10
U.S. Healthcare	HMO	1.55
U.S. Surgical	Surgical supplies	1.30

Source: Value Line Investment Survey, 1995 and 1996 reports.

Illustration of the CAPM Approach

To illustrate the CAPM approach, consider Puget Sound Health Systems, which has a beta coefficient, b_{PS}, of 1.10. Furthermore, assume that the current yield on 20-year T-bonds, the proxy for k_{RF}, is 6.5 percent and that a brokerage firm estimate for the current required rate of return on the market, k_M, is 12.5 percent. Taken together, these two values imply a market risk premium of $(k_M - k_{RF}) = 12.5\% - 6.5\% = 6.0$ percentage points. With all the required input parameters estimated, the SML equation can be completed as follows:

$$k_{s(PS)} = k_{RF} + (k_M - k_{RF})b_{PS}$$
$$= 6.5\% + (12.5\% - 6.5\%)1.10$$
$$= 6.5\% + (6.0\%)1.10 = 13.1\%$$

Thus, according to the CAPM, Puget Sound's required rate of return on equity is 13.1 percent.

In words, what does the 13.1 percent estimate for k_s imply? In essence, equity investors believe that Puget Sound's stock, with a beta of 1.10, is slightly more risky than an average stock, with a beta of 1.00. With a risk-free rate of 6.5 percent, and a market risk premium of 6.0 percentage points, an average stock, with b = 1.0, has a required rate of return on equity of 12.5 percent.

$$k_{s(A)} = k_{RF} + (k_M - k_{RF})b_A$$
$$= 6.5\% + (6.0\%)1.00 = 12.5\%$$

Thus, equity investors require 60 basis points (0.6 percentage points) more return for investing in Puget Sound Health Systems, with b = 1.10, than they require on an average stock, with b = 1.00.

It should be obvious to you that there is a great deal of uncertainty in the CAPM estimate of k_s. Some of this uncertainty stems from the fact that there is no assurance that the CAPM is correct, that is, that the CAPM accurately describes the risk/return choices of stock investors. Additionally, there is a great deal of uncertainty in the input parameter estimates, especially the required rate of return on the market and the beta coefficient. Because of these uncertainties, it is highly unlikely that Puget Sound's true, but unobservable, k_s is precisely 13.1 percent. Thus, instead of picking single values for each parameter, it may be better to develop high and low estimates and then to combine all the high estimates and all the low estimates to develop a range, rather than a point estimate, for k_s. If this approach had been taken, the conclusion might be that Puget Sound's required rate of return on equity was in the range of 12.6 to 13.6 percent.

Discounted Cash Flow (DCF) Approach

The second procedure for estimating a firm's cost of equity is the Discounted Cash Flow (DCF) method. We know that the intrinsic value of a stock, $E(P_0)$, is the present value of its expected dividend stream. If the dividend is expected to grow each year at a constant rate [constant $E(g)$], the constant growth model can be used to value the stock.

$$E(P_0) = \frac{E(D_1)}{k_s - E(g)}$$

Stock prices are generally in equilibrium, which means that the stock price, P_0, is the same as its intrinsic value, $E(P_0)$, so we can rewrite the equation as

$$P_0 = \frac{E(D_1)}{k_s - E(g)}$$

Finally, the above equation can be solved for k_s, giving this equation:

$$k_s = \frac{E(D_1)}{P_0} + E(g)$$

This is the form of the DCF model that often is used to estimate a firm's cost of equity. (There are many possible forms of the DCF model, including the quarterly growth model, which considers quarterly dividends rather than assuming annual dividends, and the nonconstant growth model, which permits different dividend growth rates in future periods. Even so, many analysts still use the constant growth model because more complex models do not necessarily give better answers when the input parameters are so uncertain.)

Estimating the Current Stock Price

As in the CAPM approach, there are three input parameters in the DCF model. Current stock price is readily available for firms that are actively traded. Puget Sound Health Systems' stock is traded in the over-the-counter (OTC) market, so its stock price generally can be found in *The Wall Street Journal*. At the time of the analysis, Puget Sound's stock price was $30.

Estimating the Next Dividend Payment

Next year's expected dividend payment, $E(D_1)$, is also relatively easy to estimate. If you are one of Puget Sound's managers, you can look in the firm's five-year financial plan for the dividend estimate. If you are an outsider, dividend data on larger publicly traded firms are available from brokerage houses and investment advisory services. Also, current (D_0) dividend information is published in *The Wall Street Journal*, and it can be used as a basis for estimating next year's dividend. Puget Sound Health Systems is followed by Value Line, which estimates next year's dividend to be $1.50, so for purposes of this analysis, $E(D_1) = \$1.50$.

Estimating the Dividend Growth Rate

The expected constant dividend growth rate, $E(g)$, is the most difficult of the DCF model parameters to estimate. Here are several methods for estimating $E(g)$.

Historical Growth Rates

If growth rates in earnings and dividends have been relatively stable in the past, and if investors expect these trends to continue, the past realized growth rate may be used as an estimate of the expected future growth rate. To illustrate, consider Table 6–3, which gives earnings per share (EPS) and dividends per share (DPS) data from 1987 to 1996 for Puget Sound Health Systems.

Table 6–3 shows 10 years (nine growth periods) of data, but it could have contained 15 years or 5 years or some other historical time period. There is no rule as to the appropriate number of years to analyze when calculating historical growth rates. However, the period chosen should reflect, to the extent possible, the conditions expected in the future.

The easiest historical growth rate to calculate is the compound rate between two dates, called the point-to-point rate. For example, EPS grew at an annual rate of 6.8 percent from 1987 to 1996, and DPS grew at a 7.2 percent rate during this same period. Note that the point-to-point growth rate could change radically if different

TABLE 6-3

Puget Sound Health Systems: Historical EPS and DPS Data

Year	EPS	DPS
1987	$2.95	$1.24
1988	3.07	1.32
1989	3.22	1.32
1990	3.40	1.52
1991	4.65	1.72
1992	5.12	1.92
1993	5.25	2.00
1994	5.20	2.20
1995	5.12	2.20
1996	5.35	2.32

historical periods are used. For example, the five-year EPS growth rate from 1990 to 1995 is only 2.8 percent.

To alleviate the problem of sensitivity to starting and ending years, some analysts use the average-to-average method, which reduces the sensitivity of the growth rate to beginning- and ending-year values. The 1987–1989 average EPS is ($2.95 + $3.07 + $3.22)/3 = $3.08; the average 1994–1996 EPS is ($5.20 + $5.12 + $5.35)/3 = $5.22; and the number of years of growth between the two averages is 1988 to 1995 = 7. The average-to-average DPS growth rate is 8.2 percent, and the average-to-average EPS growth rate is 7.8 percent. Note that the focus all along has been on compound annual growth rates, which are much easier to interpret than a single growth rate over the entire period.

If earnings and dividends are growing at different rates, there is a problem. The DCF model calls for the expected dividend growth rate, but if EPS and DPS are growing at different rates, something is going to have to change: These two series cannot grow at different rates indefinitely. There is no rule for handling differences in historical g_{EPS} and g_{DPS}, and when they differ, this simply demonstrates in yet another way the problems with using historical growth as a proxy for expected future growth. As in many aspects of financial decision making, judgment is required when estimating growth rates.

It is obvious that one can take a given set of historical data and, depending on the years and the calculation method used, obtain a large number of quite different growth rates. Therefore, the use of historical growth rates in a DCF analysis must be applied with judgment and also used in conjunction (if at all) with other growth estimation methods.

Retention Growth Model

The retention growth model is another method for estimating the constant growth rate in dividends.

$$E(g) = \text{Expected retention ratio} \times \text{Expected return on equity}$$

Here the retention ratio is the proportion of net income retained for reinvestment in the firm (not paid out as dividends), and return on equity is the ratio of net income to total equity. The retention growth model requires four assumptions: (1) The payout ratio, and thus the retention ratio, is expected to remain constant; (2) the return on equity is expected to remain constant; (3) the firm is not expected to issue new common stock, or, if it does, it will be sold at a price equal to its book value; and (4) future projects are expected to have the same degree of risk as the firm's existing assets.

Puget Sound Health Systems has had an average return on equity of about 14 percent over the past 10 years. This return has been relatively steady, but even so it has ranged from a low of 8.9 percent to a high of 17.6 percent during this period. In addition, the firm's dividend payout ratio has averaged 0.45 over the past 10 years, so its retention ratio has averaged 1.0 − 0.45 = 0.55. Using these data as the best estimate of future dividend payouts and returns on equity, the retention growth method gives an E(g) estimate of 7.7 percent.

$$E(g) = 0.55(14\%) = 7.7\%$$

This figure, together with the historical EPS and DPS growth rates examined earlier, might lead an analyst to conclude that Puget Sound Health System's expected dividend growth rate is in the range of 7.0 to 8.0 percent.

Analysts' Forecasts

A third growth-rate estimation technique calls for using brokerage and investment advisory firms' forecasts. Many such firms forecast and then publish growth-rate estimates for most of the larger publicly owned companies. For example, Value Line provides such forecasts on about 1,700 companies, and all of the larger brokerage houses provide similar forecasts. Furthermore, several companies compile analysts' forecasts on a regular basis and provide summary information such as the median and range of forecasts on widely followed companies. These growth-rate summaries, such as the one compiled by Lynch, Jones & Ryan in its *Institutional Brokers Estimate System* (IBES), can be ordered for a fee and obtained either in hardcopy format or as on-line computer data.

However, many of these forecasts assume nonconstant growth. For example, William Trible and Company forecasted that Puget Sound Health Systems would have a 20 percent annual growth rate in earnings and dividends over the next five years, followed by a steady-state growth rate of 6 percent. A simple way to handle this situation is to use the nonconstant growth forecast to develop a proxy constant growth rate. Computer simulations indicate that dividends beyond Year 50 contribute almost nothing to the value of any stock—the present value of dividends beyond Year 50 is virtually zero. So, for practical purposes, dividends beyond that point can be ignored. Using a 50-year horizon, it is easy to develop a weighted average growth rate and use it as a constant growth rate for cost of equity purposes. For Puget Sound Health Systems, a growth rate of 20 percent for five years followed by a growth rate of 6 percent for 45 years produces an average annual growth rate of $5/50(20\%) + 45/50(6\%)$ $= 0.10(20\%) + 0.90(6\%) = 7.4\%$.

Illustration of the DCF Approach

To illustrate the DCF approach, again consider Puget Sound Health Systems. The company's current stock price, P_0, is \$30, and its next expected annual dividend, $E(D_1)$, is \$1.50. Thus, the firm's DCF estimate of its cost of equity, k_s, is

$$k_s = \frac{E(D_1)}{P_0} + E(g)$$

$$= \frac{\$1.50}{\$30} + E(g) = 5.0\% + E(g)$$

With an E(g) estimate range of 7 to 8 percent, a reasonable single value estimate is the midpoint, 7.5 percent. Thus, the final DCF point estimate for Puget Sound Health System's cost of equity is 5.0% + 7.5% = 12.5%.

Comparison of the CAPM and DCF Methods

Two methods have been presented for estimating the required rate of return on equity: CAPM and DCF. The CAPM estimate was 13.1 percent, and the DCF estimate was 12.5 percent. In this case, there is sufficient consistency in the results to warrant the use of the average of the two estimates, (13.1% + 12.5%)/2 = 12.8% as the final estimate of the cost of equity for Puget Sound Health Systems. If the two methods had produced widely different estimates, Puget Sound's managers would have had to use their judgment as to the relative merits of each estimate and then chosen the estimate that seemed most reasonable under the circumstances. In general, this choice would be made on the basis of the managers' confidence in the input parameters of each approach.

COST OF FUND CAPITAL

Not-for-profit firms raise equity (fund capital) in two basic ways: (1) by receiving contributions and government grants and (2) by earning an excess of revenues over expenses (retained earnings). In recent years, there has been considerable controversy over the "cost" of this capital to not-for-profit firms. This section first discusses some views regarding the cost of fund capital and then illustrates how the cost might be estimated.

What Is the Cost of Fund Capital?

The primary purpose of this chapter is to develop an overall cost of capital that can be used in capital investment decisions. Thus, the estimated "costs" represent the cost of using capital to purchase fixed assets rather than for alternative uses. What is the cost of using fund capital for real asset investment? There are at least four positions that can be taken on this question.

1. It has been argued that fund capital has a zero cost. The rationale here is that (1) contributors do not expect a monetary return on their contributions, and (2) the firm's stakeholders, especially the patients who pay more for services than warranted by the firm's tangible costs, do not require an explicit return on the capital retained by the firm.

2. The second position is that fund capital has some cost, but that the cost is not very high. When a not-for-profit firm receives contributions or retains earnings, it can always invest these funds in marketable securities (highly liquid, safe securities) rather than purchase real assets. Thus, fund capital has an opportunity cost that should be acknowledged, and this cost is roughly equal to the return available on a portfolio of short-term, low-risk securities such as T-bills.

3. The third position rests not so much on the inherent cost of fund capital but more on the correct premise that a not-for-profit firm must earn a return on its fund capital if it is to expand its services over time. For example, assume that a hospital in a growing city must increase its total assets by 5 percent per year to keep pace with increased patient demand. To purchase the required assets without increasing the percentage of debt used to finance the assets, it must grow its fund capital at a 5 percent rate. In this way, it can finance asset growth by growing both debt and equity at the same 5 percent rate and hence can hold the relative amount of debt constant. If the hospital earned zero return on its fund capital, its equity base would remain constant over time, and the only way it could add new assets would be to take on additional debt without matching equity and hence drive up its debt ratio. Of course, at some point, lenders would be unwilling to provide additional debt financing, so no new assets could be added.

If inflation exists, a not-for-profit firm must earn a return on its fund capital just to replace its existing asset base as assets wear out or become obsolete. The return is required because new assets will cost more than the old ones being replaced, so depreciation cash flow in itself will not be sufficient to replace assets as needed. The bottom line here is that not-for-profit firms must earn a return on fund capital, and the greater the growth rate in total assets, including that caused by inflation, the greater the return that must be earned.

4. Finally, others have argued that fund capital to not-for-profit firms has about the same cost as the cost of retained earnings to similar investor-owned firms. The rationale here also rests on the

opportunity cost concept as discussed earlier in point 2, but the opportunity cost is now defined as the return available from investing fund capital in alternative investments of similar risk.

Which of the four positions is correct? Think about it this way. Suppose St. Sebastian's Hospital, a not-for-profit corporation, received $500,000 in unrestricted contributions in 1996 and also retained $4,500,000 in earnings, so it had $5 million of new fund capital available for investment. The $5 million could be used to purchase assets related to its core business, such as an outpatient clinic, diagnostic equipment, or operating rooms; or it could be temporarily invested in securities with the intent of purchasing healthcare assets some time in the future; or the $5 million could be used to retire debt; or it could be used to pay management bonuses; or it could be placed in a non-interest-bearing account at the bank; and on and on. By using this capital to invest in real healthcare assets (plant and equipment), St. Sebastian's is deprived of the opportunity to use this capital for other purposes, so an opportunity cost must be assigned.

What opportunity cost should be assigned? The answer is that the hospital's fund (equity) investment in real assets should return at least as much as the return available on alternative investments of similar risk. (Note that I do not mean to imply here that not-for-profit firms should never invest in a project that will "lose" money. Not-for-profit firms do invest in negative profit projects that benefit its stakeholders, but managers must be aware of the financial opportunity costs inherent in such investments. This issue will be addressed in more detail in Chapter 7.) What return is available on investments similar to fund capital investments in hospital assets? The answer is the return that is expected from investing in the stock of an investor-owned hospital company, such as Puget Sound Health Systems. After all, instead of using the new fund capital to purchase real healthcare assets, St. Sebastian's could always delay the real asset investment until some time in the future and use the funds to buy the stock of a hospital company such as Puget Sound Health Systems, which would have the same risk.

In general, the opportunity cost concept applies to all fund capital: It has a cost to the firm that equals the cost of equity to similar investor-owned firms. However, if contributions are made for a specific purpose, such as a children's wing to a hospital, those funds do indeed have zero cost. Since their use is restricted to a particular project, the hospital does not have the opportunity to invest those funds in other alternatives. (Note, though, that when a hospital solicits funds for a particular purpose, it is really placing the restriction on the contribution instead of the donor, so an opportunity cost may be relevant in that situation.)

Measuring the Cost of Fund Capital

The cost of fund capital to not-for-profit firms is the return available on the stocks of similar investor-owned companies. Thus, if St. Sebastian's Hospital and Puget Sound Health Systems were equivalent in all respects, the 12.8 percent final estimate for Puget Sound's cost of equity could also be used as the estimate for St. Sebastian's cost of fund capital. However, it is impossible to find identical investor-owned and not-for-profit firms; even when they are in the same line of business and about the same size, they will often use different amounts of debt financing, and one is taxable and the other is not. Because of these dissimilarities, it is necessary to adjust for-profit cost-of-equity estimates before they can be used by not-for-profit organizations.

The adjustment is accomplished by using Hamada's equation, which was developed by Robert Hamada in 1969.

$$b_{Stock} = b_{Stock\ with\ no\ debt}[1 + (1 - T)(D/S)]$$

Here b_{Stock} is the beta coefficient of the stock of the firm, assuming that the firm uses some debt financing; $b_{Stock\ with\ no\ debt}$ is the inherent beta of the stock if the firm used no debt financing; T is the tax rate; D is the market value of the firm's debt; and S is the market value of the firm's equity.

To illustrate the use of Hamada's equation, remember that the market beta of Puget Sound Health Systems is 1.10, and its tax rate is 40 percent. Also, assume that Puget Sound's capital structure (mix of debt and equity financing) consists of 60 percent debt and 40 percent equity. To begin the adjustment, use Puget Sound's known market-determined beta of 1.10 to obtain its beta assuming the hospital system used no debt financing.

$$
\begin{aligned}
b_{Stock} &= b_{Stock\ with\ no\ debt}[1 + (1 - T)(D/S)] \\
1.10 &= b_{Stock\ with\ no\ debt}[1 + (1 - 0.40)(0.60/0.40)] \\
1.10 &= b_{Stock\ with\ no\ debt}(1.90) \\
b_{Stock\ with\ no\ debt} &= 1.10/1.90 = 0.58
\end{aligned}
$$

Now, if 0.58 is the inherent stock beta of hospital assets assuming no debt financing, what is the beta of the fund capital of St. Sebastian's Hospital, which uses 50 percent debt financing and is tax exempt? To find the answer, again use Hamada's equation, but this time solve for the stock's beta assuming debt financing is used, and the values for T, D, and S reflect the values for St. Sebastian.

$$
\begin{aligned}
b_{Stock} &= b_{Stock\ with\ no\ debt}[1 + (1 - T)(D/S)] \\
&= 0.58[1 + (1 - 0)(0.50/0.50)] \\
&= 0.58(2.0) = 1.16
\end{aligned}
$$

Thus, the estimated beta of St. Sebastian's fund capital is 1.16. The difference between St. Sebastian's 1.16 beta and Puget Sound's 1.10 beta reflects capital structure and tax rate differentials.

Finally, remembering that the risk-free rate is 6.5 percent and the required rate of return on the market is 12.5 percent, the CAPM is used to estimate St. Sebastian's cost of fund capital, k_f.

$$
\begin{aligned}
k_f &= k_{RF} + (k_M - k_{RF})b \\
&= 6.5\% + (12.5\% - 6.5\%)1.16 \\
&= 6.5\% + (6.0\%)1.16 = 13.5\%
\end{aligned}
$$

Because of tax and leverage (debt financing) differences, St. Sebastian's cost of fund capital, 13.5 percent, is slightly greater than Puget Sound's cost of equity, which is 13.1 percent when estimated using the CAPM.

Before closing this section, a word of caution is in order. There are a lot of issues that cast doubt, not only on the accuracy of the adjustment process just described, but also on the entire concept of looking to a for-profit firm's cost of equity to set the opportunity cost inherent in the use of fund capital. Here are just a few: (1) Beta measures the risk to an investor-owned firm's stockholders, which is not the same as the risk to a not-for-profit firm's stakeholders, so using betas to measure the risk inherent in fund capital can only be considered a very rough approximation. (2) There is no market value of a not-for-profit firm's fund capital, so the market value of equity is not really defined for not-for-profit firms. (3) The derivation of Hamada's equation requires many unrealistic assumptions. (4) In general, stock betas are available only for very large companies, and the risk inherent in the stock ownership of a large, well-diversified company is typically less than the riskiness of an equity investment in a smaller, less-diversified company.

Thus, the cost of fund capital estimate for not-for-profit firms must be viewed as being very rough. Nevertheless, the estimate is the best that finance theory can muster, and a cost of capital developed in this way is better than ignoring the fact that there is an opportunity cost inherent in the use of fund capital. Note also that an alternative approach would be to use Puget Sound's cost of equity as a proxy for St. Sebastian's cost of fund capital without going through the Hamada adjustment process. This simpler approach would result in an estimate for St. Sebastian's cost of fund capital that is almost identical to the more complicated Hamada-adjusted estimate.

THE OVERALL COST OF CAPITAL

Thus far, the chapter has discussed how to estimate the costs of debt, equity, and fund capital. Now it is necessary to combine these component costs to form an overall cost of capital. Each firm has in mind a target capital structure, defined as that mix of debt and common equity (or fund capital) that causes its cost of capital to be minimized. (Capital structure decisions will be discussed in Chapter 10.) When the firm raises new capital, it generally tries to finance so as to keep the actual capital structure reasonably close to its target over time. The general formula for the overall cost of capital is

$$\text{Cost of capital} = w_d k_d (1 - T) + w_s (k_s \text{ or } k_f)$$

Here, w_d and w_s are the target weights for debt and equity (or fund capital), respectively. The cost of the debt component, k_d, will reflect the type of debt most commonly used for long-term financing, while the cost of equity used in the calculation will be either the cost of equity, k_s, or, for not-for-profit firms, the cost of fund capital, k_f.

To illustrate, Puget Sound Health Systems has a target capital structure calling for 60 percent debt and 40 percent common equity. As estimated earlier, the company's before-tax cost of debt, k_d, is 10.0 percent; its tax rate, T, is 40 percent; and its cost of equity, k_s, is 12.8 percent. Now suppose the firm needs to raise $100. Conceptually, to keep its capital structure on target, it must obtain $60 as debt and $40 as common equity. In any one year, the firm may raise all its required capital by issuing debt or by retaining earnings. But, over the long run, Puget Sound plans to use 60 percent debt financing and 40 percent equity financing, and these weights must be used in the firm's cost of capital estimate regardless of the actual financing plans for the near term. The overall cost of the $100 is calculated as follows:

$$\text{Cost of capital} = w_d k_d (1 - T) + w_s(k_s)$$
$$= 0.60(10.0\%)(1 - 0.40) + 0.40(12.8\%)$$
$$= 8.7\%$$

Every dollar of new capital that Puget Sound obtains consists, at least conceptually, of 60 cents of debt with an after-tax cost of 6.0 percent, and 40 cents of common equity with a cost of 12.8 percent. The average cost of each new dollar is 8.7 percent.

Could Puget Sound Health Systems raise an unlimited amount of new capital at the 8.7 percent cost? The answer is no. As companies raise larger and larger sums during a given time period, the costs of both the debt and the equity components begin to rise. As this occurs, the overall cost of new dollars also rises. Thus, just as hospitals cannot hire unlimited numbers of nurses at a constant wage, neither can they raise unlimited amounts of capital at a constant cost. At some point, the cost of each new dollar will increase above 8.7 percent. However, this point is very difficult to define, so most firms use a single cost of capital—8.7 percent for Puget Sound—unless the amount of new capital required is very large, in which case a subjective upward adjustment is made to the cost of capital estimate.

Cost of Depreciation-Generated Funds

Although not mentioned previously, the very first increment of internal funds used to finance any year's investment in new assets is depreciation-generated funds. Of course, depreciation is an allowance for the annual reduction in value of a firm's fixed assets due to wear and tear and obsolescence, and it is deducted from revenues as an expense of doing business. But, since depreciation is a noncash charge, the amount of depreciation expense is available to the firm for investment in fixed assets. For an ongoing firm, depreciation-generated funds would be used first to replace worn-out and obsolete assets. Any remaining funds would be available to purchase new assets or to return to investors.

For cost of capital purposes, should depreciation-generated funds be considered "free" capital, should they be ignored completely, or should a charge be assessed against them? The answer is that a charge should indeed be assessed against depreciation-generated funds, and the cost used should be the firm's overall cost of capital. The reasoning here is that the firm could, if it so desired, distribute depreciation-generated funds to its stockholders and creditors, the parties who financed the assets in the first place; so these funds definitely have an opportunity cost. Remember that depreciation is a return *of* capital, rather than a return *on* capital; so depreciation cash flow "belongs" to the original capital suppliers, which includes both stockholders and debtholders.

For example, suppose Puget Sound Health Systems has $10 million of depreciation-generated funds available. Suppose further that the firm has no projects available to it, not even projects that replace worn-out equipment, that return 8.7 percent or more. It obviously should not raise new capital, and it should not even retain any earnings for internal investment because stockholders would be better off receiving the earnings as dividends and investing the funds themselves. Going on, Puget Sound should not even invest its depreciation-generated $10 million. If it did, it would receive a return less than 8.7 percent and hence could not pay its investors their required rates of return. If it distributed the $10 million to investors, with $4 million going to stockholders and $6 million to bondholders, these investors could invest the funds received in alternative investments of similar risk and earn their required rates of return. The conclusion is that depreciation-generated capital has a cost that is equal to the firm's overall cost of capital. Since depreciation-generated funds have the same cost as the firm's cost of new capital, it is not necessary to consider them separately when estimating a firm's cost of capital—funds generated from depreciation have the same cost to the firm as funds raised from new debt and equity financing, including retained earnings.

The Overall Cost of Capital for Not-for-Profit Firms

The cost of capital for not-for-profit firms is developed in the same way as for investor-owned firms. To illustrate, the cost of capital for St. Sebastian's Hospital, assuming a 50 percent debt/50 percent fund capital optimal capital structure, and using the values for the other variables that were developed earlier (6.0 percent for tax-exempt debt and 13.5 percent for the cost of fund capital), is 9.8 percent.

Cost of capital = 0.50(6.0%) + 0.50(13.5%) = 9.8%

Thus, for St. Sebastian's depreciation cash flow, and for all reasonable amounts of new capital, the cost of capital is 9.8 percent.

AN ECONOMIC INTERPRETATION OF THE COST OF CAPITAL

This chapter focused on the methodologies for estimating a firm's cost of capital. In closing, it is worthwhile to step back from the mathematics of the process and examine the interpretation of the cost of capital.

First, note that the component cost estimates that make up a firm's cost of capital (the costs of debt and equity) are based on the returns that investors require to supply capital to the firm. Investors' required rates of return, in turn, are based on the opportunity costs borne by investing in the debt and equity of the firm in question rather than in alternative investments of similar risk.

The opportunity costs to investors, when combined into the firm's cost of capital, establish the opportunity cost to the firm. If the firm cannot earn this rate of return on new capital investments, the capital should be returned to investors for reinvestment elsewhere.

The required rates of return set by investors are based on perceptions regarding the riskiness of their investments (the riskiness of their expected cash flow streams), which, in turn, are based on the inherent riskiness of the business and the amount of debt financing used by the firm. (More debt usage leads to more risk to both debtholders and equityholders and hence to higher component required rates of return.) Thus, the firm's inherent business risk and capital structure are embedded in the cost-of-capital estimate.

The primary purpose for estimating a firm's cost of capital is to help make capital budgeting decisions. That is, the cost of capital will be used as the capital budgeting hurdle rate, or minimum return necessary for a project to be attractive financially. The firm can always earn its cost of capital by investing in similar-risk stocks and bonds, so it should not invest in real assets unless it can earn at least as much. Remember, though, that the cost of capital has embedded in it the aggregate risk and capital structure of the firm, or put another way, the risk and capital structure of the firm's average project. Thus, the firm's cost of capital can be used as a hurdle rate without modification only on those projects under consideration that have average risk and average debt capacity, where *average* is defined as that applicable to the firm's currently held assets in the aggregate. If a new project under consideration has risk or debt capacity that differs significantly from that of the firm's average asset, the firm's cost of capital must be adjusted to account for this differential when the project is being evaluated.

To illustrate the concept, St. Sebastian's cost of capital, 9.8 percent, is probably appropriate for use in evaluating a new outpatient clinic, which is in the same line of business as most of the firm's assets and hence has risk and debt capacity similar to the hospital's average project. However, it would not be appropriate to apply St. Sebastian's cost of capital, without adjustment, to a new project that involves establishing a for-profit food management subsidiary because this project does not have the same risk or debt capacity as the hospital's average asset. Risk and capital structure adjustments to a firm's cost of capital are discussed in Chapter 8.

At the end of her healthcare finance course, Sister Mary Margaret had a much better understanding of the estimation and use of St. Sebastian's cost of capital. Most importantly, she learned that the hospital's 9.8 percent cost of capital is only valid for projects having the same risk and debt capacity as the hospital's average project. Furthermore, she learned (as you will in the next chapter) that proposed projects that provide social value to the community should get "extra credit" when being evaluated.

Sister Mary Margaret was able to demonstrate that the neonatal care unit she had championed was a relatively low-risk project and hence should face a hurdle rate lower than the hospital's 9.8 percent overall cost of capital. In addition, she convinced the board that the neonatal care unit would produce a large amount of social value. When the lower hurdle rate and social value were factored into the financial analysis, the neonatal care unit became financially attractive, and the board of trustees approved the project. It is now in its second year of operation and running well in the black. Guess what it is named: The Sister Mary Margaret Neonatal Care Unit.

SELF-ASSESSMENT EXERCISES

6–1   a. What capital components are typically included in a firm's overall cost-of-capital estimate?

       b. Write out the generic cost of capital formula and briefly explain each term.

       c. Should the cost of debt reflect the tax benefits inherent in debt financing? Why?

       d. Should the component cost estimates reflect historical (embedded) costs or future (marginal) costs? Explain.

6–2   a. What are some of the ways that a firm can estimate its cost of debt?

       b. What are flotation costs? Should flotation costs be considered in the cost-of-debt estimate?

6–3   a. Why is there a cost associated with the retained earnings of investor-owned firms?

       b. What are the two most common methods used to estimate a firm's cost of equity?

       c. Briefly explain the Capital Asset Pricing Model (CAPM) approach. In particular, indicate the potential sources of input data.

       d. Briefly explain the discounted cash flow (DCF) approach. Again, indicate the potential sources of input data.

6–4   a. Discuss the main arguments concerning the cost of fund capital to not-for-profit firms.

       b. What is Hamada's equation? How is it used to help estimate a not-for-profit firm's cost of fund capital?

       c. What is the cost associated with depreciation-generated cash flow?

       d. What is the economic interpretation of a firm's cost of capital?

6–5   New England Health Corporation (NEHC) currently has a bond issue outstanding that has annual coupon payments of $100, 20 years remaining to maturity, and sells in the market for $789.26 per $1,000 par value. The firm's beta coefficient is 1.2, the risk-free rate is 10 percent, and the required rate of return on the market is 15 percent. NEHC's next dividend, $E(D_1)$, is estimated to be $2.00, and it is growing at a constant rate of 5 percent. The firm's stock is currently selling for $20.00. NEHC's target capital structure is 40 percent debt and 60 percent common stock. The firm's tax rate is 40 percent.

a. What is the firm's component cost of debt?
b. What is the firm's cost of equity? (Use both the CAPM and DCF methods.)
c. What is the firm's overall cost of capital?

SELECTED REFERENCES

For one of the classic works on the cost of fund capital, see Douglas A. Conrad. "Returns on Equity to Not-For-Profit Hospitals: Theory and Implementation." *Health Services Research*, April 1984, pp. 41–63.

Also, see the follow-up articles by Pauly; Conrad; and Silvers and Kauer in the April 1986 issue of *Health Services Research*.

Other articles pertaining to the cost of capital include

Boles, Keith E. "Implications of the Method of Capital Cost Payment on the Weighted Average Cost of Capital." *Health Services Research*, June 1986, pp. 191–211.

Cleverley, William O. "Return on Equity in the Hospital Industry: Requirement or Windfall?" *Inquiry*, Summer 1982, pp. 150–59.

Sloan, Frank A., Joseph Valvona, and Mahmud Hassan. "Cost of Capital to the Hospital Sector." *Journal of Health Economics*, March 1988, pp. 25–45.

Smith, Dean G. and John R.C. Wheeler. "Accounting Based Risk Measures for Not-for-Profit Hospitals." *Health Services Management Research*, November 1989, pp. 221–26.

Wheeler, John R.C. and Dean G. Smith. "The Discount Rate for Capital Expenditure Analysis in Healthcare." *Health Care Management Review*, Spring 1988, pp. 43–51.

7

CHAPTER

Capital Investment Decisions: The Basics

Janet Washington is one of 15 family practice physicians with Family Healthcare, Inc., a large group practice in Birmingham. Last winter, she saw a patient who was feeling poorly, exhibiting some of the symptoms associated with a particularly virulent version of the flu that had been devastating the area over the past several weeks. After thoroughly examining her patient, Janet concluded that he probably had some other illness, but she needed a blood test to confirm her suspicions.

The group practice had no laboratory capabilities, so its patients are referred to an outpatient lab run by a large national chain. The tests are typically run at night, so the results are available the following day. When Janet saw the blood workup, especially the white blood cell and electrolyte values, she immediately admitted her patient to the hospital. It turned out that the patient had pseudomembranous colitis, a bacterial infection of the intestine that can, under certain conditions, be fatal. Although the patient fully recovered, the whole incident renewed Janet's concerns about not having on-site lab services. "After all" she explained to the practice director, "if we had the capability of running routine tests here, we could diagnose serious problems much more quickly and potentially avert a disaster."

*Although the director agreed with Janet, his major concern was finan-
cial. "If the lab would just break even," he said, "I would support it because
it would be good for our patients. However, you are going to have to convince me." At the end of the chapter, you will see if Janet was successful.*

INTRODUCTION

Chapter 6 described how managers estimate a firm's cost of capital, which establishes the opportunity cost of providing new
healthcare services. Now, it is time to see how the cost of capital is
used to make investment decisions. Although some investment
decisions, such as the decision to expand the operating hours of a
walk-in clinic, involve only the expenditure of operating funds,
most investment decisions entail the acquisition of new facilities
and/or equipment. Thus, decisions of this type are often called
capital investment, or capital budgeting, decisions.

A number of factors combine to make capital investment decisions the most important ones managers make. First and foremost,
capital investment decisions chart the strategic direction of the
business. Since the results of capital investment decisions may continue for an extended period, the impact of the decision is often not
known for years. For example, the decision by a nursing home
director to add a new wing influences the costs and capacity of the
facility for a prolonged period. If the nursing home invests too
heavily in fixed assets, it will have too much capacity, and its costs
will be too high. On the other hand, a nursing home that invests too
little in operating assets may not be able to offer the latest in medical technology or may not have the capacity to meet the demand
for its services. In either case, it is likely that the business will lose
a portion of its market share to competitors.

Effective capital investment procedures improve both the timing of asset acquisitions and the cost and quality of the assets purchased. A firm that forecasts its needs for capital assets well in
advance will have the opportunity to carefully plan the acquisition
and thus will be able to negotiate the best assets at the best prices.

Finally, capital investment is also important because asset
expansion typically involves substantial expenditures, and large
amounts of investment capital are not usually available. A firm

with major capital expenditures should plan for its financing several years in advance to be sure of having the funds available when they are needed.

The discussion of capital investment is divided into three chapters. Chapter 7 provides an overview of the capital investment process, discusses the key elements of cash flow estimation, and explains the basic techniques used to assess a project's break-even points and profitability. Chapter 8 considers the very important topic of capital investment risk analysis and incorporation. Finally, Chapter 9 covers mergers and acquisitions, a special category of capital investment decision making in which entire firms combine assets.

THE ROLE OF FINANCIAL ANALYSIS IN HEALTHCARE INVESTMENT DECISIONS

For-profit healthcare firms have the primary goal of shareholder wealth maximization. For these firms, the importance of financial analysis is clear because such analysis identifies those projects that contribute to shareholder wealth.

Most hospitals, however, and many other healthcare providers, are not-for-profit firms that do not have shareholders. In such firms, the appropriate goal is generally expressed in terms of providing quality, cost-effective service to the communities served. In this situation, capital investment decisions must consider many factors besides a project's profitability. For example, noneconomic factors such as the needs of the medical staff and the good of the community must also be taken into account and, in some instances, these factors will outweigh financial considerations.

Nevertheless, good decision making, and hence the future viability of the organization, requires that the financial impact of capital investments be fully recognized. If a firm takes on several highly unprofitable projects that are not offset by other profitable projects, the firm's financial condition will deteriorate. If this situation persists over time, the firm will lose its financial viability and may be forced into bankruptcy and eventual closure. Bankrupt firms cannot meet a community's needs, so a project's potential impact on the firm's financial condition must be carefully considered, even by managers of not-for-profit firms. Capital investment analysis accomplishes this.

OVERVIEW OF CAPITAL INVESTMENT ANALYSIS

The financial analysis of capital investment proposals typically involves the following five steps:

1. First, the capital outlay, or cost, of the project must be estimated.

2. Second, the operating and termination cash flows of the project must be forecasted. Steps 1 and 2 constitute the cash flow estimation phase, which is discussed in the next section.

3. Next, the riskiness of the estimated cash flows must be assessed. Risk assessment will be discussed in Chapter 8.

4. Then, given the riskiness of the project, the project's cost of capital is estimated. As discussed in Chapter 6, the firm's cost of capital reflects the aggregate risk and debt capacity of the firm's assets, that is, the riskiness and optimal capital structure inherent in the firm's "average project." If the project being evaluated does not have average risk and debt capacity, the firm's cost of capital must be adjusted to reflect these differentials, resulting in a project cost of capital. This step in the analysis, called risk incorporation, is also discussed in Chapter 8.

5. Finally, the profitability of the project is assessed. There are several measures that can be used for this purpose; this chapter will discuss two commonly used measures. Additionally, two types of break-even measures will be introduced.

Cash Flow Estimation

The most important, but also the most difficult, step in evaluating capital investment proposals is cash flow estimation—estimating the investment outlays, the annual operating cash flows expected when the project goes into operation, and any cash flows associated with project termination. Many variables are involved in cash flow forecasting, and many individuals and departments participate in the process. It is often difficult to make accurate projections of the costs and revenues associated with a large, complex project, so forecast errors can be quite large. Thus, it is essential that risk analyses be performed on prospective projects. One manager with a good sense of humor developed the following five principles of capital investment cash flow estimation:

1. It is very difficult to forecast cash flows, especially those that occur in the future.
2. Those who live by the crystal ball soon learn how to eat ground glass.
3. The moment you forecast cash flows, you know that you are wrong—you just don't know by how much and in what direction.
4. If you are right, never let your bosses forget.
5. An expert is someone who has been right at least once.

It is almost impossible to overstate the difficulties one can encounter in cash flow estimation. However, if the principles discussed in the next sections are observed, errors that often arise in the cash flow estimation process can be minimized.

Cash Flow versus Accounting Income

Accounting income statements are in some respects a mix of apples and oranges. For example, accountants deduct labor costs, which are cash outflows, from revenues, which may not be entirely cash. (In the provider sector of the healthcare industry, most of the collections are from third-party payers, and payment may not be received until several months after the service is provided.) At the same time, the income statement does not recognize capital outlays, which are cash flows, but it does deduct depreciation expense, which is not a cash flow. The end result is a "bottom line" that does not generally reflect the actual cash generated by the business.

In capital investment decisions, it is critical that the decision be based on the actual dollars that flow into and out of the firm because a firm's true profitability, and hence its financial viability, depends on its cash flows, not on its income as reported in accordance with generally accepted accounting principles. Note, however, that accounting items can influence cash flows because items such as depreciation can affect tax or reimbursement cash flows. The key here is that capital investment analyses must focus on a proposed project's cash flows rather than its impact on accounting statements.

Identifying the Relevant Cash Flows

The relevant cash flows to consider when evaluating a new capital investment are the project's incremental cash flows, which are defined as the difference in the firm's cash flows in each period if the project is undertaken versus the firm's cash flows if the project is not undertaken:

$$\text{Incremental CF}_t = \text{CF}_t(\text{Firm with project})$$
$$- \text{CF}_t(\text{Firm without project})$$

Here, the subscript t specifies a time period, often years. If years are used, CF_0 is the cash flow during Year 0, which is generally assumed to end today, CF_1 is the cash flow during the first year, CF_2 is the cash flow during Year 2, and so on. In practice, the early cash flows, and Year 0 in particular, are usually cash outflows, or costs. Then, as the project is placed into operation and begins to generate revenues in excess of operating expenses, the cash flows turn positive. Finally, most projects have termination cash flows that occur when the project is closed down.

Cash Flow Timing

The cash flow estimation process must account properly for the timing of the cash flows. Accounting income statements are for periods such as years or quarters, so they do not reflect exactly when, during the period, revenues and expenses occur. In theory, capital investment cash flows should be analyzed exactly as they occur. Of course, there must be a compromise between accuracy and practicality. A time line with daily cash flows would, at least in theory, provide the most accuracy; but daily cash flow estimates would be costly to construct, unwieldy to use, and, because of the uncertainties involved, probably no more accurate than annual cash flow estimates. Thus, in most cases, analysts simply assume that all project cash flows occur at the end of each year. However, for some projects, it may be useful to assume that cash flows occur every six months or even to forecast quarterly or monthly cash flows.

Project Life

One of the first decisions that must be made in forecasting a project's cash flows is the life of the project: Do we need to forecast cash flows for 20 years, or is five years sufficient? Many projects, such as a new hospital wing or an ambulatory care clinic, potentially have very long lives, perhaps 50 years or more. In theory, a cash flow forecast should extend for the full life of a project, yet most managers clearly would have very little confidence in any cash flow forecasts beyond the near term. Thus, most organizations set a limit on project life, often 5 or 10 years. If the forecasted life is less than the arbitrary limit, the forecasted life is used to develop the cash flows, but if the forecasted life exceeds the limit, project life is truncated and all cash flows beyond the limit are left off of the time line.

Although cash flow truncation is a practical solution to a difficult problem, it does create another problem: The value inherent in the cash flows beyond the truncation point is lost to the project. This problem can be addressed either objectively or subjectively. The standard procedure at some organizations is to estimate the project's terminal, or truncation, value, which is the estimated value of the cash flows beyond the truncation point. Often, the terminal value is estimated as the liquidation value of the project at the truncation point. If the terminal value is too difficult to estimate, the fact that some portion of the project's cash flow value is being ignored should, at a minimum, be subjectively recognized by decision makers. The saving grace in all this is that cash flows well into the future typically contribute a relatively small amount to a project's profitability. For example, a $100,000 terminal value projected to occur 10 years into the future contributes only about $38,500 to the project's current value when the cost of capital is 10 percent.

Sunk Costs

A sunk cost refers to an outlay that has already occurred (or has been irrevocably committed), so it is an outlay that is unaffected by the accept/reject decision under consideration. To illustrate, suppose that in 1997 Forest View Memorial Hospital is evaluating the purchase of a lithotripter system. To help perform the analysis, in 1996 the hospital hired and paid $5,000 to a consultant to conduct a marketing study for the system. Is this 1996 cash flow relevant to the 1997 capital investment decision? The answer is no. The $5,000 is a sunk cost; Forest View cannot recover it whether or not the lithotripter is purchased. The cash flow is not incremental to the decision at hand. Sometimes, a project appears to be unprofitable when all associated costs, including sunk costs, are considered. However, on an incremental basis, the project may be profitable and should be undertaken. Thus, the correct treatment of sunk costs may be critical to the decision.

Opportunity Costs

All relevant opportunity costs must be included in a capital investment analysis. One opportunity cost involves the use of the capital. If the firm uses its capital to invest in Project A, it cannot use the capital to invest in Project B, and so on. The opportunity cost associated with capital use is accounted for in the project's cost of capital, which is used to discount the project's expected cash flows.

Another type of opportunity cost often arises in capital investment decisions. To illustrate, assume that Forest View's lithotripter would be installed in a yet-to-be-built freestanding facility and that the hospital currently owns the land upon which the facility would be constructed. In fact, the hospital purchased the land 10 years ago at a cost of $25,000, but the current market value of the property is $45,000, and the hospital would net $40,000 after legal and realtor fees if the land were sold. When evaluating the lithotripter, should the value of the land be disregarded because no cash outlay is necessary?

The answer is no because there is an opportunity cost inherent in the use of the property. Using the property for the lithotripter facility deprives Forest View of its use for anything else. Although the property might be used for a walk-in clinic rather than sold, the best measure of its value to the hospital, and hence the opportunity cost inherent in its use, is the cash flow that could be realized from selling the property. Thus, the lithotripter project should have a $40,000 opportunity cost charged against it. Note that the opportunity cost is the property's $40,000 net market value, irrespective of whether the property was acquired for $25,000 or $50,000.

Effect on Other Parts of the Firm

Capital investment analyses must consider the effect of the project on other parts of the firm. When the effect is negative, it is sometimes called cannibalization. To illustrate, assume that some of the patients who are expected to use Forest View's new lithotripter would have been treated surgically, so some surgical revenues will be lost if the lithotripter facility goes into operation. The incremental revenues to Forest View are the revenues attributable to the lithotripter, less the revenues lost from foregone surgery services.

On the other hand, new patients who use the lithotripter may use other services provided by the hospital. In this situation, the incremental cash flows generated by the new patients' utilization of other services should be credited to the lithotripter project. If possible, both positive and negative effects should be quantified; but, at a minimum, they should be noted so that the final decision maker will be aware of their existence.

Shipping and Installation Costs

When a firm acquires fixed assets, it often incurs substantial costs for shipping and installing the equipment. Because these charges are a real cost to the firm, they are added to the invoice price of the equipment to determine the overall cost of the project. Also, the full cost of the equipment, including shipping and installation charges, is typically used as the basis for calculating depreciation charges. Thus, if Forest View Memorial Hospital purchases intensive care monitoring equipment that costs $150,000, but another $30,000 is required for shipping and installation, the full cost of the equipment would be $180,000. This amount would be the project's initial cash outflow as well as the starting point for depreciation calculations.

Changes in Current Assets and Liabilities

Normally, expansion projects require additional inventories, and expanded sales usually lead to additional receivables. The increase in these current asset accounts must be paid for, or financed, just as an increase in fixed assets must be financed. (Increases on the asset side of the balance sheet have to be matched with increases on the liabilities and equity side.) However, some current liabilities such as accounts payable and accruals will probably also increase as a result of the expansion, and these incremental funds will reduce the net cash needed to finance the increase in inventories and receivables. If the increase in current assets attributable to a project exceeds the increase in current liabilities, which is typically the case, the net required financing is as much a cash cost to the project as is the cost of plant and equipment. Such projects must be charged an additional amount above the cost of the new fixed assets to reflect the net financing needed for the current asset accounts. Similarly, if the increase in current liabilities exceeds the increase in current assets, which is rare, the project will generate a positive cash flow from current account changes.

As the project approaches the end of its life, inventories will be sold off and not replaced, and receivables will be collected and hence converted to cash without new receivables being created. In effect, the firm will recover its net investment in current assets when the project is terminated. This will result in a cash flow that is equal but opposite to the current account cash flow that arises at the beginning of a project. For service organizations, such as hospitals, where inventories often represent a very small part of the investment in new projects, the cash flow arising from current account changes can often be ignored without materially affecting the results of the analysis. However, when a project is expected to produce large current account changes, failure to consider the net investment in current assets will typically result in an overstatement of the project's profitability.

Inflation Effects

Because inflation seems to be ever present in our economy and because it can have a considerable influence on a project's cash flows and hence profitability, inflation effects must be considered in any sound capital investment analysis. As discussed in Chapter 6, a firm's cost of capital is a weighted average of its costs of debt and equity. These costs are estimated on the basis of investors' required rates of return, and investors incorporate an inflation premium into their required returns. For example, a debt investor might require a 5 percent return on a 10-year bond in the absence of inflation. However, if inflation is expected to average 6 percent over the coming 10 years, the investor would require an 11 percent return on the bond. Thus, investors add inflation premiums to their required rates of return to help protect them against the loss of purchasing power that stems from inflation.

Since inflation effects are already embedded in the firm's cost of capital, and since the project's cost of capital will be used to discount the cash flows to assess the project's profitability, inflation effects must also be built into the project's estimated cash flows. If cash flows are estimated that do not include inflation effects (real cash flows), and then a discount rate is used that does include inflation effects (nominal discount rate), the profitability of the project will be understated.

The most effective way to deal with inflation is to build inflation effects directly into each cash flow element—revenues, labor costs, supply costs, and so on—using the best available information about how each element will be affected. For example, if a hospital's labor costs are expected to increase at an annual rate of 5 percent, labor costs attributed to a new project must reflect this expectation. Since it is impossible to estimate future inflation rates with much precision, errors are bound to be made. Often, inflation is assumed to be neutral; that is, it is assumed to affect revenues and costs (except depreciation) equally. However, situations can arise where costs may be rising faster than charges, or vice versa. When such situations are expected to occur, different inflation rates should be applied to each cash flow element. For example, because of increased pressures by managed care plans, a hospital's net revenues might be expected to increase at a 2 percent rate, while labor costs might be expected to increase at a 5 percent rate. Inflation adds to the uncertainty, or riskiness, of capital investments, as well as to their complexity. Fortunately, computers and spreadsheet programs are available to help with inflation analysis, so the mechanics of inflation adjustments are relatively easy, in spite of the forecasting difficulty.

Salvage Value

Most assets have positive values at the end of their useful lives. In some situations, the value may be substantial because the asset can be used productively by some other business. In other situations, the value may be solely for scrap and hence relatively small. In rare instances, the value may be negative because the cost of removal and/or disposal exceeds any inherent value the asset might have. The projected value of an asset at the end of its useful life to its current owner is called the asset's salvage value. Salvage values reflect incremental cash flows to a project and hence must be recognized in any capital investment analysis. To avoid potential confusion, note that salvage value reflects the value of an asset at the end of its useful life, while terminal value reflects the value of an asset at the point that its cash flows have been arbitrarily truncated.

Cash Flow Estimation Bias

As stated previously, cash flow estimation is the most critical, and the most difficult, part of the capital investment process. Cash flow components such as price per procedure and volume often must be forecasted many years into the future, and estimation errors are bound to occur, some of which can be quite large. However, large firms evaluate and accept many projects every year, and as long as the cash flow estimates are unbiased and the errors are random, the estimation errors will tend to offset one another. That is, the cash flow estimates on some projects will be too high and on other projects will be too low, but in the aggregate for all projects, the realized cash flows will be very close to the estimates.

Unfortunately, there are strong indications that capital investment cash flow forecasts are not unbiased; rather, managers tend to be overly optimistic in their forecasts, and, as a result, revenues tend to be overstated and costs tend to be understated. The end result is an upward bias in estimated profitability. This bias may result because managers are often rewarded on the basis of the size of their divisions or departments, so they have an incentive to maximize the number of projects accepted rather than the profitability of the projects. Or managers may become emotionally attached to their projects and become unable to objectively assess a project's potential.

There are two procedures that senior managers can use to identify cash flow estimation bias. First, if a project is judged to be highly profitable, this question should be asked: What is the underlying economic basis for this project's high profitability? If the firm has some inherent economic advantage, such as a monopoly position in a managed care market or a superior reputation in providing a specific service, such as organ transplants, there may be a logical rationale supporting high estimated profitability. If no such unique factor can be identified, senior management should be concerned about the possibility of estimation bias. Even when these unique factors exist, at some point in the future it is likely that the project's profitability will be eroded by competitive pressure from firms that seek to capture some of the high profitability inherent in the project today.

Second, continuous review of the historical performance of projects will help to identify divisions and departments that habitually overstate (or understate, but this is rare) project profitability. Many firms are now identifying managers and divisions that typically submit cash flow estimates that are optimistically biased. Then, the project forecasts are adjusted for bias either by reducing cash inflows that are thought to be too rosy or by increasing the cost of capital to such projects.

Strategic Value

The previous section discussed the problem of cash flow estimation bias, which can result in overstating a project's profitability. Another problem that can occur in cash flow estimation is underestimating a project's true profitability by not recognizing its strategic value, which is the value of future investment opportunities that can be undertaken only if the project under consideration is accepted.

To illustrate this concept, consider a hospital management company that is considering a management contract for a hospital in Hungary, its first move into Eastern Europe. A straight cash flow analysis might indicate that this contract is unprofitable, but the project could provide entry into the Eastern European market and unlock the door to a whole range of highly profitable follow-on projects. Or consider Forest View Memorial Hospital's decision to start a kidney transplant program. The financial analysis of this project showed the program to be unprofitable, but Forest View's managers considered kidney transplants to be the first service offered in an aggressive transplant program that would not only be profitable in itself but would enhance the hospital's reputation for technological and clinical excellence. Enhanced reputation, in turn, would contribute to both physician recruitment and patient capture and hence increase the hospital's overall profitability.

In theory, the best approach to dealing with strategic value is to forecast the cash flows from the follow-on projects, estimate their probabilities of occurrence, and then add the expected cash flows from the follow-on projects to the cash flows of the project under consideration. In practice, however, this approach is usually impossible to implement: Either the follow-on cash flows are too nebulous to forecast or the potential follow-on projects are too numerous to quantify. Nevertheless, decision makers must recognize that some projects have strategic value, and, at a minimum, this value should be qualitatively considered when making capital investment decisions.

CASH FLOW ESTIMATION EXAMPLE

Up to this point, the chapter has discussed several critical aspects of cash flow estimation. This section presents a simple example that illustrates some of the concepts already covered and then introduces several others that are important to good cash flow estimation.

The Basic Data

Consider the situation faced by Forest View Memorial Hospital in its evaluation of a new magnetic resonance imaging (MRI) system. The system costs two million dollars and the hospital would have to spend another $500,000 for site preparation and installation. The system would be installed in the hospital, and the space to be used has a very low, or zero, market value to outsiders. Thus, no opportunity cost has been estimated to account for the value of the space.

The MRI is expected to generate weekly usage (volume) of 30 scans. Each scan would, on average, cost the hospital $25 in supplies. The MRI is expected to operate 50 weeks a year, with the remaining 2 weeks devoted to maintenance. The estimated average charge per scan is $1,000, but 40 percent of this amount, on average, is expected to be lost because of nonpaying patients, managed care discounts and other allowances, and bad debt losses.

The MRI would require two technicians and a secretary, resulting in an incremental increase in annual labor costs of $90,000, including fringe benefits. Overhead cash costs would increase by $20,000 annually if the MRI site is activated. The equipment would require maintenance, which would be furnished by the manufacturer for an annual fee of $150,000, payable at the end of each year of operation. For book purposes, the MRI will be depreciated by the straight-line method over a five-year life.

The MRI is expected to be in operation for five years, at which time the hospital's master plan calls for a brand new imaging facility. The hospital plans to sell the MRI system at that time for an estimated $500,000 salvage value, net of removal costs. The operating revenue and cost estimates are for the first year of operation (Year 1), but inflation is estimated to average 5 percent over the life of the project. Furthermore, inflation is expected to equally impact all revenues and costs except depreciation.

Forest View's managers initially assume that projects under evaluation have average risk; thus, the hospital's 10 percent cost of capital is the appropriate starting project cost of capital. Later, as discussed in Chapter 8, the risk assessment process may indicate a higher or lower cost of capital for the project.

Although the MRI project is expected to take some patients away from the hospital's other imaging systems, new MRI patients are expected to generate revenues for some of the hospital's other departments. On net, the two effects are expected to balance out; that is, the cash-flow loss from other imaging systems is expected to be offset by the cash flow gain from other services used by new MRI patients.

Cash Flow Analysis

The first step in the financial analysis of the MRI project is to estimate the project's net cash flows. This analysis is presented in Table 7–1.

Here are the key points of the analysis by line number:

Line 1

Line 1 contains the estimated cost of the MRI system, $2,000,000. In general, capital investment analyses assume that the first cash flow, normally an outflow, occurs today, or at t = 0, even if the project would not be undertaken immediately. Note that expenses, or cash outflows, are shown in parentheses.

Line 2

The related installation expense, $500,000, is also assumed to occur at t = 0.

Line 3

Gross revenues = (Weekly volume)(Weeks of operation)(Charge per scan) = (30)(50)($1,000) = $1,500,000 in the first year. The 5 percent inflation rate is applied to all charges and costs that would likely be affected by inflation,

TABLE 7-1

Forest View Memorial Hospital: MRI Project Cash Flow Analysis

	0	1	2	3	4	5
			Cash Revenues and Costs			
1. System cost	($2,000,000)					
2. Installation expense	(500,000)					
3. Gross revenues		$1,500,000	$1,575,000	$1,653,750	$1,736,438	$1,823,259
4. Less: allowances		600,000	630,000	661,500	694,575	729,304
5. Net revenues		$ 900,000	$ 945,000	$ 992,250	$1,041,863	$1,093,956
6. Less: labor costs		90,000	94,500	99,225	104,186	109,396
7. Maintenance costs		150,000	157,500	165,375	173,644	182,326
8. Supplies		37,500	39,375	41,344	43,411	45,581
9. Incremental overhead		20,000	21,000	22,050	23,153	24,310
10. Depreciation		400,000	400,000	400,000	400,000	400,000
11. Operating income		$ 202,500	$ 232,625	$ 264,256	$ 297,469	$ 332,343
12. Taxes		0	0	0	0	0
13. Net operating income		$ 202,500	$ 232,625	$ 264,256	$ 297,469	$ 332,343
14. Plus: depreciation		400,000	400,000	400,000	400,000	400,000
15. Plus: net salvage value						500,000
16. Net cash flow	($2,500,000)	$ 602,500	$ 632,625	$ 664,256	$ 697,469	$1,232,343

Note: The cash flows were constructed using a spreadsheet model, so some differences due to rounding appear in the table.

so the $1,000 charge per scan, and hence Line 3 gross revenues, increases by 5 percent over time. Although most of the operating revenues and costs would occur more or less evenly over the year, it is very difficult to forecast exactly when during the year most of the flows would occur. Furthermore, there is significant potential for large errors in cash flow estimation. For these reasons, operating cash flows are often assumed to occur at the end of each year. Also, the operating cash flow estimates assume that the MRI system could be placed in operation quickly. If this were not the case, the first year's operating flows would be reduced. In some situations, it might take several years from the first investment cash flow to the point when the project is operational and begins to generate positive operating cash flows.

Line 4

Indigent care losses and other allowances are estimated to average 40 percent of gross revenues, so in Year 1, 0.40($1,500,000) = $600,000 of gross revenues would be uncollectible. This amount increases each year by the 5 percent inflation rate.

Line 5

Line 5 contains the net revenues in each year, Line 3 – Line 4.

Line 6

Labor costs are forecasted to be $90,000 during the first year, but increase over time at the 5 percent inflation rate.

Line 7

Maintenance costs must be paid to the manufacturer at the end of each year of operation. These costs are assumed to increase at the 5 percent inflation rate.

Line 8

Each scan uses $25 of supplies, so supply costs in the first year total 30(50)($25) = $37,500, and they are expected to increase each year by the inflation rate.

Line 9

If the project is accepted, cash overhead costs will increase by $20,000 in the first year. Note that the $20,000 are cash costs that are related directly to the acceptance of the MRI project. Existing overhead costs that might be arbitrarily allocated to the MRI project are not incremental cash flows and thus should not be included in the analysis. Overhead costs are also assumed to increase over time at the inflation rate.

Line 10

Book (accounting) depreciation in each year is calculated by the straight-line method, assuming a five-year depreciable life. The depreciable basis is equal to the capitalized cost of the project, which is the cost of the asset plus installation charges, less the estimated salvage value. Thus, the depreciable basis = ($2,000,000 + $500,000) − $500,000 = $2,000,000. Then, the straight-line depreciation in each year of the project's five-year depreciable life is (1/5)($2,000,000) = $400,000.

Note that depreciation is based solely on acquisition costs, so it is unaffected by inflation. Also note that depreciation expense is not a cash flow but an accounting convention to recognize the reduction in the value of fixed assets over time caused by wear and tear and obsolescence. Since Forest View Memorial Hospital is tax-exempt, depreciation expense has no impact on the project's operating cash flows, so it is not necessary to explicitly include it on Line 10. However, the Table 7–1 cash flows are presented in a generic format that can be used by both investor-owned and not-for-profit hospitals. Since we have included depreciation, an unnecessary step, we will readjust the cash flows in Line 14.

Line 11

Line 11 shows the project's operating income in each year, which is merely the net revenues less all operating expenses.

Line 12

Line 12 is blank for Forest View's analysis, since the hospital is not-for-profit and does not pay taxes.

Line 13

Forest View pays no taxes, so the project's net operating income equals its operating income.

Line 14

Since depreciation, a noncash expense, was included on Line 10, it must be added back to the project's net operating income in each year to obtain each year's net cash flow. If depreciation were not shown on Line 10, Line 14 could be omitted.

Line 15

Finally, the project is expected to be terminated after five years, at which time the MRI system would be sold for an estimated $500,000. This salvage value cash flow is shown as an inflow at the end of Year 5 on Line 15.

Line 16

The project's net cash flows are shown on Line 16. The project requires a $2,500,000 investment at Year 0 but then generates cash inflows over its five-year operating life.

Note that the Table 7–1 cash flows do not include any allowance for interest expense. On average, Forest View Memorial Hospital will finance new projects in accordance with its target capital structure, 50 percent debt financing and 50 percent equity (fund) financing. The costs associated with this financing mix, including interest expense, are incorporated into the firm's 10 percent cost of capital. Since the cost of debt financing is included in the discount rate that will be applied to the cash flows, recognition of interest expense in the cash flows would be double counting.

Taxable Organizations

The Table 7–1 cash flow analysis can be easily modified to reflect tax implications if the analyzing firm is taxable. To illustrate, assume that the MRI project is being evaluated by Deseret Regional Health Systems, an investor-owned hospital chain based in Salt Lake City. Further, assume that all of the project data presented earlier apply to Deseret, except (1) the MRI falls into the five-year class for tax depreciation, and (2) the firm has a 40 percent tax rate. Table 7–2 contains Deseret's cash flow analysis.

Note the following differences:

Line 10

First, the depreciation expense on Line 10 must be modified to reflect tax depreciation rather than book depreciation. Taxes must be calculated on the basis of tax laws, not accounting convention, so taxable firms must use tax depre-

TABLE 7-2

Deseret Regional Health Systems: MRI Project Cash-Flow Analysis

	0	1	2	3	4	5
			Cash Revenues and Costs			
1. System cost	($2,000,000)					
2. Installation expense	(500,000)					
3. Gross revenues		$1,500,000	$1,575,000	$1,653,750	$1,736,438	$1,823,259
4. Less: allowances		600,000	630,000	661,500	694,575	729,304
5. Net revenues		$ 900,000	$ 945,000	$ 992,250	$1,041,863	$1,093,956
6. Less: labor costs		90,000	94,500	99,225	104,186	109,396
7. Maintenance costs		150,000	157,500	165,375	173,644	182,326
8. Supplies		37,500	39,375	41,344	43,411	45,581
9. Incremental overhead		20,000	21,000	22,050	23,153	24,310
10. Depreciation		500,000	800,000	475,000	300,000	275,000
11. Operating income		$ 102,500	($ 167,375)	$ 189,256	$ 397,469	$ 457,343
12. Taxes		41,000	(66,950)	75,703	158,988	182,937
13. Net operating income		$ 61,500	($ 100,425)	$ 113,554	$ 238,481	$ 274,406
14. Plus: depreciation		500,000	800,000	475,000	300,000	275,000
15. Plus: net salvage value						360,000
16. Net cash flow	($2,500,000)	$ 561,500	$ 699,575	$ 588,554	$ 538,481	$ 909,406

Note: The cash flows were constructed using a spreadsheet model, so some differences due to rounding occur in the table.

ciation to calculate taxes in their project cash flow analyses. It is impossible to turn you into a tax depreciation expert here, but note that (1) depreciation for tax purposes must be in accordance with the Modified Accelerated Cost Recovery System (MACRS) prescribed by the Internal Revenue Service (IRS), (2) all assets fall into one of several classes roughly based on usable life, and (3) each class has a set of factors that are multiplied by the asset's depreciable basis (cost) to get the depreciation expense for each year. In this example, the depreciable basis is $2,500,000, and the MRI system falls into the MACRS five-year class, so the MACRS factors are 0.20, 0.32, 0.19, 0.12, 0.11, and 0.06, in Years 1–6 respectively. (Only partial deprecation can be taken in the first year, so depreciation of five-year property actually extends over six years.) Thus, tax depreciation in Year 1 is 0.20($2,500,000) = $500,000; in Year 2, depreciation is 0.32($2,500,000) = $800,000; and so on.

Line 12

Taxable firms must reduce the operating income on Line 11 by the amount of taxes. Taxes, which appear on Line 12, are computed by multiplying the Line 11 pretax operating income by the firm's marginal tax rate. For example, Deseret's taxes for Year 1 are 0.40($102,500) = $41,000. Note that the taxes shown for Year 2 are a negative $66,950. In this year, the project is expected to have negative income of $167,375; hence, Deseret's taxable income (assuming its existing assets are profitable and hence generating taxable income to the firm) will be reduced by this amount if the project is undertaken. This reduction in taxable income would lower the firm's tax bill by T(Taxable income reduction) = 0.40($167,375) = $66,950. If Deseret did not have taxable income to offset in Year 2 and had no taxable income to offset in the three previous years, the loss would have to be carried forward; hence, the tax benefit would not be immediately realized. In this situation, the tax shield value of the loss would be reduced because it would be pushed into the future.

Line 14

The tax depreciation is added back in Line 15. Note that, as Deseret is a taxable firm, it was necessary for its managers to include depreciation in the analysis because the firm's taxes are reduced by the amount of depreciation in each year. However, depreciation expense is a noncash charge, so it must be added back to determine the project's annual net cash flow.

Line 15

Investor-owned firms will normally incur a tax liability on the sale of an asset at the end of a project's life. According to the IRS, the value of the MRI system at the end of Year 5 is the tax book value, which is the depreciation that remains on the tax books. In the illustration, five-years worth of depreciation would be taken, so only one year of depreciation remains. The MACRS factor for Year 6 is 0.06; so by the end of Year 5, Deseret has expensed 0.94 of the MRI's depreciable basis, and the remaining tax book value is 0.06($2,500,000) = $150,000. Thus, according to the IRS, the value of the MRI system is $150,000. When Deseret sells the system for its estimated salvage value of $500,000, it realizes a "profit" of $500,000 − $150,000 = $350,000, and it must repay the IRS an amount equal to 0.40($350,000) = $140,000. The $140,000 tax bill recognizes that Deseret took too much depreciation on the MRI system, so it represents a "recapture" of the excess tax benefit taken over the system's five-year life. The $140,000 in taxes reduces the cash received from the sale of the asset, so the salvage value net of taxes is $500,000 − $140,000 = $360,000.

As can be seen by comparing Line 16 in Tables 7–1 and 7–2, all else the same, the taxes paid by investor-owned firms tend to reduce a project's net cash inflows and hence reduce the project's profitability.

Replacement Analysis

The MRI project was used to illustrate how the cash flows from an expansion project are analyzed. All firms, including Forest View Memorial Hospital and Deseret Regional Health Systems, also make replacement decisions, in which a new asset is being considered to replace an existing asset that could, if not replaced, continue in operation. The cash flow analysis for a replacement decision is somewhat more complex than for an expansion decision because the cash flows from the existing asset must be considered.

Again, the key to cash flow estimation is to focus on the incremental cash flows. If the new asset is acquired, the existing asset can be sold, so the current market value of the existing asset is a cash inflow in the analysis. When considering the operating flows, the incremental flows are the cash flows expected from the replacement asset less the flows that the existing asset produces. By applying the incremental cash flow concept, the correct cash flows can be estimated for replacement decisions.

BREAK-EVEN MEASURES

Once a project's net cash flows have been estimated, the next step is to analyze the flows. There are two types of information that can be gleaned from a project's net cash flows: breakeven and profitability. Break-even analysis is used to gain some insights into the potential riskiness of a project, and it can also shed some light on a project's profitability, although that is not its primary purpose. Furthermore, break-even analysis is useful in evaluating projects that do not require capital investment, such as expanding the hours of operation of a clinic, since there is no initial investment on which to judge profitability. Although break-even analysis can be applied in many different ways, two types of breakeven are most common: (1) volume (unit sales) breakeven and (2) time breakeven.

Volume (Unit Sales) Breakeven

To illustrate volume breakeven, let's alter the assumptions used thus far in the Forest View Memorial Hospital MRI illustration. Assume that the equipment is already in place, but, for one reason or another, it has not been placed into service. Now, the $2,500,000 expended on the project is a sunk cost and thus irrelevant to the decision as to whether to operate the equipment. Further, let's confine our analysis to a single year of operation, Year 1 in Table 7–1.

Table 7–1 indicates that 30 scans a week would produce a net cash flow in Year 1 of $602,500. But, a logical question to ask would be this: How many scans per week would be necessary to break even in Year 1? That is, how many scans per week are required to generate a positive cash flow in Year 1? With the basic analysis performed using a spreadsheet program, it is very easy to do break-even analysis. Table 7–3 contains the Year 1 net cash flow at different volume levels and, as indicated by the data, the project breaks even in Year 1 if the hospital performs 10 scans per week.

Volume breakeven can also be applied to the entire project rather than focusing on just one year. Here we want to know the answer to this question: What weekly usage, over the life of the project, would allow the hospital to recover all the costs associated with the project, including capital costs? Again, if a spreadsheet is used for the analysis, answers to these types of questions are very easy to develop. As discussed in a later section, total breakeven in the profitability sense occurs for a project when its net present value (NPV) equals zero (or just turns positive). In Forest View's MRI project, this occurs at an average weekly usage of 27.4 scans. Thus, the project in its entirety just breaks even when the hospital averages 27.4 scans per week over the five-year forecasted life of the project. This is clearly useful information to Forest View's decision makers. If they feel strongly that volume will exceed 27.4 scans per week, it is highly likely that the project will be profitable. Conversely, if they believe volume will be less than 27.4 scans, the project will probably be unprofitable.

TABLE 7–3

Forest View Memorial Hospital: MRI Site Year 1 Break-Even Analysis

Number of Scans per Week	Year 1 Net Cash Flow
0	($260,000)
5	(116,250)
6	(87,500)
7	(58,750)
8	(30,000)
9	(1,250)
10	27,500
20	315,000
30	602,500
40	890,000

Time Breakeven (Payback)

The payback, or payback period, measures time breakeven. Payback is defined as the expected number of years required to recover the investment in the project. To illustrate, consider the net cash flows for the MRI project contained in Table 7–1. The best way to determine the project's payback is to construct the project's cumulative cash flows, as shown in Table 7–4. The $2,500,000 investment in the MRI would be recovered sometime during Year 4 because the cumulative cash flow is first positive in that year. (Because $600,619 remains to be recovered at the beginning of Year 4 and the project generates $697,469 during the year, a surplus of $96,850 occurs at the end of the year.) If the project's cash flows are assumed to come in evenly during the year, breakeven would occur $600,619 / $697,469 = 0.86 of the way through Year 4, so the MRI project's payback is 3.86 years.

If cash flows come in at the expected rate until payback, the project will break even in the sense that the initial investment will be recovered. Thus, the shorter the payback, the more quickly the funds invested in the project will become available for other purposes and hence the more liquid the project. Also, cash flows expected in the distant future are generally regarded as being riskier than near-term cash flows. Therefore, payback is often used as a rough measure of a project's riskiness. Note, though, that payback does not consider the opportunity cost of the capital employed in the project; that is, it does not consider capital costs. Another measure, the discounted payback, is similar to the standard payback, except that the cash flows in each year are discounted to Year 0 by the project's cost of

TABLE 7–4

Forest View Memorial Hospital: MRI Site Cumulative Cash Flows

Year	Annual Cash Flows	Cumulative Cash Flows
0	($2,500,000)	($2,500,000)
1	602,500	(1,897,500)
2	632,625	(1,264,875)
3	664,256	(600,619)
4	697,469	96,850
5	1,232,343	1,329,193

capital prior to calculating the payback. Thus, the discounted payback solves the standard payback's problem of not considering the project's cost of capital in the payback calculation.

PROFITABILITY MEASURES

Up to this point, the chapter has focused on cash flow estimation and break-even analysis. Perhaps the most important piece of information stemming from a capital investment financial analysis is the project's expected profitability. In general, the expected profitability of capital investments can be measured either in dollars or in percentage rate of return. In the next sections, we present one dollar measure: net present value; and one rate of return measure: internal rate of return.

Net Present Value (NPV)

Net present value (NPV) is a profitability measure that uses the discounted cash flow (DCF) techniques discussed in Chapter 4, so it is often referred to as a DCF measure. NPV is calculated as follows:

1. Find the present (t = 0) value of each net cash flow, including both inflows and outflows, discounted at the project's cost of capital.
2. Sum the present values. This sum is defined as the project's NPV.
3. If the NPV is positive, the project is profitable. The higher the NPV, the more profitable the project. If the NPV is zero, the project just breaks even. If the NPV is negative, the project is unprofitable.

   With a project cost of capital of 10 percent, the NPV calculation of Forest View's MRI project can be visualized as follows:

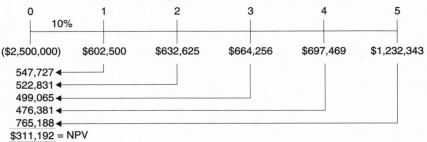

The actual calculation will typically be done using a spreadsheet program's NPV function. Alternatively, NPV can be calculated using a financial calculator after the project's cash flows have been entered into the calculator's cash flow registers. (For more detail on the actual calculation, see Self-Assessment Exercises 7–4 and 7–5, and their solutions.)

Once a project's NPV has been calculated, it is easy for decision makers to interpret its significance. An NPV of zero signifies that the project's cash inflows are just sufficient to (1) return the capital invested in the project and (2) provide investors with their required rates of return on that invested capital (the capital's opportunity cost). If a project has a positive NPV, it is generating excess cash flows. These excess cash flows are available to management to reinvest in the firm and, for investor-owned firms, to pay dividends. If a project has a negative NPV, its cash inflows are insufficient to compensate the firm for the capital invested, so the project is unprofitable and acceptance would cause the financial condition of the firm to deteriorate.

The NPV of the MRI project is $311,192, so on a present value basis, the project is projected to generate a value of more than $300,000 above its costs. Thus, the project is profitable, and its acceptance would have a positive impact on Forest View's financial condition.

Internal Rate of Return (IRR)

Whereas NPV measures a project's dollar profitability, internal rate of return (IRR) measures a project's percentage profitability, or its expected rate of return. Mathematically, the IRR is defined as that discount rate that equates the present value of the project's expected cash inflows to the present value of the project's expected cash outflows. Thus, IRR is simply that discount rate that forces the NPV of the project to equal zero.

IRRs can be calculated in two ways. First, trial and error can be used. Here, the discount rate is changed until the project's NPV equals zero. Obviously, this method is neither quick nor efficient. Second, financial calculators and computer spreadsheet programs have IRR functions that calculate IRRs very rapidly once the cash flows are developed. (Again, for more details on the actual calculation, see Self-Assessment Exercises 7–4 and 7–5.)

For Forest View's MRI project, the IRR is that discount rate that forces the sum of the present values of the cash inflows to equal the $2,500,000 cost of the project:

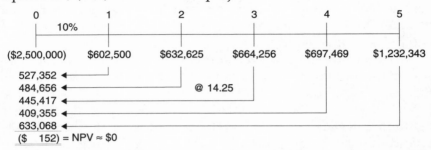

When all of the MRI project's cash flows are discounted at 14.25 percent, the NPV of the project is approximately zero. Thus, the MRI project's IRR is about 14.2 percent. Put another way, the project is expected to generate a 14.2 percent rate of return on its $2,500,000 investment.

If a project's IRR exceeds its cost of capital, a surplus remains after returning the investment and paying for the capital, and this surplus accrues to the firm's stockholders (in Forest View's case, to its noncreditor stakeholders). On the other hand, if the IRR is less than the project's cost of capital, taking on the project imposes a cost on the firm's stockholders (or stakeholders). The MRI project's 14.2 percent IRR exceeds the project's 10 percent cost of capital. Thus, as measured by IRR, the MRI project is profitable and its acceptance would enhance Forest View's financial condition.

Comparison of the NPV and IRR Methods

Consider a project with a zero NPV. In this situation, the project's IRR must equal its cost of capital. The project has zero profitability, and acceptance would neither enhance nor diminish the firm's financial condition. In order to have a positive NPV, the project's IRR must be greater than its cost of capital, and a negative NPV signifies a project with an IRR less than its cost of capital. Thus, projects deemed profitable by the NPV method will also be deemed profitable by the IRR method. In the MRI example, the project would have a positive NPV for all costs of capital less than 14.2 percent. If the cost of capital is greater than 14.2 percent, the project would have a negative NPV. In effect, the NPV and IRR are perfect substitutes for one another in measuring whether a project is profitable or not.

Many financial experts favor NPV over IRR because NPV is a direct measure of the dollar value of a project to the firm. However, nonfinancial executives—particularly members of boards of directors and boards of trustees—often are more comfortable dealing with percentage rates of return because that is what they deal with in their personal investments. Thus, it is often useful to calculate and present both NPV and IRR when conducting a project's financial analysis so that decision makers have both measures available to them for interpretation. Similarly, virtually all capital investment decisions of financial consequence are analyzed by computer; hence, it is easy to calculate and list numerous break-even measures along with NPV and IRR. Since each measure contributes slightly different information about the financial consequences of a project, it would be foolish for decision makers to focus on a single financial measure. Thus, a thorough financial analysis of a proposed project includes numerous financial measures because capital investment decisions are clearly enhanced if all information inherent in the cash flow forecast is considered.

CAPITAL RATIONING

Standard capital investment procedures assume that firms can raise virtually unlimited amounts of capital to meet capital investment needs. Presumably, as long as the firm is investing the funds in profitable (positive NPV) projects, it should be able to raise the capital needed to fund an almost unlimited number of projects. Of course, the firm must raise both debt and equity capital so that its debt usage does not become dangerously high over time.

This picture of a firm's capital financing/capital investment process is probably appropriate for most investor-owned firms. However, not-for-profit firms do not have unlimited access to capital. Their equity (fund) capital is limited to retentions, contributions, and grants, and their debt capital is limited to the amount supported by the equity (fund) capital base. Thus, it is likely that not-for-profit firms will face periods in which the capital needed for investment in new projects will exceed the amount of capital available. This situation is called capital rationing because available capital must be "rationed" among the multitude of available projects.

If capital rationing occurs, and hence the firm has more acceptable projects than capital, then from a purely financial perspective, the firm should accept that set of capital projects that maximizes aggregate NPV and still meets the capital constraint. This approach could be called "getting the most bang from the buck," and it picks those projects that have the most positive impact on the firm's financial condition. In the healthcare industry, firms will often be motivated to accept some negative NPV projects because of their values to the medical staff and community. This is not irrational, but any unprofitable projects undertaken must be offset by the selection of profitable projects, which prevents the unprofitable projects from eroding the firm's financial condition.

SOCIAL VALUE

Except for our discussion of strategic value, the financial analysis techniques discussed thus far have focused exclusively on the cash flow implications of a proposed project. Some healthcare firms, particularly not-for-profit providers, have the goal of producing social services along with commercial, or money-making, services. For these firms, the proper analysis of proposed projects must systematically consider the social value of a project along with its pure financial, or cash flow, value.

When social value is considered, the total net present value (TNPV) of a project can be expressed as follows:

$$TNPV = NPV + PVSV$$

Here, NPV is the net present value of the project's cash flow stream (developed as discussed earlier), and PVSV is the present value of the project's social value. The second term of the above equation clearly differentiates capital investment in not-for-profit firms from that in investor-owned firms. PVSV represents managers' assessment of the social value of the project as opposed to its pure financial value measured by NPV.

A project is acceptable if the sum of its financial and social values is greater than zero. In other words, when both facets of value are considered, the project has positive, or at least nonnegative, worth. Note that all projects will probably not have social value, but if a project does, it is considered formally in this decision model.

To ensure the financial viability of the firm, the sum of the NPVs of all projects initiated in a planning period must equal or exceed zero. If this restriction were not imposed, social value could displace financial value over time; a firm cannot continue to provide social value unless its financial integrity is maintained.

PVSV can be defined as the sum of the present values of the social value in each Year t, quantified in some way, that occurs if the project is accepted. In essence, the suppliers of fund capital to a not-for-profit firm never receive a cash return on their investment. Instead, they receive a return on their investment in the form of social dividends such as charity care, medical research and education, and a myriad of other services that, for one reason or another, are not financially self-supporting. Services provided to patients that generate revenues equal to or greater than the full cost of production do not create social value. Similarly, if governmental entities purchase care directly for beneficiaries of a program or support research, the resulting social value is created by the sponsoring governmental entity, not by the provider of the services.

In estimating a project's PVSV, it is necessary to (1) quantitatively estimate the social value of the services provided by the project in each year and (2) determine the discount rate to apply to those services. When a project produces services to individuals who are willing and able to pay for those services, the value of those services is captured by the amount they actually pay. Thus, the value of the services provided to those who cannot pay, or to those who cannot pay the full amount, can be approximated by the average net price paid by those individuals who are able to pay. This approach to valuing social services has intuitive appeal, but there are five points that merit further discussion.

1. Price is a fair measure of value only if the payer has the capacity to judge the true value of the service provided. Many observers of the healthcare industry would argue that information asymmetries between the provider and the purchaser reduce the ability of the purchaser to judge true value.

2. Because most payments for healthcare services are made by third-party payers, price distortions may occur. For example, insurers may be willing to pay more for services than an individual would pay in the absence of insurance; or the presence of strong purchasing power, say, by Medicare, might result in a net price that is less than individuals actually would be willing to pay.

3. The amount that an individual is willing to pay may be more or less than the amount that a contributor or other fund supplier would be willing to pay for the same service.

4. There is a great deal of controversy over the true value of treatment in many healthcare situations. If patients are entitled to any treatment that is available, regardless of cost, and if patients are not individually required to pay for the care (even though society, as a whole, must pay), patients may demand a level of care that is of questionable value. For example, should $100,000 be spent to keep a comatose 87-year-old person alive for an extra five days? If the true social value of such an effort is zero, it makes little sense to assign a $100,000 value to the care just because that is its "monetary value."

5. Finally, the issue of interpersonal values also arises. Is the value of a heart transplant the same to a 75-year-old in poor health as to a 16-year-old in otherwise good health?

In spite of these potential problems, it still seems reasonable to assign a social value to many (but not all) healthcare services on the basis of the price that others are willing to pay for those services.

The second element required to estimate the PVSV of a project is the discount rate to apply to the annual social-value stream. Like the cost of fund capital to not-for-profit firms, there has been considerable controversy over the proper discount rate to apply to future social values. However, it is clear that contributors of fund capital can capture social value in two ways. First, as is commonly done, contributions can be made directly to not-for-profit organizations. Second, contributors could always invest the funds in a portfolio of securities and then use the proceeds to purchase the healthcare services directly. Since the second alternative exists, providers should require a return on their social-value stream that approximates the return available on similar-risk securities investments, that is, on the equity investment in for-profit firms offering the same services.

The social value model formalizes the capital investment decision process applicable to not-for-profit healthcare firms. Although few organizations attempt to quantify PVSV, at a minimum not-for-profit firms should subjectively consider the social value inherent in projects under consideration.

Janet Washington was not about to give up on her idea of an in-house laboratory for Family Healthcare. In fact, when the practice director said, "You will have to convince me," he might as well have been waving a red flag in front of a bull. Fortunately, Janet's husband was a financial analyst at Alabama Power Company, so he was very familiar with how to analyze potential capital investments. With his knowledge of financial analysis, and her knowledge of the potential costs and revenues associat-

ed with an in-house clinical laboratory, they were able to develop a sound financial analysis of the project.

They concluded that a laboratory, which would handle 80 percent of the practice's tests, could be installed and profitably operated in an unused area of the office. In fact, the laboratory had an NPV of $45,000 and an IRR of 13.5 percent compared to the group's cost of capital of 11 percent. Furthermore, even under pessimistic assumptions, it looked as though the laboratory would be a shoo-in to break even.

When the analysis was presented to the clinic director and other physicians in the group, it was apparent to them that installing an in-house lab was the right thing to do. Janet ultimately prevailed, and both her patients and her colleagues benefitted.

SELF-ASSESSMENT EXERCISES

7–1   a. What is capital investment? Why are capital invest-
          ment decisions so important to businesses?
        b. Should financial analysis play the dominant role in
           capital investment decisions? Explain.
        c. What are the five steps of capital investment analysis?
        d. Briefly define the following cash flow estimation
           concepts:
           (1) Cash flow versus accounting income.
           (2) Incremental cash flow.
           (3) Project life.
           (4) Sunk cost.
           (5) Opportunity cost.
           (6) Current account effects.
           (7) Cash flow estimation bias.
           (8) Strategic value.
           (9) Inflation effects.
           (10) Salvage value.

7–2   Describe the following project break-even and prof-
        itability measures. Be sure to include each measure's
        economic interpretation.
        a. Volume (unit sales) breakeven.
        b. Time breakeven (payback).

c. Net present value (NPV).

d. Internal rate of return (IRR).

7–3 Describe how not-for-profit firms could incorporate social value into their capital-budgeting process.

7–4 Assume that you are the chief financial officer at Regency Clinics. The CEO has asked you to analyze two proposed capital investments, Project X and Project Y. Each project requires a net investment outlay of $10,000, and the cost of capital for each project is 12 percent. The expected net cash flows of the projects are as follows:

	Expected Net Cash Flow	
Year	Project X	Project Y
0	($10,000)	($10,000)
1	6,500	3,000
2	3,000	3,000
3	3,000	3,000
4	1,000	3,000

a. Calculate each project's payback period, net present value (NPV), and internal rate of return (IRR).

b. Which project (or projects) is acceptable financially? Explain.

7–5 Diagnostic Services, Inc., a for-profit firm that owns and operates outpatient diagnostic centers, is evaluating the purchase of some new diagnostic equipment. The equipment, which costs $600,000, has an expected life of five years and an estimated pretax salvage value of $200,000 at the end of the project's life. The equipment is expected to be used 15 times a day for 250 days a year for each year of the project's life. On average, each procedure is expected to generate $80 in collections, net of bad debt losses and contractual allowances, in its first year of use. Thus, net revenues for Year 1 are estimated at 15(250)($80) = $300,000.

Labor and maintenance costs are expected to be $100,000 during the first year of operation; while utilities will cost another $10,000, and cash overhead will increase by $5,000 in Year 1. The cost for expendable supplies is expected to average five dollars per procedure during the first year. All costs, except depreciation and net collections, are expected to increase at a 5 percent inflation rate after the first year.

The equipment falls into the five-year class for tax depreciation and hence is subject to the following depreciation allowances:

Year	Allowance
1	0.20
2	0.32
3	0.19
4	0.12
5	0.11
6	0.06
	1.00

The hospital's tax rate is 40 percent, and its cost of capital for this project is 10 percent.

a. Estimate the project's net cash flows over its five-year estimated life. (Hint: Use the following format as a guide.)

	Year					
	0	1	2	3	4	5
Equipment cost						
Net revenues						
Less: labor/maint. costs						
Utilities costs						
Supplies						
Incremental overhead						
Depreciation						
Income before taxes						
Taxes						
Project net income						
Plus: depreciation						
Plus: equip salvage value						
Net cash flow						

b. What are the project's NPV and IRR?

c. What are financial implications of the project for the firm?

SELECTED REFERENCES

Allen, Robert J. "Proper Planning Reduces Risk in New Technology Acquisitions." *Healthcare Financial Management,* December 1989, pp. 48–56.

Bergman, Judson T. and Brett J. McIntyre. "Valuation Analysis." *Topics in Health Care Financing,* Summer 1989, pp. 32–40.

Campbell, Claudia. "Hospital Plant and Equipment Replacement Decisions: A Survey of Hospital Financial Managers." *Hospital and Health Services Administration,* Winter 1994, 538-56.

Carroll, John J. and Gerald D. Newbold. "Inflation, Risk, Replacement, Closure: Concerns in Capital investment." *Healthcare Financial Management,* December 1986, pp. 64–68.

———. "NPV versus IRR: With Capital investment, Which do You Choose?" *Healthcare Financial Management,* November 1986, pp. 62–68.

Chow, Chee W. and Alan H. McNamee. "Watch for Pitfalls of Discounted Cash Flow Techniques." *Healthcare Financial Management,* April 1991, pp. 34–43.

Chow, Chee W., Kamal M. Haddad, and Adrien Wong-Boren. "Improving Subjective Decision Making in Healthcare Administration." *Hospital and Health Services Administration,* Summer 1991, pp. 191–210.

Cleverley, William O. and Joseph G. Felkner. "The Association of Capital investment Techniques with Hospital Financial Performance." *Health Care Management Review,* Summer 1984, pp. 45–55.

Gapenski, Louis C. "A Better Approach to Internal Rate of Return." *Healthcare Financial Management,* April 1989, pp. 93–99.

———. "Analysis Provides Test for Profitability of New Services." *Healthcare Financial Management,* November 1989, pp. 48–58.

———. "Capital Investment Analysis: Three Methods." *Healthcare Financial Management,* August 1993, pp. 60–66.

Gordon, David C. and Douglas F. Londal. "Guidelines to Capital Investment." *Topics in Health Care Financing,* Summer 1989, pp. 9–17.

Horowitz, Judith L. "Contribution Margin Analysis: A Case Study." *Healthcare Financial Management,* June 1993, pp. 129–33.

Kamath, Ravindra R. and Julie Elmer. "Capital Investment Decisions in Hospitals: Survey Results." *Health Care Management Review,* Spring 1989, pp. 45–56.

Mellen, Chris M. "Valuing a Long-Term Care Facility." *Healthcare Financial Management,* October 1992, pp. 20–25.

Meyer, Alan D. "Hospital Capital investment: Fusion of Rationality, Politics and Ceremony." *Healthcare Management Review,* Spring 1985, pp. 17–27.

Ryan, J. Bruce, Mathews E. Ward, and Deborah S. Kolb. "Capital Management Balances Charitable, Financial Goals." *Healthcare Financial Management,* March 1990, pp. 32–40.

Schramm, Carl J. and George D. Pillari. "Investing in the Wrong Future for Hospitals." *Healthcare Management Review,* Fall 1987, pp. 31–37.

Straley, Peter F. and Carol R. Swaim. "Financial Analysis of Medical Office Buildings." *Topics in Health Care Financing,* Spring 1993, pp. 76–85.

Topics in Health Care Financing, Fall 1992, entitled "Capital Management," J. Bruce Ryan and Matthews E. Ward, editors.

Watts, Dave, Donna L. Finney, and Brian Louie. "Integrating Technology Assessment into the Capital Budgeting Process." *Healthcare Financial Management*, February 1993, pp. 21–29.

Wedig, Gerald J., Mahmud Hassan, and Frank A. Sloan. "Hospital Investment Decisions and the Cost of Capital." *Journal of Business*, 1989, pp. 517–37.

8

CHAPTER

Capital Investment Decisions: Risk Considerations

*T*oday was a sad day for George Fernandez, chief executive officer of Palm Bay Community Hospital, for today he reluctantly approved the plan to close the hospital's only freestanding ambulatory care clinic, which the hospital called the Palm Bay Urgent Care Center. George really had no choice, for the urgent care center had become a financial drag on the hospital.

George remembers as though it were yesterday the meeting of the board of trustees three years ago when the urgent care center was approved. The primary proponent for the ambulatory care center was the chief of emergency medicine, a well-respected member of the medical staff and a pillar of the community. Additionally, the urgent care center received a great deal of support from the hospital's CFO, who was convinced that it would be a big moneymaker because it was located across a main thoroughfare from Southgate Mall, the area's largest shopping center. George even remembers the overhead charts that showed the expected usage of the clinic along with expected reimbursements; and when projected costs were subtracted out of projected revenues, the urgent care center appeared to be a financial winner.

With such a positive outlook, why is the urgent care center being closed? The answer is simple: Revenues did not live up to expectations, while costs were higher than projected. In hindsight, George now realizes that everyone at that fateful meeting accepted the projections as cast in stone and assumed that, because the numbers on the overhead looked very polished and precise, the urgent care center was a sure winner. What the decision makers did not properly account for was the undisputable fact that we live in a world of uncertainty.

It is now clear to George that the initial analysis should have recognized that projections are uncertain and that some type of risk analysis should have been performed. While you are reading this chapter, think about how the risk of the urgent care center could have been assessed. In the meantime, George requested Palm Bay's CFO to prepare a point paper on risk assessment. The main points are summarized at the end of the chapter. See if you and Palm Bay's CFO agree.

INTRODUCTION

The last chapter discussed the basics of capital investment decision making, including cash flow estimation and profitability measures. Now, our discussion turns to capital investment risk analysis, which includes three elements: (1) defining the type of risk relevant to the project, (2) measuring the project's risk, and (3) incorporating the risk assessment into the decision process. Although risk analysis is a key element in all financial decisions, the importance of capital investment decisions to a healthcare organization's success or failure makes risk analysis vital.

We know that the higher the risk associated with an investment, the higher its required rate of return. This principle is just as valid for healthcare organizations making capital investment decisions as it is for individuals making personal investment decisions. Thus, the ultimate goal in project risk analysis is to ensure that the cost of capital used in a project's profitability analysis properly reflects the riskiness of that project. Chapter 6 discussed how to estimate a firm's cost of capital. This value reflects the cost of capital to the organization based on its aggregate risk and debt capacity, that is, based on the riskiness and debt capacity of the firm's "average project." In project risk analysis, decision makers assess a project's risk relative to the firm's average project—does the project have average risk, below-average risk, or above-average risk? Then, the firm's overall cost of capital is modified to reflect the project's differential risk. Higher-than-average risk projects are assigned a project cost of capital that is higher than the firm's cost of capital, average risk projects are evaluated at the overall cost of capital, and lower-than-average risk projects are assigned a discount rate that is less than the firm's cost of capital.

At the same time that risk adjustments are being made, the project's debt capacity—its ability to be financed with debt—is also evaluated. If the project's debt capacity is significantly different from the firm's average project, additional cost of capital adjustments must be made.

TYPES OF PROJECT RISK

As discussed in Chapter 2, three separate and distinct types of project risk can be defined: (1) stand-alone risk, which views the risk of a project as if it were held in isolation and hence which ignores portfolio effects both within the firm and among equity investors; (2) corporate risk, which views the risk of a project within the context of the firm's portfolio of projects; and (3) market risk, which views a project's risk from the perspective of a shareholder who holds a well-diversified portfolio of stocks. The type of risk that is most relevant to a particular capital-budgeting decision depends on the number of projects that the firm holds and the firm's ownership structure. The following sections describe each of the three types of project risk in detail.

Stand-Alone Risk

Conceptually, stand-alone risk is only relevant in one situation: when a not-for-profit firm (which has no shareholders) is evaluating its first project. In this situation, the project will be operated in isolation, and no portfolio diversification is present: The firm does not have a collection (portfolio) of different projects nor does the firm have stockholders who hold portfolios of stocks of different companies. Although stand-alone risk is generally not relevant in real-world decision making, the other types of risk, which are more relevant, are very difficult, if not impossible, to measure. Thus, in practice, most project risk analyses measure stand-alone risk, and then subjective adjustments are applied to convert the project's assessed stand-alone risk to either corporate risk or market risk.

Stand-alone risk is present whenever there is some chance of a return on the project that is less than the expected return. In effect, a project is risky whenever its cash flows are not known with certainty. Furthermore, the greater the probability of a return far below the expected return, the greater the stand-alone risk. In this context, risk is often measured by the standard deviation of the project's profitability, typically net present value (NPV) or internal rate of return (IRR). Since standard deviation measures the dispersion of a distribution about its expected value, the larger the standard deviation, the greater the dispersion and hence the greater the probability of a project's profitability (NPV or IRR) being far below that expected.

Corporate Risk

Most firms actually offer a myriad of different products or services and thus can be thought of as having a large number (hundreds or even thousands) of individual projects. For example, most HMOs offer healthcare services to a large number of diverse groups in numerous service areas, and each group could be considered a separate project. In this situation, the stand-alone risk of a project under consideration is not relevant because the project will not be held in isolation. Here, the relevant risk of a new project is its contribution to the firm's overall risk, or the impact of the project on the variability of the overall profitability of the firm. This type of risk, which is relevant when the project is part of a not-for-profit firm's portfolio of projects, is called corporate risk.

Conceptually, a project's corporate risk is measured by its corporate beta coefficient, which reflects the volatility of the project's profitability relative to that of the firm as a whole, which has a corporate beta of 1.0. A project with a high corporate beta, say, 1.5, has returns that are more volatile than the firm's average project and hence has high corporate risk. Similarly, a project with a low corporate beta, say, 0.5, has returns that are less volatile than the aggregate firm and hence has low corporate risk. Note that a project's corporate risk depends on the context (the firm's other projects), so a project may have high corporate risk to one firm, but low corporate risk to another, particularly when the two firms operate in widely different business lines.

Market Risk

Market risk is generally viewed as the relevant risk for projects under consideration by investor-owned firms. The goal of shareholder wealth maximization implies that a project's returns, as well as its risk, should be defined and measured from the shareholders' perspective. The riskiness of an individual project, as seen by a well-diversified shareholder, is not the riskiness of the project as if it were owned and operated in isolation (its stand-alone risk), nor is it the contribution of the project to the riskiness of the firm (its corporate risk). Most shareholders hold a large diversified portfolio of stocks of many firms, which can be thought of as a very large diversified portfolio of individual projects. Thus, the risk of any single project as seen by a firm's stockholders is its contribution to the riskiness of a well-diversified portfolio, which is measured by the project's market beta.

A project's market beta measures the volatility of the project's returns relative to the returns on a well-diversified portfolio of stocks. Note that a project's absolute market risk, as measured by its market beta, is the same to all firms (assuming that the project's cash flows firm independent), but the market risk of a project relative to the firm's other projects depends on the market risk of the firm. To managers of investor-owned firms, a project's market risk relative to the market risk of the firm's other projects is measured by comparing the project's market beta to the firm's market beta. A project with a market beta higher than the firm's market beta has higher-than-average market risk, where average is measured by the market risk of the firm's stock.

Relationships among the Three Project Risk Types

Once one understands the three different types of project risk and the situations in which each is relevant, it is tempting to say that (1) stand-alone risk is almost never important, (2) not-for-profit firms should focus on a project's corporate risk, and (3) investor-owned firms should concentrate on a project's market risk. Unfortunately, things aren't quite that simple.

It is almost impossible in practice to quantify a project's corporate or market risk because it is extremely difficult (some practitioners would say impossible) to estimate the corporate and market betas for a project. If these betas cannot be estimated, it is impossible to precisely quantify the project's corporate or market risk.

Fortunately, as will be demonstrated in the next section, it is possible to get a feel for the relative stand-alone risk of a project. Thus, managers can make statements such as Project A has above-average risk, Project B has below-average risk, or Project C has average risk, all in the stand-alone sense. Once a project's stand-alone risk has been assessed, the primary factor in converting stand-alone risk to either corporate or market risk is the correlation, or movement relationship, between the project's returns and returns on the firm's other assets. If a project's profitability is highly correlated with the firm's profitability, that is, if the project will do well when the firm does well, and vice versa, then high stand-alone risk translates into high corporate risk. Similarly, if the firm's returns are highly correlated with the stock market's returns, high corporate risk translates into high market risk. The same analogies hold when the project is judged to have average or low stand-alone risk.

Most projects under consideration will be in a firm's primary line of business and hence will be in the same line of business as the firm's average project. Since all projects in the same line of business are generally impacted by the same economic factors, such projects' returns are usually highly correlated. When this situation exists, a project's stand-alone risk is a good proxy for its corporate risk. Furthermore, most projects' returns are also positively correlated with the returns on other assets in the economy: Most assets have high returns when the economy is strong and low returns when the economy is weak. When this situation holds, a project's stand-alone risk is a good proxy for its market risk.

Thus, for most projects, the stand-alone risk assessment also gives good insights into a project's corporate and market risk. The only exception is when the project's returns are expected to be independent of or negatively correlated to the firm's average project or to the market. In these situations, considerable judgment is required because a project's stand-alone risk will overstate the project's corporate or market risk.

A second problem arises with for-profit healthcare firms. Finance theory specifies that investor-owned firms should focus on market risk when making capital investment decisions. However, most healthcare firms, even proprietary ones, have corporate goals that focus on the provision of quality healthcare services along with the goal of shareholder wealth maximization. Furthermore, a proprietary healthcare firm's stability and financial condition, which primarily depends on corporate risk, is important to all the firm's other stakeholders—managers, physicians, patients, community, and so on. Some financial theorists even argue that stockholders, including those that are well diversified, consider factors other than market risk when setting required returns. Considering all this, it may be reasonable for managers of investor-owned healthcare firms to be just as concerned about corporate risk as are managers of not-for-profit firms. Fortunately, in most real-world situations, a project that has high (or low) corporate risk will also have high (or low) market risk.

PROJECT RISK ANALYSIS

To illustrate project risk analysis, consider Forest View Memorial Hospital's evaluation of a new magnetic resonance imaging (MRI) system that was first presented in Chapter 7. Table 8–1 contains the project's cash flow analysis.

The starting point for analyzing a project's stand-alone risk involves estimating the uncertainty inherent in the project's cash flows. Most of the individual cash flows in Table 8–1 are subject to uncertainty. For example, weekly volume was projected at 30 scans per week to obtain the gross revenues listed on Line 3. However, volume would almost certainly be higher or lower than the 30-scan forecast, so realized revenues will almost certainly be different from their Line 3 values. In effect, the volume estimate, and hence revenues, is really an expected value taken from some probability distribution, as are many of the other values listed in Table 8–1. The input variable distributions could be relatively "tight," reflecting small standard deviations and low risk, or they could be relatively "flat," denoting a great deal of uncertainty in the variable in question and hence a high degree of risk.

The nature of the component cash flow distributions, and their correlations with one another, determine the nature of the

TABLE 8-1

Forest View Memorial Hospital: MRI Project Cash Flow Analysis

	0	Cash Revenues and Costs 1	2	3	4	5
1. System cost	($2,000,000)					
2. Installation expense	(500,000)					
3. Gross revenues		$1,500,000	$1,575,000	$1,653,750	$1,736,438	$1,823,259
4. Less: allowances		600,000	630,000	661,500	694,575	729,304
5. Net revenues		$ 900,000	$ 945,000	$ 992,250	$1,041,863	$1,093,956
6. Less: labor costs		90,000	94,500	99,225	104,186	109,396
7. Maintenance costs		150,000	157,500	165,375	173,644	182,326
8. Supplies		37,500	39,375	41,344	43,411	45,581
9. Incremental overhead		20,000	21,000	22,050	23,153	24,310
10. Depreciation		400,000	400,000	400,000	400,000	400,000
11. Operating income		$ 202,500	$ 232,625	$ 264,256	$ 297,469	$ 332,343
12. Taxes		0	0	0	0	0
13. Net operating income		$ 202,500	$ 232,625	$ 264,256	$ 297,469	$ 332,343
14. Plus: depreciation		400,000	400,000	400,000	400,000	400,000
15. Plus: net salvage value						500,000
16. Net cash flow	($2,500,000)	$ 602,500	$ 632,625	$ 664,256	$ 697,469	$1,232,343

Net present value (NPV): $ 311,192
Internal rate of return (IRR): 14.25%

project's profitability distribution and thus the project's stand-alone risk. The following sections discuss three alternative techniques for assessing a project's stand-alone risk: (1) sensitivity analysis, (2) scenario analysis, and (3) Monte Carlo simulation.

Sensitivity Analysis

Intuitively, we know that many of the variables that determine a project's cash flows are subject to some type of probability distribution rather than known with certainty. We also know that if a key input variable such as volume changes, so will the project's cash flows and hence projected profitability. Sensitivity analysis is a technique that indicates exactly how much a project's profitability (NPV or IRR) will change in response to a given change in a single input variable, other things held constant.

Sensitivity analysis begins with a base case cash flow analysis such as that contained in Table 8–1, which is developed using expected (point) values for all uncertain variables. For example, assume Forest View's managers believe that the project's volume could be as low as 20 scans per week or as high as 40 scans per week and that the most likely volume is 30 scans per week. Furthermore, there is a 25 percent chance of the extreme values occurring and a 50 percent chance of the most likely value. With these estimates, the expected value for volume is 0.25(20) + 0.50(30) + 0.25(40) = 30 scans per week, which is used to calculate gross revenues in the base case analysis.

To illustrate sensitivity analysis, assume that all of the MRI project's input variables are known with certainty except for weekly volume, salvage value, and cost of capital. The expected, or base case, values for these variables result in a base case NPV of $311,192. Sensitivity analysis is designed to provide decision makers the answers to such questions as: What if volume is less than the expected level? What if salvage value is more than expected? What if the cost of capital is higher than estimated?

In a sensitivity analysis, each uncertain variable is usually changed by fixed percentage amounts above and below its expected value, holding all other uncertain variables constant at their expected values. The resulting NPVs (or IRRs) are recorded and plotted. Table 8–2 presents the sensitivity analysis for the MRI project, con-

TABLE 8–2

MRI Project Sensitivity Analysis

	Net Present Value (NPV)		
Change from Base Value	Volume	Salvage Value	Cost of Capital
–30%	($ 762,774)	$218,054	$568,613
–20	(404,785)	249,100	478,925
–10	(46,797)	280,146	393,191
0	311,192	311,192	311,192
+10	669,180	342,238	232,724
+20	1,027,169	373,284	157,594
+30	1,385,157	404,330	85,624

sidering three uncertain variables: volume, salvage value, and cost of capital. Figure 8–1 plots the results on a single graph.

The slopes of the lines in Figure 8–1 show how sensitive the MRI project's NPV is to changes in each of the three designated uncertain input variables: The steeper the slope, the more sensitive NPV is to a change in the variable's value. We see that the MRI project's NPV is very sensitive to changes in volume, fairly sensitive to changes in the cost of capital, and relatively insensitive to changes in salvage value. Note also that the cost of capital sensitivity plot has a negative slope because increases in the cost of capital have a negative impact on NPV. If we were comparing two projects, the one with the steeper sensitivity lines would be regarded as riskier because a relatively small error in estimating a variable such as volume would produce a large error in the project's projected NPV. That is, if actual volume turns out to be less than projected in the analysis, the project's realized profitability would be much less than forecasted.

Although sensitivity analysis is widely used in project risk analysis, it does have severe limitations. Suppose that Forest View Memorial Hospital had a contract with a Blue Cross HMO that guaranteed a minimum MRI usage at a fixed reimbursement rate. In that situation, the project might not be very risky at all, in spite of the fact that the sensitivity analysis showed NPV to be highly

FIGURE 8–1

MRI Project Sensitivity Analysis

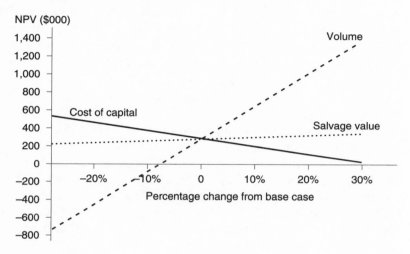

sensitive to changes in volume. In general, a project's stand-alone risk depends on both the sensitivity of its profitability to changes in key input variables and the ranges of likely values of these variables. Because sensitivity analysis considers only the first factor, it can give misleading results. Furthermore, sensitivity analysis does not consider any interactions among the uncertain input variables—it considers each variable independent of the others.

In spite of the shortcomings of sensitivity analysis as a risk measure, it does provide decision makers with valuable information. First, it provides profitability break-even information for the uncertain variables. For example, Table 8–1 tells us quickly that a 30 percent decrease in volume (21 scans per week) makes the project unprofitable, while the project remains profitable under 30 percent negative changes in salvage value and cost of capital. Even a 10 percent reduction in volume below the expected value results in an unprofitable project. Second, sensitivity analysis tells decision makers which input variables are most critical to the project's profitability. In the MRI example, volume is clearly the key input variable (of the ones that were examined), so Forest View's managers should ensure that the volume estimate is the best possible.

Scenario Analysis

Scenario analysis is a stand-alone risk analysis technique that considers (1) the sensitivity of NPV to changes in key input variables, (2) the likely range of variable values, and (3) the interactions among variables. To conduct a scenario analysis, the managers pick a "bad" set of circumstances (low volume, low salvage value, and so on); an average, or "most likely" set; and a "good" set. The resulting input values are then used to create a probability distribution of NPV (or IRR).

To illustrate scenario analysis, assume that Forest View's managers regard a drop in weekly volume below 20 scans as very unlikely, and a volume value above 40 is also improbable. On the other hand, salvage value could be as low as $0, in which case the cost of removal equals the scrap value of the machine, or as high as $1,000,000. The most likely values are 30 scans per week for volume and $500,000 for salvage value. Thus, volume of 20 and a zero salvage value define the lower bound, or worst-case (pessimistic) scenario, while volume of 40 and a salvage value of $1,000,000 define the upper bound, or best-case (optimistic) scenario. Forest View's managers can now use the worst-, most likely-, and best-case values for the input variables to obtain the corresponding NPVs.

A spreadsheet model was used to conduct a scenario analysis, and Table 8–3 summarizes the results. We see that the most likely case results in a positive NPV; the worst case results in a large negative NPV; and the best case results in a large positive NPV. We can

TABLE 8–3

MRI Project Scenario Analysis

Scenario	Probability of Occurrence	Volume	Salvage Value	NPV
Worst	0.25	20	$ 0	($1,192,564)
Most likely	0.50	30	500,000	311,192
Best	0.25	40	1,000,000	1,814,948
Expected value		30	$ 500,000	$ 311,192
Standard deviation				$1,063,316
Coefficient of variation				3.4

now use these results to determine the expected NPV, standard deviation of NPV, and coefficient of variation of NPV. For this, we need an estimate of the probabilities of occurrence of the three scenarios. Suppose Forest View's managers estimate there is a 25 percent chance of the worst case occurring, a 50 percent chance of the most likely case, and a 25 percent chance of the best case. Of course, it is very difficult to estimate scenario probabilities with any confidence.

Table 8–3 contains a discrete distribution of returns, so we can find the MRI project's expected NPV as follows:

$$E(NPV) = 0.25(-\$1,192,564) + 0.50(\$311,192) + 0.25(\$1,814,948)$$
$$= \$311,192$$

Note that the expected NPV in the scenario analysis is the same as the base case NPV, $311,192. If the base case expected values for the uncertain input variables are consistent with the expected values used in the scenario analysis (in this case 30 for volume and $500,000 for salvage value), the results will be consistent.

The standard deviation of NPV is $1,063,316, while the coefficient of variation of NPV is 3.4.

$$CV = \frac{\sigma}{E(NPV)} = \frac{\$1,063,316}{\$311,192} = 3.4$$

The MRI project's standard deviation and coefficient of variation of NPV measure its stand-alone risk. (Remember that the coefficient of variation standardizes risk and hence compensates for the fact that different projects may have widely varying values of expected NPV.) Suppose, when a similar scenario analysis is applied to Forest View's average project (the hospital in the aggregate), it has a coefficient of variation of NPV somewhere in the range 1.0–2.0. Then, on the basis of its stand-alone risk as measured by coefficient of variation of NPV, Forest View's managers would conclude that the MRI project is riskier than the hospital's average project, so it would be classified as a high-risk project.

Scenario analysis is also often used in a less mathematical way. The worst case NPV, about negative $1.2 million in the MRI illustration, represents an estimate of the worst possible financial consequences of the project. If Forest View can absorb such a loss without much impact on its financial condition, the project doesn't represent a significant financial danger to the hospital. Conversely, if such a loss would mean financial disaster for the hospital, its managers might be unwilling to undertake the project, regardless of its profitability under the most likely and best case scenarios.

While scenario analysis provides useful information about a project's stand-alone risk, it is limited in two ways. First, it only considers a few discrete states of the economy, and hence profitability outcomes (NPVs or IRRs), for the project. In reality, there is an almost infinite number of possibilities. Although the illustrative scenario analysis contained only three scenarios, it could be expanded to include more states of the economy, say five or seven. However, there is a practical limit on how many scenarios can be included in a scenario analysis.

Second, scenario analysis—at least as normally applied in practice—implies a very definite relationship among the uncertain variables. That is, the analysis assumed that the worst value for volume (20 scans per week) would occur at the same time as the worst value for salvage value ($0) because the worst-case scenario was defined by combining the worst possible value of each uncertain variable. Although this relationship (all worst values occurring together) may hold in some situations, in others it may not.

For example, if volume is low, maybe the MRI will have less wear and tear and hence be worth more after five years of use. Then, the worst value for volume should be coupled with the best salvage value. Conversely, poor volume may be symptomatic of poor medical acceptance of the MRI and hence lead to limited demand for used equipment and a low salvage value. Regardless of the actual relationships among input variables, scenario analysis generally creates extreme profitability values for the worst and best cases because it combines all worst and all best input values even though these extremes often have little chance of actually occurring simultaneously. The next section describes a method of assessing a project's stand-alone risk that deals with these two problems.

Monte Carlo Simulation

Monte Carlo simulation, so named because it grew out of work on the mathematics of casino gambling, describes uncertainty in terms of continuous probability distributions rather than just a few values; hence, it provides a more realistic view of a project's stand-alone risk than does scenario analysis. Although the use of Monte Carlo simulation in capital investment decisions was first proposed over 30 years ago, it had not been used extensively in practice, primarily because it required a mainframe computer along with relatively powerful financial planning or statistical software. Recently, however, Monte Carlo simulation software has become available for personal computers as an add-in to spreadsheet software. Since more and more financial analysis is being done with spreadsheets, Monte Carlo simulation is now accessible to almost all healthcare organizations.

The first step in a Monte Carlo simulation is to create a spreadsheet model that calculates the project's net cash flows and profitability measures, just as Forest View's managers have done for the hospital's MRI project. For the Monte Carlo simulation, the relatively certain input variables are estimated as single, or point, values in the model, while continuous probability distributions are used to specify the uncertainty inherent in the uncertain variables. Once the model has been created and the distributions for the uncertain variables specified, the simulation software automatically executes the following steps:

1. The Monte Carlo program chooses a single random value for each uncertain input variable on the basis of its specified probability distribution.

2. The value selected for each uncertain variable, along with the point values for the relatively certain variables, are combined in the model to calculate the net cash flow for each year.

3. Using the net cash flow data, the model calculates the project's profitability, say, as measured by NPV. A single completion of Steps 1, 2, and 3 constitutes one iteration, or "run," in the Monte Carlo simulation.

4. The Monte Carlo software repeats the above steps many times, say 5,000, and records the resulting NPVs. Since the values for the uncertain variables will almost always be different in each run, the end result will be a probability distribution of NPV with 5,000 individual "scenarios" that reflect the underlying uncertainty of the project.

Monte Carlo software displays the results of the simulation (the probability distribution of NPV) in both tabular and graphical forms, and automatically calculates summary statistical data such as expected value, standard deviation, and the probability of a positive NPV.

To illustrate Monte Carlo simulation, again consider Forest View Memorial Hospital's MRI project. As in the scenario analysis, the illustration has been simplified by focusing on only two uncertain variables, weekly volume and salvage value. Assume that Forest View's managers believe that weekly volume will not vary by more than ±10 scans from its expected value of 30 scans. Since this is a symmetrical situation, the normal distribution can be used to represent the uncertainty inherent in volume. In a normal distribution, the expected value plus or minus three standard deviations will encompass almost the entire distribution. Thus, a normal distribution with an expected value of 30 scans and a standard deviation of $10/3 = 3.33$ scans is a reasonable description of the uncertainty inherent in weekly volume. This distribution can be visualized as a bell-shaped curve, with 30 scans in the center of the curve and sides extending to 20 scans on the left and 40 scans on the right.

Since the project's salvage value is not likely to fall below zero, a normal distribution is not a good way to express its uncertainty. (The normal distribution is unbounded, but we want to set absolute limits on the salvage value distribution.) Thus, salvage value was specified by a triangular distribution with a lower limit of $0, a most likely value of $500,000, and an upper limit of $1,000,000. This distribution looks like a pyramid, with $500,000 at the center (highest point) and $0 and $1,000,000 at the left and right limits where the pyramid touches the ground. The inputs to the basic MRI spreadsheet model were changed so that all inputs were set at their expected values except volume and salvage value, which were specified by the continuous distributions described above.

A spreadsheet add-in program (@RISK) was used to run the Monte Carlo simulation with 5,000 iterations. The output is summarized in Table 8–4, and the resulting probability distribution of NPV is plotted in Figure 8–2. The mean, or expected, NPV, $311,172, is about the same as the base-case NPV and expected NPV indicated in the scenario analysis, $311,192. In theory, all three results should be the same because the expected values for all input variables are the same in the three analyses. However, there is some randomness in the Monte Carlo simulation, and this leads to an expected NPV that is slightly different from the others. The

TABLE 8-4

Monte Carlo Simulation Results Summary

Expected NPV	$ 311,172
Minimum NPV	($1,729,008)
Maximum NPV	$2,111,034
Probability of a positive NPV	77.2%
Standard deviation	$ 418,680
Coefficient of variation	1.3

more iterations that are run, the more likely the Monte Carlo NPV will be the same as the base case NPV.

Note that the minimum and maximum NPVs are farther from the mean in the Monte Carlo simulation than in the scenario analysis. This occurs because the normal distribution allows values for weekly volumes that are less than 20 or greater than 40, although the chances of picking these values are very low. In spite of larger extremes for NPV, the Monte Carlo standard deviation and coefficient of variation of NPV are significantly lower than in the scenario analysis. This results because the NPV distribution in the simulation contains values within the entire range of possible outcomes; whereas, the NPV distribution in the scenario analysis contains only the most likely value and best and worst case extremes, and the extremes are given relatively high probabilities of occurrence, 25 percent.

In this illustration, volume uncertainty was held constant across the entire life of the project; that is, the value chosen by the Monte Carlo software for volume in Year 1, say 34 scans, was used as the volume input for the remaining four years in that iteration of the simulation analysis. As an alternative, the normal distribution for Year 1 could be respecified in each succeeding year so that volume would be estimated separately for each year of the project. Then, each year would have its own uncertainty, and the Monte Carlo software might choose 34 as the Year 1 weekly volume, 23 as the Year 2 input, 31 for Year 3, and so on. But does this independence of volume uncertainty over time seem reasonable? Probably not—a high usage in the first year presumably means strong acceptance of MR imaging and hence high usage in the remaining years.

FIGURE 8–2

MRI Project Monte Carlo Simulation Results

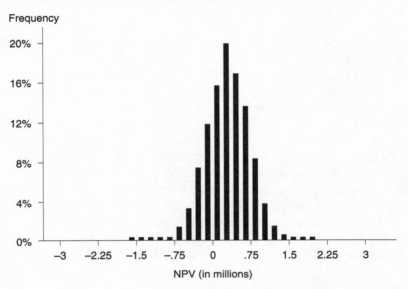

Similarly, low usage in the first year probably portends low usage in future years.

Finally, note that the volume and salvage value variables were treated as independent in the illustration; that is, the value chosen from the salvage value distribution was not related to the value chosen from the volume distribution. Thus, a low volume could be coupled with a high salvage value in the first iteration, a low volume could be coupled with a low salvage value in the next iteration, and a high volume could be coupled with a low salvage value in the third iteration. If Forest View's managers believed that high MRI volume at the hospital indicated a strong national demand for such systems, they might specify a positive correlation between these variables. This would tend to increase the riskiness of the project, since low volume could not be offset by a high salvage value, and low salvage value could not be offset by high volume. Conversely, if the salvage value is more a function of the technological advances that occur over the next five years than local usage, it might be best to specify the variables as being independent, as was done in our illustration. Mechanically, it is easy to (1) specify the distributions for each uncertain variable, (2) incorporate the correlations of the different variable probability distributions in each year, and (3) incorporate the correlations of single variables over time. However, it is much more difficult to realistically estimate what the distributions and their correlations should be.

As in scenario analysis, the simulation results provide valuable information about the stand-alone riskiness of the MRI project. For example, it tells Forest View's managers that the project has a 77.2 percent chance of being profitable, and hence it has a 22.8 percent chance of being unprofitable. Additionally, Monte Carlo simulation can be used to make judgments about the project's stand-alone risk relative to the hospital's other projects. If Forest View's average project has a Monte Carlo simulation coefficient of variation of NPV in the range of 0.4–0.6, the MRI project, with a coefficient of variation of 1.3, would be judged by Monte Carlo simulation to have above-average, or high, stand-alone risk.

INCORPORATING RISK INTO THE DECISION PROCESS

In most cases, it is impossible to assess quantitatively a project's corporate or market risk, and, as with Forest View's MRI project, managers are left with only an assessment of the project's stand-alone risk. However, like the MRI project, most projects being evaluated by a firm are in the same line of business as the firm's other projects. For example, most projects being evaluated by Forest View Memorial Hospital directly involve providing healthcare services to patients, typically inpatient services. Thus, most of the hospital's projects are affected similarly by healthcare reform, demographic trends, the movement towards more managed care patients with corresponding pressures for higher discounts, and so on. Furthermore, most firms' profitability is highly correlated with the national economy, although the relationship for healthcare firms is probably not a strong as for many other industries, especially producers and retailers of consumer durables such as automobiles and appliances.

Because of these generally positive correlations, a project's relative stand-alone, corporate, and market risk are usually the same. This suggests that managers can get a feel for the relative risk of most projects on the basis of sensitivity, scenario, and/or Monte Carlo analyses conducted to assess the project's stand-alone risk. In Forest View's case, its managers concluded that the MRI project had above-average stand-alone risk, and that the returns on the project were highly correlated with the hospital's other projects. Thus, the project was categorized as having high corporate risk, and for a not-for-profit hospital, corporate risk is the most relevant risk.

A firm's overall cost of capital provides the basis for estimating a project's differential risk-adjusted discount rate: Average-risk projects are discounted at the firm's cost of capital, high-risk projects are discounted at a higher cost of capital, and low-risk projects are discounted at a rate below the firm's cost of capital. Unfortunately, there is no good way of specifying exactly how much higher or lower these discount rates should be. Given the present state of the art, risk adjustments are necessarily judgmental, and somewhat arbitrary. Forest View Memorial Hospital's standard procedure is to add 4 percentage points to its 10 percent cost of capital when evaluating high-risk projects, and to subtract 3 percentage points when evaluating low-risk projects. Thus, to estimate the high-risk MRI project's differential risk-adjusted NPV, the project's expected (base-case) cash flows shown in Table 8–1 are discounted at 10% + 4% = 14%. This rate is called the project's cost of capital, as opposed to the firm's cost of capital, since it reflects the risk characteristics of the project rather than the risk of the firm. The resultant NPV is $16,645, so the project remains profitable, but just barely, after adjusting for differential project risk.

Differences in the amount of debt financing applicable to a project should also be taken into account in capital investment analyses. Some projects are able to support more debt financing than others and hence would be financed (at least constructively) with a higher proportion of debt. For example, a hospital holding company might have one subsidiary that invests primarily in medical services real estate, while another subsidiary runs an HMO. The assets held by the real estate subsidiary are well suited as collateral for loans, so this subsidiary can easily obtain large amounts of debt financing at a relatively low cost. Conversely, the HMO subsidiary has very few tangible assets, so it has little to pledge as collateral. The real estate subsidiary is said to have a relatively high "debt capacity," and its optimal capital structure would contain a large percentage of debt financing, perhaps as high as 80 percent, while the HMO's optimal capital structure might contain only 20 percent debt. Furthermore, the HMO subsidiary probably has significantly more risk than the real estate unit before any financing differentials are even considered.

The process of accounting for differences in risk and debt capacity is especially important when a firm has subsidiaries that operate in widely different lines of business. Although the process is not exact, many firms use a two-step procedure to develop project discount rates:

1. Subsidiary costs of capital are established for each of the major subsidiaries on the basis of its estimated riskiness and debt capacity. Risk differentials are handled by using different costs of equity for the subsidiaries (but typically not different costs of debt unless each subsidiary issues its own debt), and differential debt capacities are incorporated into the subsidiary costs of capital by using different weights for debt and equity.

2. Within each subsidiary, all projects are classified into three categories—high risk, average risk, and low risk—and then the subsidiary's cost of capital is adjusted to reflect the riskiness of each project.

This procedure, which is illustrated in Figure 8–3, is far from precise, but it does at least recognize that different subsidiaries have different debt capacities and riskiness and that different projects within each subsidiary can have different riskiness. In Figure 8–3, the firm has three subsidiaries, one with high risk (HR), one with average risk (AR), and one with low risk (LR). The overall corporate cost of capital is 10 percent, and the firm's policy is to add three percentage points for increased risk and subtract two percentage points for decreased risk. The end result is a range of project costs of capital from 16 percent for a high-risk project in the high-risk subsidiary to 6 percent for a low-risk project in the low-risk subsidiary.

It is possible, although infrequent, for projects within the same subsidiary to have different debt capacities as well as different risks, but debt capacity differences are usually very difficult to measure for individual projects, and the adjustment process is even

FIGURE 8-3

Project Costs of Capital for a Firm with Three Subsidiaries

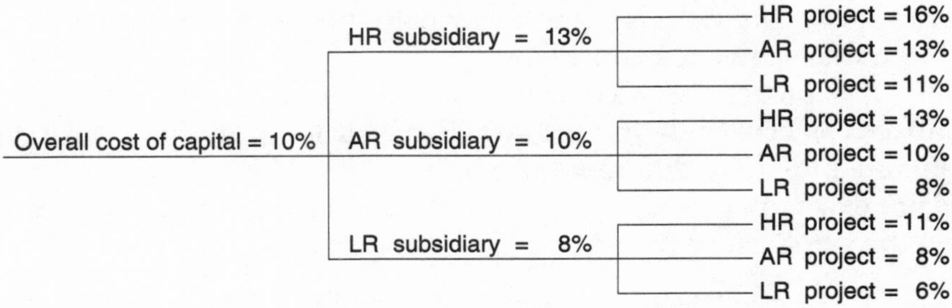

```
                                       HR subsidiary = 13%   ┌───── HR project = 16%
                                                             ├───── AR project = 13%
                                                             └───── LR project = 11%
                                                             ┌───── HR project = 13%
Overall cost of capital = 10%      AR subsidiary =  10%      ├───── AR project = 10%
                                                             └───── LR project =  8%
                                                             ┌───── HR project = 11%
                                       LR subsidiary =   8%  ├───── AR project =  8%
                                                             └───── LR project =  6%
```

Note: HR = High risk
AR = Average risk
LR = Low risk

more difficult. For example, even though Forest View Memorial Hospital may be able to obtain a secured loan for nearly the entire cost of the MRI equipment, the equipment does not have a debt capacity of 100 percent. The willingness of lenders to furnish 100 percent debt capital for the MRI project is based more on the overall profitability of all of Forest View's assets than it is on the MRI project since all of the hospital's operating cash flow, less interest payments on already-outstanding debt, would be available to pay the lender. Think of it this way: Would lenders provide 100 percent financing if Forest View were a start-up hospital with the MRI project as its sole source of income?

The end result of the risk assessment and incorporation process is a project cost of capital that incorporates, to the extent possible, each project's own debt capacity and riskiness. However, managers also must consider other possible risk factors that may not have been included in the quantitative analysis. For example, could the MRI project significantly increase the liability exposure of the hospital? Conversely, does the project have any strategic value or social value that could impact its profitability and riskiness? Such additional factors must be considered, at least subjectively, before a final decision can be made. Typically, if the project involves new products or services and is large relative to the firm's average project, the additional subjective factors will be very important to the final decision—one large mistake can bankrupt a firm, and "bet-the-business" decisions are not made lightly. On the other hand, the decision on a small replacement project would be made mostly on the basis of the numerical analysis.

Ultimately, capital budgeting decisions require an analysis of a mix of objective and subjective factors such as profitability, risk, debt capacity, strategic value, medical staff needs, and social value. The process is not precise, and often there is a temptation to ignore one or more important factors because they are nebulous and difficult to measure. Despite the imprecision and subjectiveness, a project's risk, as well as other attributes, should be assessed and incorporated into the capital budgeting decision process. Anything less would be tantamount to ignoring one of the basic principles of finance: Investments with higher risk require higher expected returns.

RISKY CASH OUTFLOWS

Some mutually exclusive projects are evaluated on the basis of minimizing the present value of future costs rather than on the basis of the projects' NPVs. (Projects are mutually exclusive when only one project out of a set of projects will be undertaken.) This is done because (1) it is often impossible to allocate revenues to competing projects, and (2) it is easier to focus on comparative costs when two projects will produce the same revenue stream. For example, suppose that Crescent City Clinics, which operates eight primary care clinics in New Orleans, must choose one of two ways for disposing of its medical waste materials. There is no question about the need for the project, and the clinic's revenue stream is unaffected by which method is chosen. Thus, from a financial perspective, the best way to analyze the decision is to estimate the present value of each alternative's expected future cost stream. Then, the method with the lower present value of costs would be the preferred alternative.

Table 8–5 contains the projected costs associated with each method. The in-house system would require a large expenditure ($300,000) at Year 0 to upgrade the clinic's current centralized disposal system, but the operating costs are relatively low. Conversely, if the firm contracts for disposal services with an outside contractor, it only would have to pay $15,000 up front to initiate the contract, but the annual contract fee would be $100,000 a year. (For simplicity,

TABLE 8–5

Crescent City Clinics: Waste Disposal Cash Flows

Year	In-House System	Outside Contract
0	($300,000)	($ 15,000)
1	(25,000)	(100,000)
2	(25,000)	(100,000)
3	(25,000)	(100,000)
4	(25,000)	(100,000)
5	(25,000)	(100,000)
PV of Costs at k =		
10%	($394,770)	($394,079)
14%	—	($358,308)
6%	—	($436,236)

inflation effects have been ignored.) Crescent City's cost of capital is 10 percent, which it applies to average-risk projects, and it uses a ±4 percentage point adjustment to account for differential risk.

If both methods were judged to have average risk, Crescent City's 10 percent cost of capital would be applied to each alternative's cash flows to obtain the present value (PV) of costs. Under the assumption of average risk for both methods, the PV of costs for the in-house system is $394,770, and for the contract method the PV of costs is $394,079. So from a financial standpoint, Crescent City's managers are, for all practical purposes, indifferent as to which method should be chosen.

However, Crescent City's managers believe that the contract method is much riskier than the in-house method. The cost of modifying the current system is known almost to the dollar, and operating costs can be predicted fairly well. Furthermore, with the in-house system, operating costs are under the control of Crescent City's managers. Conversely, once the clinic relies on an outside contractor for its waste disposal, it would become very difficult to discontinue the contract because the clinic would lose its in-house capability. The contractor was only willing to guarantee the price for the first two years, so maybe this bid was lowballed to get the contract, with the expectation of large price increases in later years.

Since the two methods have about the same PV of costs when both are considered to have average risk, which method should be chosen if the contract method is judged to have high risk? Clearly, if the costs are about the same, the lower-risk alternative should be chosen.

Now, let's try to incorporate our intuitive differential risk assessment into the quantitative analysis. Conventional wisdom is to increase the project cost of capital for high-risk projects, so we would discount the contract method's cash flows using a project cost of capital of 14 percent, the rate that Crescent City applies to high-risk projects. But, at a 14 percent discount rate, the contract method has a PV of costs of only $358,308, which is about $36,000 lower than that for the in-house method. If we upped the discount rate to 20 percent on the contract method, it would appear to be even more attractive than the in-house method. Thus, the riskier the contract method is judged to be, the better it looks!

Something is obviously wrong in our risk adjustment. If we want to penalize a cash outflow for higher-than-average risk, that outflow must have a higher, not lower, present value. Therefore, a cash outflow that has higher-than-average risk must be evaluated with a lower-than-average cost of capital. Recognizing this, Crescent City's managers actually applied a 10% − 4% = 6% discount rate to the high-risk contract method's cash flows. This produced a PV of costs for the contract method of $436,236, which is about $41,000 more than the PV of costs for the average-risk in-house method. From this example, we conclude that the risk adjustment for cash outflows is the opposite of the adjustment for cash inflows; higher-risk flows must now be discounted at a lower rate, and lower-risk flows must be discounted at a higher rate.

The appropriate risk adjustment for cash outflows is also applicable to other situations. For example, the City of New York offered Empire State Health Systems the opportunity to use a city-owned building in one of the city's blighted areas for a walk-in clinic. The city would pay to refurbish the building and furnish it rent free, and all clinic revenues, including some large taxpayer subsidies, would accrue to Empire State. However, after 10 years, Empire State would have to buy the building from the city at the then current market value. The value estimate that Empire State used in its financial analysis was two million dollars, but the realized cost could be much greater or much less, depending on the economic condition of the neighborhood after 10 years. The rest of the project's cash flows were of average risk, but this single outflow had high risk; so, in the analysis, Empire State's managers used the corporate cost of capital on all other cash flows but lowered the discount rate that it applied to this one cash outflow.

In his memo to George Fernandez, Palm Bay's CFO indicated that three techniques could have been used to assess the financial riskiness of the urgent care center. Essentially, these techniques would recognize that usage could be lower than projected for many reasons and that increased pressure from managed care organizations could lead to less-than-expected per-visit reimbursement. Furthermore, operating costs could prove to be higher than expected. If these factors resulted in realized net cash flows that were less favorable than projected, the urgent care center could end up being a money loser rather than a moneymaker. Of course, the three techniques the CFO mentioned were sensitivity analysis, scenario analysis, and Monte Carlo simulation.

Consideration of the uncertainty, or risk, inherent in the urgent care center may not have affected the initial decision to go ahead with the project, but, at a minimum, it would have waved some red flags for the board to consider. The risks may even have been judged too great for the hospital to bear; hence, George might have been saved today's unpleasantness.

SELF-ASSESSMENT EXERCISES

8–1 a. Why is risk analysis so important to capital investment decision making?

b. Describe the three types of project risk. Under what situations is each of the types most relevant to the capital investment decision?

c. Which type of risk is easiest to measure in practice?

d. Are the three types of project risk usually highly correlated? Explain. Why is the correlation among project risk measures important?

8–2 a. Briefly describe sensitivity analysis. What are its strengths and weaknesses?

b. Briefly describe scenario analysis. What are its strengths and weaknesses?

c. Briefly describe Monte Carlo simulation. What are its strengths and weaknesses?

8–3   a. How is a project's risk incorporated into the capital investment decision process?

b. Suppose you were evaluating two mutually exclusive projects on the basis of cash costs. How would risk adjustments be applied in this situation?

8–4   How do differential debt capacities affect capital investment analyses?

8–5   Consider the project contained in question 7–5.

a. Think about how to perform a sensitivity analysis to see how NPV is affected by changes in the number of procedures per day. What do you think the sensitivity diagram would look like? Examine the answer in Appendix A to see if you are on the right track.

b. Now think about performing a scenario analysis. Suppose the firm's staff concluded that the three most uncertain variables were number of procedures per day, average collection amount, and the equipment's salvage value. Further, assume the following data were developed.

Scenario	Prob.	Number of Procedures	Average Collection	Equipment Salvage Value
Worst	0.25	10	$ 60	$100,000
Most likely	0.50	15	80	200,000
Best	0.25	20	100	300,000

What information would the scenario analysis provide? Examine the answer in Appendix A to see if you are on the right track.

c. Finally, assume that the firm's average project has a coefficient of variation (CV) in the range of 1.0–2.0.

(1) If the project had a CV of 3.1, would it be classified as low risk, average risk, or high risk?

(2) Assume that the firm adjusts for risk by adding or subtracting three percentage points to its 10 percent cost of capital. After adjusting for differential risk, is the project still profitable?

d. What type of risk was measured and accounted for in Parts b and c above? Should this be of concern to the firm's managers?

SELECTED REFERENCES

Allen, Robert J. "Proper Planning Reduces Risk in New Technology Acquisitions." *Healthcare Financial Management*, December 1989, pp. 48–56.

Ang, James S. and Wilbur G. Lewellen. "Risk Adjustment in Capital Investment Project Evaluations." *Financial Management*, Summer 1982, pp. 5–14.

Capettini, Robert, Chee W. Chow, and James E. Williamson. "Breakdown Approach Helps Managers Select Projects." *Healthcare Financial Management*, November 1990, pp. 48–56.

Gapenski, Louis C. "Accuracy of Investment Risk Models Varies." *Healthcare Financial Management*, April 1992, pp. 40–52.

———. "Project Risk Definition and Measurement in a Not-for-Profit Setting." *Health Services Management Research*, November 1992, pp. 216–24.

———. "Using Monte Carlo Simulation to Help Make Better Capital Investment Decisions." *Hospital and Health Services Administration*, Summer 1990, pp. 207–19.

Gup, Benton E. and S. W. Norwood III. "Divisional Cost of Capital: A Practical Approach." *Financial Management*, Spring 1981, pp. 20–24.

Hastie, K. Larry. "One Businessman's View of Capital Budgeting." *Financial Management*, Winter 1974, pp. 36–43.

Hertz, David B. "Risk Analysis in Capital Investments." *Harvard Business Review*, January–February 1964, pp. 96–106.

Lewellen, Wilbur G. and Michael S. Long. "Simulation versus Single-Value Estimates in Capital Expenditure Analysis." *Decision Sciences*, October 1972, pp. 19–33.

Ryan, J. Bruce and Joseph L. Gocke. "Incorporating Risk into the Investment Decision." *Topics in Health Care Financing*, Fall 1988, pp. 49-65.

Topics in Health Care Financing, Fall 1992, entitled "Capital Management," J. Bruce Ryan and Matthews E. Ward, editors.

Weaver, Samuel C., Peter J. Clemmens III, Jack A. Gunn, and Bruce D. Danneburg. "Divisional Hurdle Rates and the Cost of Capital." *Financial Management*, Spring 1989, pp. 18–25.

9

CHAPTER

Capital Investment Decisions: Mergers and Acquisitions

*U*ntil a few years ago, the demand for inpatient services in River City, Iowa, could easily support the three local hospitals. In the "good old days," there were plenty of patients to fill the 5.6 beds per 1,000 population capacity, and a more-or-less friendly rivalry prevailed. However, with managed care penetration increasing, the situation was changing rapidly. In areas where managed care dominated, moderately aggressive case management reduced the need for hospital beds to only two per 1,000 population. Thus, it was readily apparent that the local market would not be able to support all three hospitals in the future and that some type of market rationalization would have to take place.

To add to the concern, one of the hospitals in River City was owned by a very aggressive for-profit management company, TransHealth. TransHealth had been actively pursuing merger partners in other markets, including not-for-profit hospitals, with the goal of becoming the dominant inpatient provider in those markets. When any acquisitions took place, TransHealth eliminated duplicate services and replaced excess beds with other more needed services, thereby creating low-cost powerhouses.

Although there was no indication that TransHealth would follow the same strategy in River City, the managers at the other two hospitals were nervous. If TransHealth bought one of the not-for-profit hospitals, life would become very difficult for the managers of the other. The best candidate for acquisition by TransHealth was the financially ailing 300-bed General Hospital. The likely survivor, which would then have to go head-to-head with the TransHealth System, was the 500-bed University Hospital.

For Lucy Radcliffe, CEO of University Hospital, the solution was obvious: University Hospital needed to make a preemptive strategic move—it needed to acquire General Hospital. To implement this strategy, many issues had to be resolved, but two were considered most important by University's board of trustees. First, what legal hurdles had to be over-come? General Hospital is not-for-profit, but it is owned by Midwest Health Plans, a not-for-profit managed care company. Second, how could University establish a value for the potential acquisition? After you read this chapter, you will have a better appreciation of the issues involved in mergers and acquisitions. At the end of the chapter, you will see how University Hospital handled the situation.

INTRODUCTION

Most of the growth in healthcare businesses occurs through internal expansion, which takes place when a firm's existing operations grow through normal capital investment activities. However, the most dramatic examples of growth result from mergers and acquisitions, the focus of this chapter. For legal and accounting purposes, there are distinctions between a merger and an acquisition, but those distinctions do not affect the fundamental business and financial considerations involved. Thus, we will not distinguish between the two, but rather we will refer to all combinations in which a single business unit is formed from two or more existing units as a merger.

MERGERS IN THE HEALTHCARE INDUSTRY

Prior to the mid-1980s, mergers in the healthcare industry were not as frequent nor as large as mergers in other industries. First, the healthcare industry, at least in its current form, is relatively new, not having really developed until after World War II. Second, the motivations that fueled mergers in other industries—primarily low stockholder valuations—only partially applied to healthcare, so the industry was not one of the major merger participants. However, in recent years, the healthcare industry has become a hotbed of merger activity, as evidenced by the following recent deals:

1. Aetna bought U.S. Healthcare for $8.9 billion in cash and stock. The deal linked the insurance giant with an aggressive HMO operator, creating the nation's largest managed care company.

2. Columbia/HCA Healthcare acquired Healthtrust for $5.6 billion. The deal added 116 hospitals to Columbia/HCA, giving the combined firm over 300 hospitals.

3. National Medical Enterprises acquired American Medical International for $3.3 billion. The combined company, which is now the second largest hospital chain in the United States, was renamed Tenet Healthcare.

4. American Healthcare Systems and Premier Health Alliance, two major hospital alliances, merged to create an alliance that serves over 1,400 hospitals, or about one-fourth of all community hospitals. The alliance is expected to buy about $8 billion annually in goods and services for its member hospitals.

5. Eli Lilly & Co. acquired PCS Health Systems, a unit of McKesson Corporation, for $4 billion. PCS is a management company that oversees the drug benefits programs of major employers and health plans. The deal gives Lilly, a major drug manufacturer, entree to a growing business with potentially valuable information on prescription patterns. The acquisition also gives Lilly a captive distribution channel, although the Federal Trade Commission indicated that any anticompetitive behavior would cause the merger to be reviewed.

6. Abbey Healthcare Group and Homedco Group merged to form Apria Healthcare Group, a powerhouse in home healthcare. The $1.1 billion merger created a company that is the largest provider of home respiratory care and the second largest provider of home infusion services.

The deal frenzy in the healthcare industry is occurring because providers are convinced that size is the key to success in the evolving healthcare market. This view is based on the trend towards managed care, in which buyers are grouping together as never before. HMOs are growing rapidly, worker groups are forming consortia to contract with plans as single entities, and insurers are combining to form increasingly formidable alliances. In response, providers are seeking greater size and scope of services to spread overhead, shift risk, and most importantly, to offer the full range of services required by large payers. Current thinking mandates that providers must offer more types of services over larger geographic areas at lower prices to gain market share and hence ensure survival in changing market conditions. Furthermore, mergers fuel mergers because providers are afraid to sit on the sidelines while others are merging around them. Although healthcare megamergers are occurring on the for-profit side, all providers are subject to the same industry trends, so there has also been considerable merger activity among not-for-profit providers, including mergers between investor-owned and not-for-profit firms.

MOTIVES FOR MERGERS

There are a variety of motives behind mergers; some valid and some questionable. In this section, we take a more detailed look at some of the motives behind business mergers, along with some views regarding the validity of these motives.

Synergy

From an economic perspective, the best motivation for mergers is to increase the value of the combined enterprise. If Companies A and B merge to form Company C, and if C's value exceeds that of A and B taken separately, then synergy is said to exist. When synergy drives a merger, value is created, and society benefits. Furthermore, such a merger can be beneficial to both A's and B's stockholders if the companies are investor-owned.

Synergistic effects can arise from four sources: (1) operating economies, which result from economies of scale in management, marketing, contracting, operations, or distribution, including mergers that better position a firm strategically; (2) financial economies, including lower transactions costs, access to additional capital markets, and better coverage by security analysts; (3) differential efficiency, which implies that the management of one firm is inefficient and that the firm's assets will be used more productively after the merger; and (4) increased market power due to reduced competition. Operating and financial economies are socially desirable, as are mergers that increase managerial efficiency. To some extent, increased market power can also be beneficial to society, such as the contracting savings that results when major purchasers buy health-care services. However, dominant market power can be harmful to society and hence is both undesirable and illegal.

Availability of Excess Cash

Mergers are an easy, perhaps too easy, way for firms to get rid of excess cash. If a firm has a shortage of internal investment opportunities compared with its cash flow, it could (1) increase its dividend or repurchase stock if investor-owned, (2) pay down its debt, (3) invest in marketable securities, or (4) purchase another firm. Debt repayment and marketable securities investments often provide a good short-term solution to excess cash flow, but these actions are generally inappropriate for the long term.

Although there is nothing inherently wrong with using excess cash to buy other companies, the acquisition must create value to be economically worthwhile. Just making a company larger may benefit managers, but it does not necessarily benefit stockholders, patients, or society at large. If the return on a potential acquisition is not as high as the opportunity cost of the capital used, the capital should be used for other purposes. If the firm is investor-owned, the capital should be returned to the firm's investors, while if the firm is not-for-profit, it should be used to retire debt or invested temporarily until better uses can be found.

Purchase of Assets at Below Replacement Cost

Sometimes a firm will be touted as a possible acquisition candidate because the cost of replacing its assets is considerably higher than its market value. For example, suppose that a small, rural hospital can be acquired for $5 million, while the cost to construct a similar hospital from the ground up is $10 million. There might be a strong temptation to say that the hospital is a good buy because it can be bought for less than its replacement value.

However, the true value of any business depends on its earning power, which sets the economic value of its assets. The real question, then, is not whether the hospital can be acquired for less than its replacement cost but whether it can be acquired for less than its economic value, which is a function of the cash flows that the hospital is expected to produce in the future. If the rural hospital's earning power gives it a value of $7 million, then it is a good buy at $5 million; but this conclusion is based on economic, not replacement, value. (Of course, the rural hospital would likely have some social value that would have to be considered in the valuation process.)

Diversification

Managers often claim that diversification into other lines of business is a reason for mergers. They contend that diversification helps to stabilize the firm's earnings stream and thus benefits its owners. Stabilization of earnings is certainly beneficial to managers, employees, suppliers, customers, and other stakeholders, but its value is less certain from the standpoint of stockholders. If a stockholder is worried about the variability of a firm's earnings, he or she could diversify more easily than could the firm. Why should Firms A and B merge to stabilize earnings when a stockholder in Firm A could sell half of his or her stock and use the proceeds to purchase stock in Firm B? Stockholders can create diversification more easily than can the firm.

Also, if a stockholder is concerned about the relative performance of different industry segments, he or she can solve the problem more easily through portfolio diversification than can managers through mergers. For example, assume that a stockholder who holds primarily hospital stocks is concerned that the increased purchasing power of managed care plans will erode hospital profits, and hence value, over time. It is easier for the stockholder to purchase HMO stocks than it is for hospitals to diversify into managed care.

Of course, there are some situations where mergers for diversification do make sense from a stockholder's perspective. For example, if you were the owner-manager of a closely held firm, it might be nearly impossible for you to sell part of your stock to diversify because this would dilute your ownership and perhaps also generate a large capital gains tax liability. In this case, a diversification merger might well be the best way to achieve personal diversification. Also, as mentioned earlier, diversification mergers that better position firms to deal with future events are worthwhile because such mergers can create operating synergies.

Even though diversification, without synergy, does not benefit shareholders directly, it clearly benefits a firm's other stakeholders. Thus, diversification-motivated mergers can be beneficial to not-for-profit firms. Furthermore, stockholders can obtain indirect benefits from diversification because making the firm less risky to managers, creditors, suppliers, customers, and the like could have positive implications for shareholders' wealth.

Personal Incentives

Economists like to think that business decisions are based only on economic considerations. However, there can be no question that some business decisions are based more on managers' personal motivations than on economic analyses. Many people, business leaders included, like power, and more power is attached to running a larger corporation than a smaller one. Obviously, no executive would ever admit that his or her ego was the primary reason behind a merger, but knowledgeable observers are convinced that egos do play a prominent role in many mergers. It has also been observed that executive salaries, prestige, and perquisites are highly correlated with company size: The bigger the company, the higher these executive benefits. This too could play a role in the aggressive acquisition programs of some corporations. Of course, there is nothing wrong with executives feeling good about increasing the size of their firms or with their getting a better compensation package as a result of growth through mergers, provided the mergers make economic sense.

HOSTILE VERSUS FRIENDLY TAKEOVERS

In the vast majority of merger situations, one firm (the acquirer) simply decides to buy another company (the target), negotiates a price with the target firm's management, and acquires the company. Occasionally, the acquired firm will initiate the action, but it is much more common for a firm to seek acquisitions than to seek to be acquired.

Once an acquiring company has identified a possible target, it must establish a suitable price, or range of prices, and tentatively set the method of payment: Will it offer cash, its own common stock, bonds, or a mix of securities? Next, the acquiring firm's managers must decide how to approach the target company's managers. If the acquiring firm has reason to believe the target's management will support the merger, it will simply propose a merger and try to work out suitable terms. If an agreement is reached, the two management groups will issue statements indicating that they approve the merger and, if the firms are investor-owned, recommend that stockholders agree to the merger. Generally, the stockholders of acquiring firms must merely vote to approve the merger, but the stockholders of target firms are asked to tender (or send in) their shares to a designated financial institution, along with a signed power of attorney that transfers ownership of the shares to the acquiring firm. The target firm's stockholders then receive the specified payment, be it common stock of the acquiring company (in which case the target company's stockholders become stockholders of the acquiring company), cash, bonds, or some mix of cash and securities. This type of merger is called a friendly merger, or a friendly tender offer.

The 1993 acquisition of HCA (Hospital Corporation of America) by Columbia Healthcare typifies a friendly merger. First, the boards of directors of the two firms announced that HCA had agreed to be acquired by Columbia in a stock-swap transaction. (HCA stockholders received 1.05 shares of Columbia stock for each share held.) The merger was approved by shareholders of both companies and by the Justice Department, and then the acquisition was completed. The merger created a hospital management giant, with significant market share and scale economies in many service areas.

Another example of a friendly merger is the previously mentioned combination of Abbey Healthcare Group and Homedco Group to form Apria Healthcare Group. In the deal, each holder of Homedco stock received two shares of the new firm per share held, while each Abbey holder received 1.4 shares of the new company for each share held. Because the two companies competed in some of the same markets, about 100 of the combined 450 offices were expected to be closed, resulting in a pretax savings of between $30 million and $40 million. Analysts praised the merger as a smart combination that would add Abbey's strength in home infusion to Homedco's strength in home respiration, resulting in one company that could offer a single package contract to an increasingly cost-conscious managed care industry.

Often, however, the target company's management resists the merger. Perhaps the managers feel that the price offered for the stock is too low, or perhaps they simply want to retain their autonomy. In either case, the acquiring firm's offer is said to be hostile rather than friendly, and the acquiring firm must make a direct appeal to the target firm's stockholders. In a hostile merger, the acquiring company will again make a tender offer, and again it will ask the stockholders of the target firm to tender their shares in exchange for the offered price. This time, though, the target firm's managers will urge stockholders not to tender their shares, generally stating that the price offered (cash, bonds, or stocks in the acquiring firm) is too low.

The recent battle between Monarch Group, a Virginia-based long-term care company, and Dominion Health Holdings illustrates a failed hostile merger attempt. It began in the summer of 1995, when Monarch's stock was trading at under $10 a share. At the time, many analysts had declared that Monarch was a likely takeover candidate because of its sluggish stock performance but good earnings and spotless image in an industry that has many questionable players. Then, Dominion Health Holdings, the investment vehicle of the Robert Pettijohn family, purchased 5 percent of Monarch's stock, proposed a friendly takeover, was rebuffed, and made a $15-per-share hostile tender offer. Monarch responded to the unwanted offer (1) by selling a chunk of its stock to a newly established employee stock ownership plan (ESOP), (2) by selling another chunk to a friendly investor (a "white squire"), and (3) by buying back 30 percent of its outstanding shares at $17 a share. To finance all of this, Monarch added $40 million in bank debt. Additionally, Monarch restructured its operations by cutting its workforce by 15 percent. Dominion Health responded to these actions (1) by initiating a proxy fight to elect new directors on Monarch's board and (2) by filing a lawsuit challenging the legitimacy of Monarch's defensive maneuvers.

After nine months of heated exchanges between the companies, an accord was reached in March 1996. Monarch agreed to pay Dominion Health $5 million in compensation for expenses incurred in the battle, plus repurchase all of Monarch's shares held by Dominion Health at $15 per share. For its part, Dominion Health promised not to seek control of Monarch for 10 years. Finally, Dominion Health agreed to drop all litigation, as well as its proxy fight. Although defeated, Dominion Health ended up making about $10 million before taxes, considering both the cash settlement and the profit on the Monarch shares that it owned. Charles Pettijohn, Dominion Health's president, said that the decision to settle was sealed by a Virginia court decision that upheld Monarch's defenses. "It isn't that we went away quietly; we tried as hard as we could," he said.

Monarch ended up with more debt, although it still has a strong balance sheet, and a $12.50-per-share stock price. Monarch's president and CEO, Jerome Martin, said, "The fundamental changes and initiatives put in place during this period made us stronger, despite the pressure."

Although many hostile takeover bids fail, many others succeed. It is very difficult to defend against a hostile takeover attempt if the bidder has a large amount of resources that it is willing to spend on the battle. In such situations, the acquiring firm can offer enough cash to shareholders to overcome even the most adamant managerial resistance.

MERGER REGULATION

Merger regulation falls into two broad categories: (1) regulation concerning the procedures acquiring companies must follow in making hostile bids and (2) antitrust regulation to ensure that mergers do not lead to monopoly power.

Bid Procedure Regulation

Prior to the mid-1960s, friendly acquisitions generally took place through simple exchange-of-stock mergers, and the proxy fight was the primary weapon used in a hostile control battle. However, in the mid-1960s, corporate raiders began to operate differently. First, they noted that it took a long time to mount a proxy fight;

they had to first request a list of the target company's stockholders, then be refused, and finally get a court order forcing management to turn over the list. During that time, management could think through and then implement a strategy to fend off the raider. As a result, the instigator lost most proxy fights.

Then raiders began saying to themselves, "If we could take an action that would bring the decision to a head quickly, before management could take countermeasures, that would greatly increase the probability of a successful takeover." That led raiders to turn from proxy fights to tender offers, which have a much shorter response time. For example, the stockholders of a company whose stock was selling for $20 might be offered $25 per share and be given two weeks to accept. The raider, meanwhile, would have accumulated a substantial block of the shares in open market purchases, and additional shares might have been purchased by institutional friends of the raider who promised to tender their shares in exchange for the tip that a raid was to occur, even though such actions are illegal.

Faced with a well-planned raid, managements were generally overwhelmed. The stock might actually still be undervalued at the offered price, at least in the opinion of management of the target firm, but it simply might not have time to get this message across to stockholders or to find a friendly competing bidder (called a "white knight") or to take any other action. This situation was thought to be unfair, and as a result, Congress passed the Williams Act in 1968. This law had two main objectives: (1) to regulate the way in which acquiring firms can structure takeover offers and (2) to force acquiring firms to disclose more information about their offers. Basically, Congress wanted to put target managements in a better position to defend against hostile offers. Additionally, Congress believed that shareholders needed easy access to information about tender offers—including information on any securities that might be offered in lieu of cash—in order to make a rational decision.

The Williams Act placed the following three major restrictions on the activities of acquiring firms: (1) Acquirers must disclose their current holdings and future intentions within 10 days of amassing at least 5 percent of a company's stock, and they must disclose the source of the funds to be used in the acquisition. (2) The target firm's shareholders must be allowed at least 20 days to tender their shares; that is, the offer must be "open" for at least 20 days. (3) If the acquiring firm increases the offer price during the 20-day open period, all shareholders who tendered prior to the improved offer must receive the higher price.

In total, these restrictions were intended to reduce the ability of the acquiring firm to surprise management and to stampede target shareholders into accepting the offer. Prior to the Williams Act, offers were generally made on a first-come, first-served basis, and they were often accompanied by an implicit threat to lower the bid price after 50 percent of the shares were in hand. The legislation also gave target managements more time to mount a defense, and it gave rival bidders and white knights a chance to enter the fray and thus help a target's stockholders obtain a better price.

Many states have also passed laws designed to protect firms in their states from hostile takeovers. At first, these laws focused on disclosure requirements, but by the late 1970s, several states had enacted takeover statutes so restrictive they virtually precluded hostile takeovers. The constitutionality of state laws regulating takeover bids was challenged, and at first, the state laws were struck down. In spite of such decisions, states kept trying to protect their state-headquartered companies. In 1987, the U.S. Supreme Court upheld an Indiana law that radically changed the rules of the takeover game. Specifically, the Indiana law defined "control shares" as enough shares to give an investor 20 percent of the vote. It went on to state that when an investor buys control shares, those shares can be voted only after approval by a majority of "disinterested shareholders," defined as those who are neither officers nor inside directors of the company, nor associates of the raider. Thus, a hostile acquirer that owned 20 percent of a target company's shares could not force a takeover by gaining only 31 percent more but, rather, would have to get 51 percent of the remaining 80 percent, or 41 percent more.

The law also gives the buyer of control shares the right to insist that a shareholders' meeting be called within 50 days to decide whether the shares may be voted. The Indiana law dealt a major blow to raiders, mainly because it slowed down the action. Delaware (the state in which most large companies are incorporated) later passed a similar bill, as did New York and a number of other states.

The new state laws also have features that protect target stockholders from their own managers. Included are limits on the use of golden parachutes—lucrative compensation plans given to managers who lose their jobs as a result of takeovers—and the elimination of some types of poison pills—actions that managers of beleaguered firms can take to "kill off" their own companies to make them less attractive as targets. Since these types of state laws do not regulate tender offers per se but, rather, govern the practices of firms in the state, they have thus far withstood all legal challenges.

Antitrust Regulation

Antitrust laws are intended to ensure that no organization attains enough market power to act as a monopoly. Such laws are based on the assumption that vigorous competition is the most effective way to ensure that consumers receive the best possible goods and services at the lowest cost. Two key laws govern antitrust litigation: the Sherman Act and the Clayton Act. The Sherman Act, which dates to 1890, prohibits contracts, conspiracies, and combinations that restrain trade. The Clayton Act, passed in 1914, prohibits all mergers, acquisitions, and joint ventures that may substantially lessen competition or allow creation of a monopoly.

The two agencies that are charged with enforcing antitrust laws are the Federal Trade Commission (FTC) and the Justice Department (JD). The FTC and JD classify potential antitrust violations into two categories: per se and rule of reason. Per se violations are those so unlikely to produce redeeming consumer benefits that they are immediately presumed to be illegal. Examples would be two hospitals agreeing to fix prices for certain procedures or agreeing to allocate specific markets. Actions that are not considered per se violations are evaluated using rule-of-reason analysis. Under rule-of-reason analysis, the FTC or JD must first determine whether a merger (or other combination) will enable a firm to exercise market power in an anticompetitive manner. If so, the agency must then analyze whether the activity produces economic efficiencies that outweigh the anticompetitive effects. If the benefits outweigh the anticompetitive consequences, the merger is allowed to take place. Mergers within the healthcare industry generally fall into the rule-of-reason category, so a great deal of leeway exists in implementing the antitrust laws.

Regulators are informed of pending mergers by premerger notification laws, which require companies involved in mergers to file certain information with federal and state agencies. Such agencies, including the FTC and JD, have 30 days to request additional information, approve the application, or file suit to prevent the merger.

Clearly, the manner in which antitrust laws are enforced has a significant impact on merger activity and hence on the future structure of the healthcare system. Before the 1990s, when fee-for-service insurance prevailed, physicians competed with one another for patients, and hospitals competed for inpatient business. Today, however, the health services industry is being transformed by the growth of managed care, selective contracting, and vertical integration, in which an organization provides both insurance and medical services. This transformation means that the FTC and JD have their hands full figuring out how and when to apply antitrust laws. For example, two hospitals may merge to increase their bargaining power with insurers. If insurers now have fewer hospitals with which to negotiate, they cannot drive nearly as hard a bargain as before, so the merger may be anticompetitive. But, by merging, the hospitals may be able to reduce duplicated services and achieve other operating efficiencies that could lead to lower prices, which would be good for the insurers and ultimately for consumers. The issue becomes which policy—vigorous or lax enforcement—the FTC and JD should follow to ensure good health policy.

The answer is not easy. For example, consider the case of Ukiah Valley Medical Center, a 94-bed not-for-profit hospital company located some 120 miles north of San Francisco. The company was created by the recent merger of two rural hospitals: one with 51 beds and one with 43 beds. However, the merger was initially challenged by the FTC, which charged that it violated antitrust laws because it injured consumers by reducing competition among acute care providers. The company resisted the FTC challenge, spending two million dollars over a five-year period to save the merger. Finally, in 1994, the commission voted five to nothing to drop the lawsuit, ruling that evidence of anticompetitive effects was weak. Furthermore, the ruling stated that the creation of a larger, more efficient system would provide better medical care than could either of the two hospitals when operated separately. "Obviously, we feel great," said Ukiah's president. "However, the decision is about five years and two million dollars late."

Much of the healthcare industry, led by the American Hospital Association, has been lobbying for antitrust relief, arguing that antitrust laws and enforcement policies have thwarted beneficial collaborative arrangements among hospitals and other providers. However, federal regulators have requested additional information on only 7 percent of the proposed hospital mergers between 1981 and 1993 and stopped less than 4 percent from being consummated.

With encouragement from the Clinton administration, in late 1994 the FTC and JD issued a joint policy statement containing "safety zone" guidelines. The statement describes circumstances under which mergers between hospitals, physician/network joint ventures, and other healthcare combinations will not be challenged. For example, a hospital merger will not be challenged if one or both of the hospitals has fewer than 100 beds, less than 40 patients per day, and is more than five years old. Also, a physician network will not be contested if the network has no more than 20 percent of the physicians in a specialty in a particular geographical market. Although the guidelines have no effect on court decisions, and hence are no guarantee of legality, most industry representatives agree that the guidelines are needed and are helpful in establishing ground rules for future merger activity.

States are also involved in the antitrust field, both supporting and challenging proposed mergers. For example, four states requested information concerning the impact of the Columbia/ HCA-Healthtrust merger on individual markets, and state actions have caused hospital chains involved in large mergers to agree to sell off hospitals in particular markets to avoid antitrust actions. However, for the most part, states have been supportive of mergers in the healthcare industry. Over 20 states have used the state action immunity doctrine to pass laws that grant immunity from federal antitrust laws. However, the doctrine requires states to actively regulate anticompetitive conduct, and there is always the possibility that the FTC or JD might challenge activities permitted by state immunity doctrine legislation because of lax supervision.

The consolidation of the healthcare industry has produced different views on how aggressively antitrust laws should be enforced. Physicians and hospitals tend to support lenient enforcement, arguing that they can achieve efficiencies only through mergers, acquisitions, and joint ventures. In particular, there is concern over the fact that an insurer or HMO can sign up, say, 70 percent of the physicians in a community, while antitrust laws prohibit even 40 or 50 percent of the physicians in a market from joining together to form their own network. According to an American Medical Association spokesman, "It doesn't make any sense to prevent doctors from getting together. They won't fix prices; they will be subject to market discipline from buyers." Insurers and HMOs, however, tend to argue for strict enforcement of antitrust laws on the grounds that competition will produce maximum efficiency and innovation in the healthcare system.

MERGER VALUATION

In theory, merger analysis is quite simple. The acquiring firm simply performs an analysis to value the target company and then determines whether the target can be bought at that value or, preferably, for less than the assessed value. The target company, on the other hand, should accept the proposal if the price offered exceeds the value of the target firm if it continued to operate independently. Theory aside, however, some difficult issues are involved. In this section, we discuss valuing the target firm, the first step in merger analysis. Then, in later sections, we discuss the remainder of merger analysis: setting the bid price and structuring the bid.

Several methodologies are used to value firms, but we will confine our discussion to the two most commonly used methods in the healthcare industry: discounted cash flow analysis and market multiple analysis. However, regardless of the valuation methodology, it is crucial to recognize two factors. First, the business being valued typically will not continue to operate as a separate entity but, rather, will become part of the acquiring firm's portfolio of assets. Thus, any changes in ownership form or operations occurring as a result of the proposed merger that will impact the value of the business must be considered in the analysis. Second, the goal of merger valuation is to set the value of the target business's equity, or ownership position, because a business is acquired from its owners, not from its creditors. Thus, although we use the phrase "valuing the firm," we are really valuing the firm's equity stake rather than the total value of the firm.

Discounted Cash Flow Analysis

The discounted cash flow (DCF) approach to valuing a business involves the application of classical capital investment analysis to an entire firm rather than to a single project. To apply this method, two key items are needed: (1) a set of pro forma statements that develop the incremental cash flows expected to result from the merger and (2) a discount rate, or cost of capital, to apply to these projected cash flows.

The development of accurate postmerger cash flow forecasts is, by far, the most important step in a DCF merger analysis. In a pure financial merger, in which no synergies are expected, the incremental postmerger cash flows are simply the expected cash flows of the target firm if it were to continue to operate independently. However, even in this situation, the cash flows for a healthcare provider may be quite difficult to forecast because the nature of the industry is changing so rapidly. In an operational merger, in which the two firms' operations are to be integrated or the acquiring firm plans to change the target firm's operations in order to get better results, forecasting future cash flows is even more complex.

Table 9–1 shows the projected cash flow statements for Physicians' Hospital, an investor-owned hospital that is being eval-

TABLE 9–1

Projected Cash Flow Statements (Millions of Dollars)

	1998	1999	2000	2001	2002
1. Net revenues	$105.0	$126.0	$151.0	$174.0	$191.0
2. Patient services expenses	80.0	94.0	111.0	127.0	137.0
3. Other expenses	10.0	12.0	13.0	15.0	16.0
4. Depreciation	8.0	8.0	9.0	9.0	10.0
5. Earnings before interest and taxes (EBIT)	$ 7.0	$ 12.0	$ 18.0	$ 23.0	$ 28.0
6. Interest	3.0	4.0	5.0	6.0	6.0
7. Earnings before taxes (EBT)	$ 4.0	$ 8.0	$ 13.0	$ 17.0	$ 22.0
8. Taxes (40 percent)	1.6	3.2	5.2	6.8	8.8
9. Net income	$ 2.4	$ 4.8	$ 7.8	$ 10.2	$ 13.2
10. Plus depreciation	8.0	8.0	9.0	9.0	10.0
11. Cash flow	$ 10.4	$ 12.8	$ 16.8	$ 19.2	$ 23.2
12. Less retentions	4.0	4.0	7.0	9.0	12.0
13. Plus terminal value					89.1
14. Net cash flow to TransHealth	$ 6.4	$ 8.8	$ 9.8	$ 10.2	$100.3

uated as a possible acquisition by TransHealth, a large hospital management company. The projected data are for the postmerger period, so all synergistic effects have been included in the cash flow estimates. Physicians' Hospital currently uses 30 percent debt, but if it were acquired, TransHealth would increase Physicians' debt ratio to 50 percent. Both TransHealth and Physicians' Hospital have 40 percent marginal federal-plus-state tax rates.

Line 1 of Table 9–1 contains the forecast for Physicians' net revenues, including patient services revenue, other operating revenue, and nonoperating revenue. Note that all contractual allowances and other adjustments to charges, including collections delays, have been considered, so Line 1 represents actual cash revenues. Note also that any change in Physicians' stand-alone forecasted revenues resulting from synergies have been incorporated into the Line 1 amounts.

Lines 2 through 4 contain the expense forecasts, including depreciation. These are the cash costs (except for depreciation) that must be borne to generate the net revenues in Line 1. Again, the expense amounts pertain to the Physicians' Hospital subsidiary assuming that the merger takes place, so savings due to operational efficiencies are included. Line 5, which is merely Line 1 minus Lines 2, 3, and 4, contains the earnings before interest and taxes (EBIT) for each year.

Unlike a typical capital budgeting analysis, merger analyses usually incorporate interest expense, which is shown on Line 6, into the cash flow forecast. This is done for three reasons: (1) Acquiring firms often assume the debt of the target firm, so old debt having different coupon rates is often part of the deal; (2) the acquisition is often partially financed by debt; and (3) if the subsidiary is expected to grow in the future, new debt will have to be issued over time to support the expansion. Thus, the debt structure associated with a merger is typically much more complex than the single issue of new debt that is assumed to occur in a normal capital budgeting analysis. The easiest way to properly account for the complexities of merger debt is to explicitly include each year's expected interest expense in the cash flow forecast. In essence, this form of DCF analysis uses the equity residual, or free cash flow, method to value the target firm, since the net cash flows that are being estimated belong solely to the acquiring firm's shareholders.

Line 7 contains the earnings before taxes (EBT), and Line 8 lists the taxes based on TransHealth's 40 percent marginal rate. Note that the tax rate applied in the analysis must reflect the rate that will be applied to the combined enterprise. Line 9 lists each year's net income, but depreciation is added back in Line 10 to obtain each year's cash flow, which is shown on Line 11. Since some of Physicians' assets are expected to wear out or become obsolete, and since TransHealth plans to expand the Physicians' Hospital subsidiary should the acquisition occur, some equity funds must be retained and reinvested in the subsidiary. These retentions, which are not available for transfer from the hospital subsidiary to the TransHealth parent, are shown on Line 12.

Finally, we have projected only 5 years of cash flows, but TransHealth would likely operate Physicians' Hospital for many years, perhaps 20 or 30 or more. If the cash flows from the hospital are assumed to grow at a constant rate after 2002, the constant growth model can be used to estimate the target firm's terminal value. Assuming a constant 5 percent growth rate in net cash flow after 2002, the terminal value is estimated to be $89.1 million.

$$\text{Value of CFs beyond } 2002 = \frac{2002 \text{ Cash flow } (1 + \text{Growth rate})}{\text{Required rate of return} - \text{Growth rate}}$$

$$= \frac{(\$23.2 - \$12.0)(1.05)}{0.182 - 0.05} = \$89.1 \text{ million}$$

This terminal value of Physicians' Hospital, which represents its market value at the end of 2002, is shown on Line 13. Note that the discount rate applied in the terminal value calculation, 18.2 percent, will be estimated shortly.

The net cash flows shown on Line 14 are the flows that would be available to TransHealth's stockholders, and these are the basis of the valuation. Of course, the postmerger cash flows attributable to the target firm are extremely difficult to estimate. In a complete merger valuation, just as in a complete capital investment analysis, the component cash flow probability distributions would be specified; and sensitivity, scenario, and Monte Carlo simulation analyses would be conducted. Indeed, in a friendly merger, the acquiring firm would send a team consisting of literally dozens of accountants, financial analysts, engineers, and so forth, to the target firm to go over its books, to estimate required maintenance expenditures, to set values on assets such as real estate, and the like.

The bottom-line net cash flows shown in Line 14 of Table 9–1 belong to TransHealth's stockholders, so they should be discounted at a cost of equity rather than at an overall cost of capital. Furthermore, the cost of equity used must reflect the riskiness of the net cash flows in the table, and hence the discount rate is more closely aligned with the cost of equity of Physicians' Hospital, not that of either TransHealth or the consolidated postmerger firm.

In this illustration, as with many healthcare mergers, the target company is investor-owned but not publicly traded, so it is not possible to obtain a market beta on Physicians' stock. However, we can obtain market betas of the stocks of the major investor-owned hospital chains. Assume that the average market beta of the stock of several hospital chains is 1.28. This value reflects an average 30 percent debt ratio, while Physicians' postmerger debt ratio will be 50 percent, as well as an average 40 percent tax rate, the same as Physicians'.

Hamada's equation, which was first discussed in Chapter 8, can be used to approximate the effects of the leverage change on beta. First, we obtain the unlevered beta of the average hospital's assets, that is, the beta of an average hospital assuming that it is financed entirely with equity.

$$b_{Assets} = \frac{b_{Firm}}{1+(1-T)(D/E)} = \frac{1.28}{1+(1-0.40)(0.30/0.70)} = \frac{1.28}{1.26} = 1.02$$

Next, we relever the average hospital's asset beta to reflect the 50 percent debt ratio that would be used in the acquisition.

$$b_{Firm} = b_{Assets}\left[1+(1-T)(D/E)\right]$$
$$= 1.02\left[1+(1-0.40)(0.50/0.50)\right] = 1.02(1.6) = 1.63$$

Then, we use the Security Market Line to estimate the postmerger cost of equity for the Physicians' Hospital subsidiary. If the risk-free rate is 10 percent and the required rate of return on the market (an average stock with b = 1.0) is 15 percent, then the cost of equity of the Physicians' Hospital subsidiary, and hence the discount rate to apply to the Table 9–1 net cash flows, would be about 18.2 percent.

$$\text{Cost of equity} = k_{RF} + (k_M - k_{RF})b = 10\% + (15\% - 10\%)1.63 = 18.2\%$$

Finally, the current value of Physicians' Hospital to Trans-Health is the present value of the cash flows expected to accrue to TransHealth, discounted at 18.2 percent. The present value of the Table 9-1 net cash flows, when discounted at 18.2 percent, is $66.3 million. Thus, if TransHealth could acquire Physicians' Hospital for $66.3 million or less, the merger would appear to be acceptable from TransHealth's standpoint. Obviously, TransHealth would try to buy Physicians' at as low a price as possible, while Physicians' managers would hold out for the highest possible price. The final price is determined by negotiation, with the stronger negotiator capturing most of the incremental value. The larger the synergistic benefits, the more room for bargaining and the higher the proba-bility that the merger will actually be consummated. We will have more to say about setting the bid price in a later section.

Market Multiple Analysis

Another method of valuing a business is market multiple analysis, which applies a market-determined multiple to some measure of earnings, such as net income or earnings per share. Like the DCF valuation method, the basic premise is that the value of any busi-ness depends on the earnings that the business produces. The DCF method applies this rationale to forecasted cash flows, while mar-ket multiple analysis uses comparative data to value earnings.

The earnings measure that market multiples are most com-monly applied to when analyzing healthcare mergers is earnings before interest, taxes, depreciation, and amortization (EBITDA). To apply the EBITDA earnings multiple method to the Physicians' Hospital analysis, note that the hospital's 1998 forecasted EBITDA is $7.0 + $8.0 = $15 million. If a market analysis of publicly traded investor-owned hospitals indicates an average Stock price/EBITDA ratio of 5.0, the value of Physicians' Hospital would be set at $15(5) = $75 million, as compared to $66.3 million using the DCF method.

Clearly, the valuation of a business can only be considered a rough estimate. Although the DCF method has strong theoretical support, one has to be very concerned over the validity of the estimated cash flows and the discount rate applied to those flows. It doesn't take much variation in these estimates to create large differences in estimated value. The market multiple method has less theoretical support, but its proponents argue that earnings estimates for a single year, such as measured by EBITDA, are much more likely to be accurate than a multiple-year cash flow forecast. Furthermore, the market multiple method avoids the problem of having to estimate a discount rate. Of course, the market multiple method has problems of its own. One concern is the comparability between the firm being analyzed and the firm (or firms) that set the market multiple. Another concern is how well one year of EBITDA, or even an average of several years, captures the value of a firm that will be operated for many years into the future, and whose EBITDA could soar due to merger-related synergies.

Setting the Bid Price

Assume that TransHealth's managers concluded that the value of Physicians' Hospital was $70 million. Furthermore, assume that Physicians' Hospital has one million shares of stock outstanding and that it has sold recently in a private sale at $50 a share, so Physicians' total market value is assumed to be $50 million. With an estimated value of $70 million to TransHealth, it could offer as much as $70 per share for Physicians' without diluting the value of its own stock.

Figure 9–1 illustrates the situation facing TransHealth's managers as they set the bid price. The $70 per share maximum offer price is shown as a point on the horizontal axis, which plots bid price. If TransHealth pays less, say, $65 a share, its stockholders will gain $5 per share, or $5 million in total, from the merger. On the other hand, if TransHealth pays more than $70 per share, its stockholders will lose value. The line that shows the impact of the per-share bid price on TransHealth's stockholders is a downward sloping line that cuts the X axis at $70. The distance between this diagonal line and the X axis is the amount that TransHealth's stockholders will gain (or lose) for each share of Physicians' acquired.

The situation facing Physicians' shareholders is depicted by an upward sloping line that crosses the X axis at $50. If the hospital is

FIGURE 9–1

Evaluating the Takeover Bid

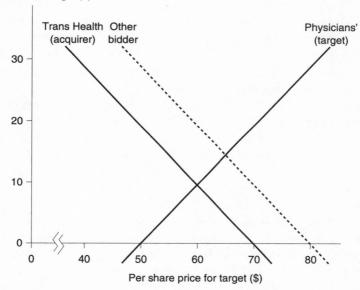

Change in wealth
per share of target ($)

Trans Health Other   Physicians'
(acquirer)   bidder   (target)

Per share price for target ($)

acquired for more than $50 per share, its shareholders will gain value, while they would lose value if the price is less than $50.

Figure 9–1 shows clearly there is a bid price range between $50 and $70 where the shareholders of both TransHealth and Physicians' Hospital benefit from the merger. The range exists because the merger has synergistic benefits that can be divided between the two sets of stockholders. The greater the synergistic benefits, the greater the range of feasible bid prices, and the greater the chance that the merger will be consummated.

The issue of how to divide the synergistic benefit is critically important in any merger analysis. Obviously, both parties will want to gain as much as possible. If Physicians' shareholders knew the maximum price that TransHealth is willing to pay, $70, it would hold out for that price. TransHealth, on the other hand, will try to acquire the hospital at a price as close to $50 a share as possible.

Where within the $50 to $70 range should TransHealth set its initial bid? The answer depends on a number of factors, including whether TransHealth will pay with cash or securities, whether the managers of TransHealth or Physicians' Hospital have the better negotiating skills, and whether another bidder is likely to enter the picture.

The likelihood of a bidding war for Physicians' Hospital plays an important role in setting the initial bid. Suppose first that no other bidder is likely. In this situation, TransHealth might make a relatively low take-it-or-leave-it offer, and Physicians' shareholders would probably take it because some gain is better than no gain. On the other hand, if Physicians' Hospital has a unique situation that makes it attractive to several competing health systems, other bidders may enter the fray, and the final price will likely be close to $70 per share. Perhaps another potential acquirer could achieve even greater synergies with Physicians' Hospital than could TransHealth, as shown in Figure 9–1 by the "Other bidder" dashed line. If so, the bid price could rise above $70, in which case TransHealth should drop out of the bidding.

TransHealth would, of course, want to keep its maximum bid secret, and it would plan its bidding strategy carefully and consistent with the situation. If TransHealth thought that other bidders would emerge, or that Physicians' management would resist a bid to protect their jobs, TransHealth might decide to make a high preemptive, or "knockout," bid in hopes of scaring off competing bids, eliminating management resistance, or both. On the other hand, if no other bidders were expected, TransHealth might make a lowball bid in hopes of stealing the hospital.

Another factor that influences the initial bid is the employment/control situation. First, consider the situation in which a small, owner-managed firm sells out to a larger concern. The owner-manager may be anxious to retain a high-status position, and he or she may also have developed a camaraderie with the employees and thus be concerned about keeping operating control of the organization after the merger. These points are often stressed during the merger negotiations. When a publicly owned firm not controlled by its managers is merged into another company, the acquired firm's management is also worried about its postmerger position. If the acquiring firm agrees to retain the old management, management may be willing to support the merger and to recommend its acceptance to the stockholders. If the old management is to be removed, it will probably resist the merger.

Structuring the Takeover Bid

The acquiring firm's offer to the target's shareholders can be in the form of cash, stock of the acquiring firm, debt of the acquiring firm, or a combination of the three. The structure of the bid is extremely important since it affects (1) the capital structure of the postmerger firm, (2) the tax treatment of both the acquiring firm and the target's stockholders, (3) the ability of the target firm's stockholders to reap the rewards of future merger-related gains, and (4) the types of federal and state regulations to which the acquiring firm will be subjected. In this section, we focus on how taxes and regulation influence the way in which acquiring firms structure their offers.

The form of payment offered to the target shareholders determines the personal tax treatment of the target's stockholders. Target shareholders do not have to pay taxes on the transaction if they maintain a substantial equity position in the combined firm, defined by the IRS to mean that at least 50 percent of the payment to target shareholders must be in shares (either common or preferred) of the acquiring firm. In such nontaxable offers, target shareholders do not realize any capital gains or losses until the equity securities they receive in the takeover are sold. However, capital gains must be taken and treated as income in the transaction year if an offer consists of over 50 percent of either cash or debt securities, or some combination of the two.

All other things being equal, target stockholders prefer nontaxable offers, especially when they believe that the combined firm will perform well, since they can (1) benefit from the continuing good performance of the combined firm and (2) postpone the realization of capital gains and the payment of taxes. Most target shareholders are thus willing to sell their stock for a lower price in a nontaxable offer than in a taxable offer. As a result, one might expect nontaxable bids to dominate; however, other factors are at work. If a firm pays more than book value for a target firm's assets in a taxable merger, it can write up those assets, depreciate the marked-up value for tax purposes, and thus lower the postmerger firm's taxes vis-à-vis the taxes of the two firms operating separately. However, if the acquiring company writes up the target company's assets for tax purposes, the target company must pay capital gains taxes in the year the merger occurs. (These taxes can be avoided if the acquiring company elects not to write up acquired assets and depreciates them on their old basis.)

Securities laws also have an effect on the construction of the offer. Whenever a corporation bids for control of another firm through the exchange of equity or debt, the entire process must take place under the scrutiny of the Securities and Exchange Commission (SEC). The time required for such reviews allows target managements to implement defensive tactics and other firms to make competing offers, and as a result, most hostile tender offers are for cash rather than securities.

Due Diligence Analysis

One of the most important aspects of a merger is due diligence analysis. The primary purposes of a due diligence analysis are (1) to uncover issues that would prevent the acquirer from pursuing the acquisition and (2) to provide the acquirer with insights into the day-to-day operations of the target firm so that an appropriate transaction can take place. Due diligence requires a uniform, disciplined approach to merger analysis, which presumably will minimize the risk of overlooking issues that are key to the acquisition.

Due diligence analysis normally takes place after a letter of intent has been signed between the acquiring and target firms but before the terms of the transaction have been completed. It is normally carried out by a team that has been specially assembled for the task. Typically, the team will include one or two top executives, plus specialists from applicable staffs such as finance, legal, medical, nursing, personnel, risk management, and engineering. The team may consist entirely of personnel from the acquiring firm, or it may contain consultants in addition to the in-house members.

The due diligence team will gather and analyze information about the acquisition. The end result is a report that summarizes the team's findings and makes recommendations as to whether or not to proceed with the acquisition and how the deal, if recommended, should be structured. The time required to conduct a due diligence analysis varies, depending on the number of individuals on the team, the nature of the acquisition, and the accessibility of information. Generally, however, due diligence analyses take about 60 to 90 days, so acquirers must allow sufficient time for due diligence analysis when developing merger timetables.

Conducting a thorough due diligence analysis is a necessary component of the acquisition process. In addition to protecting the acquirer against a poor acquisition, it can establish a relationship between acquiring and target firms' managements that not only facilitate successful negotiations but, more importantly, can help lead to a successful merger.

Mergers Involving Not-for-Profit Firms

One of the unique aspects of the healthcare industry is the large proportion of not-for-profit firms. Although the general principles discussed up to this point apply to all businesses, some unique problems arise when not-for-profit firms are involved in mergers. In general, the merger of two not-for-profit firms does not require special consideration, but the acquisition of a not-for-profit firm by an investor-owned acquirer presents two significant problems.

The first problem involves the charitable trust doctrine. This doctrine, which was first developed in English common law and has been adopted by most states, holds that assets used for charitable purposes must be held in trust. This doctrine shaped the state incorporation laws for not-for-profit firms, which require that assets being used for charitable purposes must be used for such purposes in perpetuity (forever). The end result is that the proceeds from the sale of a not-for-profit corporation to an investor-owned business must be held in trust and continue to be used for charitable purposes. These laws place two requirements on the board of trustees of a not-for-profit firm about to be acquired by an investor-owned firm. First, the trustees must ensure that the acquisition price reflects the full fair market value of the assets being acquired. This assurance is normally obtained by getting the opinion of an investment banker or professional appraiser. Second, the trustees must establish a charitable foundation to administer the proceeds from the sale for a charitable purpose. The usual vehicle for continuing the charitable purpose of the not-for-profit corporation is the tax-exempt foundation.

By the end of 1995, over 30 foundations had been spawned by the sales of not-for-profit businesses to investor-owned companies, primarily in the hospital industry and primarily as a result of acquisitions by Columbia/HCA Healthcare. Note, however, that foundations have also been created by sales of HMOs and other not-for-profit healthcare companies. To illustrate the foundation concept, Presbyterian Health Foundation was created in 1985 when Presbyterian Hospital in Oklahoma City was acquired by Hospital Corporation of America (HCA). The foundation began with $60 million in assets but now has over $110 million. By law, at least 5 percent of assets of charitable foundations must be distributed each year, and Presbyterian Health Foundation has given a total of $30 million alone for rural outreach programs at the University of Oklahoma Health Science Center.

Although merger-related foundations are clearly doing a lot of good work with their vast amount of assets, they do not escape criticism. Most of the criticism stems from the close relationships that many foundations have with the for-profit providers that funded them. Indeed, some foundations, instead of being funded entirely with cash, have ownership interests in the newly created for-profit entity, and it is easy for conflicts of interest to occur. One not-for-profit foundation has even lost its tax-exempt status because it squandered millions of dollars on overpriced clinics, excessive compensation, and extravagant spending on personal items for managers and employees. At least not-for-profit hospitals are constrained somewhat by competitive markets, whereas the burden of oversight at charitable foundations falls completely on the board of trustees.

The second major problem in the acquisition of a not-for-profit provider by an investor-owned company involves the tax-exempt, or municipal, debt that is often outstanding. Typically, such debt is issued for the sole purpose of funding plant and equipment owned by not-for-profit corporations. Furthermore, such debt usually has covenants that constrain the provider from merger activity that would lower the creditworthiness of the bonds or negatively affect the bonds' tax-exempt status. However, the issuer normally has the right to refund that debt when transactions of this nature occur. The end result is that, in most situations, the entire amount of outstanding tax-exempt debt has to be refunded coincident with the acquisition of a not-for-profit provider by a for-profit firm.

Clearly, the restrictions on mergers involving not-for-profit firms and for-profit firms make such activities much more complicated than mergers involving only for-profits or only not-for-profits. Nevertheless, as evidenced by the amount of merger activity, these kinds of mergers do occur, and their volume is likely to increase, not decrease, in the future.

To begin the acquisition process, Lucy Radcliffe talked informally with Fred McCracken, Midwest Health Plans' CEO. Fred was also concerned about the future viability of River City's three hospitals. Additionally, he believed that Midwest should divest its provider network so that it could focus its managerial efforts on running its core managed care business. Thus, Fred was receptive to the idea of a possible sale of General Hospital to University Hospital.

With the positive interest shown by Fred McCracken, Lucy and her staff at University Hospital began the difficult job of investigating the legal issues and placing a value on General. Since both entities were not-for-profit, it would not be necessary to establish a charitable foundation; the proceeds of the sale would still be used (at least by legal definition) for charitable purposes.

Regarding valuation, University's financial staff first estimated what General's earnings before interest, taxes, depreciation, and amortization (EBITDA) would be if the transaction were completed. The cash flow analysis paid special attention to the synergistic benefits of the proposed merger. Specifically, cost savings were expected from combining some services, and other savings plus additional revenues were forecasted from converting one inpatient wing to outpatient services. Then, a market value was estimated by applying a market multiple of seven to the resulting EBITDA estimate. The multiple of seven was chosen because, at the time of the analysis, Columbia/HCA, OrNda, Tenet, and Quorum all had observable market multiples of 6.9 to 7.5 times EBITDA. The end result was a valuation estimate of close to $100 million.

After further negotiation, and a due diligence analysis, a deal was struck. No objections were raised by federal or state regulators, so the acquisition was completed in 1996. It is much too early to pass judgment on the acquisition, but Lucy Radcliffe feels confident that University Hospital did the right thing. "At least," she said, "we reacted early to changing market conditions, and now we are much better positioned to deal with the realities of the marketplace."

SELF-ASSESSMENT EXERCISES

9–1 Discuss the primary motives for mergers. Which motives have merit, and which do not?

9–2 a. What is the difference between a hostile and a friendly merger?

b. Is it possible to have a hostile acquisition of a not-for-profit firm?

9–3 a. Merger regulation falls into what two categories?

b. What is the purpose of bid procedure regulation?

c. What is the purpose of antitrust regulation?

d. Who are the primary federal antitrust regulators? What special problems do they face?

9–4 Briefly explain the discounted cash flow (DCF) and market multiple approaches to merger valuation.

9–5 Continental Healthcare, a large for-profit hospital system, is evaluating the possible acquisition of Brandon Memorial Hospital, a stand-alone for-profit hospital. Continental's financial staff forecasts the following postmerger net cash flows should the acquisition take place (in millions of dollars). Note that the cash flow for 2001 includes a terminal value to account for all cash flows occurring in 2002 and beyond.

1998	$ 12
1999	19
2000	23
2001	429

The acquisition, if made, would occur on January 1, 1998. All cash flows are assumed to occur at year-end. Brandon Hospital currently has a market value capital structure of only 10 percent debt, but Continental would increase Brandon's debt to 50 percent if the acquisition were completed. Brandon's current tax rate is 30 percent, but its income would be taxed at 40 percent if it is consolidated with Continental's income. Brandon's current market-determined beta is 1.20.

All interest payments and retentions to finance growth have been incorporated into the estimated cash flows. Thus, the net cash flows listed above would accrue to Continental's stockholders should the acquisition occur.

    a. What is the appropriate discount rate for valuing the acquisition? (Assume a risk-free rate of 7 percent and a market risk premium of 6 percent.)

    b. What is the value of Brandon to Continental?

    c. What special problems would occur if Brandon were a not-for-profit hospital?

SELECTED REFERENCES

Baumann, Barbara H. and Majorie R. Oxaal. "Estimating the Value of Group Medical Practices." *Healthcare Financial Management*, December 1993, pp. 58–65.

Becker, Scott and Robert J. Pristave. "Physician-Based Transactions: The Sale of Medical Practices, Ambulatory Surgery Centers, and Dialysis Facilities." *Journal of Health Care Finance*, Winter 1995, pp. 13–26.

Boo, Michael and Paul Louiselle. "Structuring Medical Practice Acquisitions." *Healthcare Financial Management*, December 1994, pp. 23–27.

Bryant, L. Edward, Jr. "Avoiding Antitrust Compliance Difficulties in Mergers and Acquisitions." *Healthcare Financial Management*, August 1993, pp. 48–58.

Collins, Hobart and Glenda Simpson. "Avoiding Pitfalls in Medical Practice Valuation." *Healthcare Financial Management*, March 1995, pp. 20–22.

Federa, R. Danielle and Jonathan S. Ketcham. "The Valuation of Medical Practices." *Topics in Health Care Financing*, Spring 1993, pp. 67–75.

Hahn, William. "Determining a Healthcare Organization's Value." *Healthcare Financial Management*, August 1994, pp. 40–44.

Hill, John E. and Jennifer Wild. "Survey Provides Data on Practice Acquisition Activity." *Healthcare Financial Management*, September 1995, pp. 54–72.

Meiling, Terence M., editor. "Mergers and Acquisitions." *Topics in Health Care Financing*, Summer 1989.

Peregrine, Michael W. and D. Louis Glaser. "Legal Issues in Medical Practice Acquisitions." *Healthcare Financial Management*, February 1995, pp. 70–76.

Reilly, Robert F. "The Valuation of a Medical Practice." *Health Care Management Review*, Summer 1990, pp. 25–34.

Rimmer, Timothy B. "Physician Practice Acquisitions: Valuation Issues and Concerns." *Hospital & Health Services Administration*, Fall 1995, pp. 415–25.

Unland, James J. *Valuation of Hospitals and Medical Centers* (Chicago: Health Management Research Institute, 1989).

Ward, Matthews E. and Susanna E. Krentz. "Diversification: Myths versus Realities." *Topics in Health Care Financing*, Fall 1988, pp. 32–39.

Williams, Latham. "Structuring Managed Care Joint Ventures." *Healthcare Financial Management*, August 1995, pp. 32–36.

10
CHAPTER

Financing Decisions:
Capital Structure

*R*oberta Williams, the recently hired CEO of San Gabriel Memorial Hospital, knew she had a tough assignment. The not-for-profit hospital prospered during the 1970s and 1980s, but a combination of circumstances, including increasing competition, rising operating costs, and increasing managed care penetration, has led to recent poor financial performance and a current financial condition that had been termed "critical" by the local press. In fact, Roberta was hired specifically to get the hospital back on track, and her contract gave her only one year to show improvement.

Roberta believed strongly that the first thing she needed to accomplish was to gain a thorough understanding of the hospital's current financial condition. This process would give her many insights into what occurred historically and, hopefully, generate some ideas about what might be done to stem the hospital's negative momentum.

One of the elements of the hospital's current condition that bothered her most was the large amount of debt financing. San Gabriel's current debt ratio, which is defined as total debt divided by total assets, is 60 percent. That meant that every dollar of assets was financed by 60 cents

worth of debt and only 40 cents of fund capital. The debt ratio of compa-
rable hospitals, as reported by a national data service, is only 35 percent.
This startling observation prompted many questions, such as Why do
firms use debt financing in the first place? Is there some right amount of
debt usage, or doesn't it matter? Should a firm be concerned if its use of
debt is way out of line with other firms in the same line of business?

During her first year at San Gabriel, Roberta gained many new
insights, including some answers to the questions posed above. At the end
of the chapter, you can read about her conclusions regarding debt financ-
ing and see if she was successful in turning the situation around.

INTRODUCTION

In Chapter 6, in the discussion of a firm's overall cost of capital, it
was noted that the weights used in the cost of capital formula (w_d
and w_s) represent the firm's optimal, or target, mix of debt and
equity financing, which is the financing mix that the firm plans to
use for asset acquisitions over the long run. Unfortunately, setting
the optimal, or target, capital structure is one of the most perplex-
ing issues facing managers. The term *capital structure* means the
structure of the capital, or liability and equity, side of the balance
sheet, so capital structure decisions involve (1) setting the mix of
debt and equity financing and (2) given the target amount of debt
financing, setting the mix of short-term and long-term debt.

The discussion of capital structure decisions will begin by
examining the impact of debt financing on a firm's risk and return.
Then, the chapter will summarize the most important capital structure theories, which attempt to define the relationship between the
use of debt financing and firm value. Next, the discussion will
focus on how managers actually make capital structure decisions
in practice. Finally, the chapter presents some concepts relevant to
the choice between long-term and short-term debt financing.

IMPACT OF DEBT FINANCING ON RISK AND RETURN

Perhaps the most important concept in capital structure decisions
is the impact of debt financing on a business's risk and return. The
best way to present this concept is by use of an illustration. Assume
that you are about to start a new company. Let's call it Super
Health, Inc. The company requires two hundred dollars in assets to

get into operation, and there are only two financing alternatives available to you: (1) all equity (all common stock) and (2) 50 percent equity and 50 percent debt. (If you want to think big, assume that all dollar amounts are in millions.)

Table 10–1 contains the business's projected financial statements under the two financing alternatives. To begin, consider the balance sheets shown in the top portion of the table. The business will require one hundred dollars in current assets and one hundred dollars in fixed assets to begin operations. Since the asset requirement depends on the nature and size of the business rather than on how the business will be financed, the asset side of the balance

TABLE 10–1

Super Health, Inc.
Projected Financial Statements under Two Financing Alternatives

Balance Sheets:	Stock	Stock/Debt
Current assets	$100	$100
Fixed assets	100	100
Total assets	$200	$200
Debt (10% cost)	$ 0	$100
Common stock	200	100
Total claims	$200	$200
Income Statements:	Stock	Stock/Debt
Revenues	$150	$150
Operating costs	100	100
Operating income	$ 50	$ 50
Interest expense	0	10
Taxable income	$ 50	$ 40
Taxes (40%)	20	16
Net income	$ 30	$ 24
ROE	15%	24%
Total dollar return to investors	$ 30	$ 34

sheet is unaffected by the financing scheme. However, the capital, or liabilities and equity, side of the balance sheet is impacted by the type of financing. Under the all-equity alternative, you will put up the entire two hundred dollars needed to purchase the assets. If 50 percent debt financing is used, you will contribute only one hundred dollars of your own funds, and the remaining one hundred dollars will be obtained from creditors, for example, a bank loan with a 10 percent interest rate.

Now consider the impact of the two financing alternatives on the business's projected income statement. Revenues are projected to be $150, and operating costs are forecasted at $100, so the firm's operating income (earnings before interest and taxes) is expected to be $50. Since the method of financing does not impact revenues and operating costs, the operating income projection is the same under both financing alternatives. However, interest expense must be paid if debt financing is used, so the stock/debt alternative results in a 0.10($100) = $10 annual interest charge, while no interest expense occurs if the firm is financed entirely by stock. The result is taxable income of $50 under the all-equity alternative and lower taxable income of $40 under the stock/debt alternative. Since the business anticipates being taxed at a 40 percent federal-plus-state rate, the expected tax liability is 0.40($50) = $20 under the all-equity alternative and 0.40($40) = $16 for the stock/debt alternative. Finally, when taxes are deducted from the income stream, the business projects $30 in net income if all-equity financed and $24 in net income if 50 percent debt financing is used.

At first blush, debt financing appears to be the inferior alternative. After all, if you use 50 percent debt financing, the business's projected net income will fall by $30 − $24 = $6. But the conclusion that debt financing is bad requires closer examination. What is most important to you, the equity investor in Super Health, is not the business's net income but, rather, the return that you achieve on your investment. Perhaps the most meaningful measure of return to a firm's owners (stockholders) is the rate of return on equity, or just return on equity (ROE), which is defined as net income/common stock. This measure tells stock investors (owners) the percentage return on their investment. Under all-equity financing, your projected ROE is $30/$200 = 0.15 = 15%, but with 50 percent debt financing, projected ROE increases to $24/$100 = 24%. The key here is that although net income decreases with debt financing, so does the amount of capital you need to put up, and the capital requirement decreases proportionally more than does net income.

The end result is that the use of debt financing increases your rate of return on invested capital. Why does this positive result happen? There is no magic here; the key is in the tax code: Interest expense is tax deductible for investor-owned firms. To understand the impact of the tax deductibility of interest, take another look at the Table 10–1 income statements. The total dollar return to all investors, including both you and the creditor, is $30 net income if all-equity financed, but $24 net income plus $10 interest = $34 when 50 percent debt financing is used. Where did the "extra" four dollars come from? The answer is "from the tax man." Taxes are $20 if the business is all-equity financed, but only $16 when debt financing is used, and $4 less in taxes means $4 more for investors. Because debt financing reduces taxes, more of a firm's operating income is available for distribution to investors (including both stockholders and creditors).

It now appears that the financing decision on your business is clear. Given only two alternatives, you should use the 50 percent debt alternative because it provides you (the stockholder) with the higher return. Unfortunately, as with the proverbial fine print, there is a catch. The use of debt financing not only increases the return to equity holders, it also increases their risk. Table 10–2 demonstrates the risk-increasing characteristics of debt financing. Here, we recognize that your business, like all businesses, is risky. You really don't know precisely what the first year's revenues and operating costs will be. Assume, for illustrative purposes, that Revenues – Operating costs = Operating income could be as low as zero or as high as one hundred dollars in the business's first year of operation. Furthermore, assume there is a 25 percent chance of the worst and best cases occurring, and a 50 percent chance that the Table 10–1 forecast will be realized.

The assumptions regarding uncertainty in the future profitability of the business lead to three different ROEs for each financing alternative. The expected ROEs are the same as when we ignored uncertainty, that is, 15 percent if the firm is all-equity financed and 24 percent when 50 percent debt financing is used. However, the uncertainty in operating income produces uncertain-

TABLE 10–2

Super Health, Inc.
Partial Income Statements in an Uncertain World

	Stock			Stock/Debt		
Probability	0.25	0.50	0.25	0.25	0.50	0.25
Operating income	$0	$50	$100	$ 0	$50	$100
Interest expense	0	0	0	10	10	10
Taxable income	$0	$50	$100	($10)	$40	$ 90
Taxes (40%)	0	20	40	(4)	16	36
Net income	$0	$30	$ 60	($ 6)	$24	$ 54
ROE	0%	15%	30%	–6%	24%	54%
Expected ROE		15%			24%	
Standard deviation of ROE		10.6%			21.2%	

ty, hence risk, in stockholder returns. If we measure stockholders' risk by the standard deviation of ROE, we see that the return is more risky when we use 50 percent debt financing. To be precise, the risk to stockholders is twice as much in the 50 percent debt financing alternative, 21.2 percent standard deviation of ROE versus 10.6 percent in the zero debt alternative. The conclusions would be similar if we had focused on market risk: The firm's beta coefficient would be higher with 50 percent debt financing than with zero debt.

The increase in risk is apparent without doing any calculations. If you use only stock financing, the worst you can do is an ROE of zero. However, with 50 percent debt financing, you could realize an ROE of –6 percent. (Here, the assumption is made that the business's $10 loss could be used to offset your personal income, so you can realize a $4 tax savings.) In fact, with no operating income to pay the $10 interest to the bank in the worst scenario, you, as the owner, would either have to put up additional funds to pay the interest due or declare bankruptcy. Clearly, the use of 50 percent debt financing has increased the riskiness of your equity investment in the firm. This simple illustration results in two key points about the use of debt financing:

1. The use of debt financing increases the percentage return (ROE) to the firm's stockholders. (However, even here there is a catch. For the use of debt financing to increase stockholder returns, the inherent return on the business must be greater than the interest rate on the debt. The basic business return in the illustration is 25 percent [$50 in operating income from $200 in assets], and debt financing costs only 10 percent, so the use of debt financing increases ROE.)

2. At the same time that return is increased, the use of debt financing also increases the risk to stockholders. As illustrated by the example, 50 percent debt financing doubles the risk to stockholders (as measured by standard deviation of ROE).

The ultimate decision as to which financing alternative you should choose is not clear-cut. One alternative (no debt) has a lower expected ROE but also lower risk. The second alternative (50 percent debt) offers a higher expected ROE but only at the price of higher risk. Later sections will try to resolve your dilemma as to whether or not to use debt financing, but first some other topics must be introduced.

MEASURING THE AMOUNT OF DEBT FINANCING

As discussed throughout this chapter, the extent to which a firm uses debt financing has important implications. Thus, it is essential that managers be able to measure the amount of debt financing their firms use. The primary approach to measuring debt usage is to combine elements from the firm's balance sheet, or from both the income statement and balance sheet, in such a way as to express quickly and easily the amount and impact of the firm's debt. Thus, for the most part, debt usage is measured in terms of book values since the information is taken from the firm's financial statements, or "books." From a financial perspective, more meaningful measures are created for investor-owned firms when market values are examined. For example, the market value of a firm's equity is merely the number of shares outstanding multiplied by the current stock price. However, market values can fluctuate widely in short periods, and not-for-profit firms do not have equity market values, so we will confine our discussion to book-value measures.

There are two different types of ratios that measure debt usage. One type focuses on balance sheet data to determine the extent to which borrowed funds have been used to finance assets;

these ratios are called capitalization ratios. The second type uses income statement data to determine how much operating income is available to meet financial charges; these ratios are called coverage ratios. The two sets of ratios are complementary, so both types are widely used.

To illustrate some common debt-utilization measures, consider the data from the Stock/Debt column in Table 10–1, which shows the debt financing alternative for Super Health, Inc. One common capitalization ratio is the ratio of total debt to total assets, which is generally called the debt-to-assets ratio or merely the debt ratio. It measures the percentage of total funds provided by creditors.

$$\text{Debt ratio} = \frac{\text{Total debt}}{\text{Total assets}} = \frac{\$100}{\$200} = 0.500 = 50.0\%$$

Note that *debt* is defined here to include both current liabilities and long-term debt. (A variation of this ratio is defined as long-term debt divided by the sum of long-term debt plus equity; this ratio focuses on the debt proportion of permanent capital.) Creditors prefer low debt ratios, since the lower the ratio, the greater the cushion against creditors' losses in the event of liquidation. Managers, on the other hand, may seek higher debt usage either to leverage up owners' returns or to offer more services when the amount of equity is constrained. Super Health's debt ratio is 50 percent under the stock/debt alternative; this means that its creditors would supply exactly one-half of the firm's total financing.

Another capitalization ratio that is often used is the debt-to-equity ratio.

$$\text{Debt to equity ratio} = \frac{\text{Total debt}}{\text{Total equity}} = \frac{\$100}{\$100} = 1.00$$

Both ratios provide the same information, and both ratios increase as a firm of a given size (total assets) uses a greater proportion of debt, but the debt ratio rises linearly and approaches a limit of 100 percent, while the debt-to-equity ratio rises exponentially and approaches infinity. Some analysts, especially those who work for banks and other creditors, prefer the debt-to-equity ratio because it indicates explicitly the dollars of creditors' capital per dollar of owners' (or fund) capital used to finance the company's assets. For example, Super Health's debt-to-equity ratio of 1.00 indicates that creditors would supply one dollar of capital for each dollar put up by stockholders.

The times-interest-earned (TIE) ratio is an example of a coverage ratio. It is determined by dividing operating income (earnings before interest and taxes) by the interest charges.

$$\text{TIE ratio} = \frac{\text{Operating income}}{\text{Interest expense}} = \frac{\$50}{\$10} = 5.0$$

The TIE ratio uses earnings before interest and taxes (operating income) in the numerator. Because interest is a deductible (pretax) expense, the ability of investor-owned firms to pay current interest is not affected by taxes. The TIE ratio measures the extent to which operating income can decline before the firm's earnings are less than its annual interest costs. Failure to pay interest can bring legal action by the firm's creditors, possibly resulting in bankruptcy. Super Health's interest is covered five times, so it would take a dramatic decrease in the firm's operating earnings before its ability to meet its interest payments would be threatened.

Note that coverage ratios are often better measures of a firm's debt utilization than capitalization ratios because coverage ratios discriminate between low interest rate debt and high interest rate debt. For example, consider two hospitals with $30 million in assets and $2 million in operating income. One hospital might have $10 million of 4 percent debt on its balance sheet, while the other might have $10 million of 8 percent debt. Both hospitals would show the same $10/$30 = 0.333 = 33.3 percent debt ratio. However, the hospital with 4 percent debt is clearly in a better financial position; its debt burden is not as great as the hospital with the same amount of 8 percent debt. The TIE ratio provides this information, as the low-interest-rate hospital would show a TIE ratio of $2/$0.4 = 5.0 times, while the high-interest-rate hospital would have a TIE of only $2/$0.8 = 2.5 times.

Finally, note that the TIE ratio can be expanded to (1) include more categories of fixed charges and (2) recognize that a firm, because of noncash charges, typically has additional cash flow to meet its fixed charge obligations. For example, fixed charges such as lease payments and debt principal repayments can be added to the denominator, and depreciation cash flow can be added to the numerator.

BUSINESS AND FINANCIAL RISK

In earlier chapters, we discussed several dimensions of risk, including stand-alone risk, corporate risk, and market risk. Now we introduce two more dimensions: (1) business risk, or the riskiness to the firm's stockholders if it uses no debt financing and (2) financial risk, the additional risk placed on common stockholders as a result of the firm's decision to use debt (or preferred stock) financing. Note that the concepts of business and financial risk are as applicable to not-for-profit businesses as they are to for-profit businesses, but in not-for-profits the risk applies to the firm's non-creditor stakeholders rather than common stockholders.

Business Risk

Business risk is the inherent riskiness of the business as seen by its stockholders, and it is measured by the uncertainty inherent in a firm's ROE, *assuming that the firm uses no debt financing.* To illustrate the concept of business risk, consider Santa Fe Healthcare, Inc., a *debt-free,* investor-owned hospital chain that operates in the Southwestern United States. Figure 10–1 provides some insights into the company's business risk. The graph on the right side gives both security analysts and Santa Fe's management an idea of the historical variability of ROE and consequently how the firm's ROE might vary in the future. This graph also shows that Santa Fe's ROE is growing slowly, so the relevant variability of ROE is the dis-

FIGURE 10–1

Santa Fe Healthcare, Inc.: Historical and Forecasted Return on Equity (ROE)

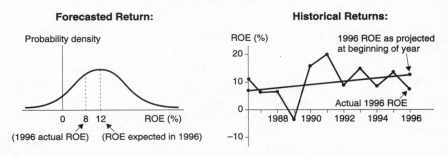

persion about the trend line rather than the overall standard deviation of historical ROE.

The graph on the left side shows the beginning-of-year subjectively estimated probability distribution of Santa Fe's ROE for 1996, based on the trend line on the right side of Figure 10–1. As both graphs indicate, Santa Fe's actual ROE in 1996 was only 8 percent, well below the expected value of 12 percent; 1996 was a bad year.

Santa Fe's past fluctuations in ROE were caused by many factors: Changes in the economy, actions by competing hospitals, payment policies of third-party payers, results of contract negotiations with managed care plans, a large liability loss at one of Santa Fe's hospitals, changing labor costs, and so on. Similar events will undoubtedly occur in the future, and when they do, Santa Fe's realized ROE will almost always be higher or lower than the projected level. Furthermore, there is always the possibility that a long-term disaster might strike, permanently depressing the company's earning power; for example, the government may move to a single-payer system with dramatically reduced hospital reimbursement rates. *Since Santa Fe uses no debt financing,* this uncertainty regarding the firm's future ROE is defined as the company's basic business risk.

Business risk varies not only from industry to industry but also among firms in a given industry. Furthermore, business risk can change over time. For example, acute-care hospitals were regarded for years as having little business risk, but events in the 1980s and 1990s (primarily the move of third-party payers to prospective payment and large discounts from charges) altered the hospitals' situation, producing sharp declines in their ROEs and greatly increasing the industry's business risk.

Business risk depends on a number of factors, including the following:

1. *Demand variability.* The more stable the demand for a firm's products or services, other things held constant, the lower its business risk.

2. *Sales price variability.* Firms whose products or services are sold in markets with highly volatile prices are exposed to more business risk than firms whose sales prices are more stable.

3. *Input cost variability.* Firms whose input costs (labor, materials, and capital) are highly uncertain are exposed to a high degree of business risk.

4. *Ability to adjust output prices when input costs rise.* Some firms are better able than others to raise their own output prices when input costs rise. The greater the ability to adjust output prices to reflect cost conditions, the lower the degree of business risk, other things held constant.

5. *Need to develop new products.* Firms in high-tech industries, such as drug manufacturers, depend on a constant stream of new products. The faster a firm's products become obsolete, the greater its business risk.

6. *Liability exposure.* Firms that have high exposure to liability losses have greater business risk than companies with limited exposure. This is especially true for firms subject to product liability or malpractice litigation.

7. *The extent to which costs are fixed: operating leverage.* If a high percentage of a firm's costs are fixed and hence do not decline when demand falls off, the firm is exposed to a relatively high degree of business risk. This factor is called operating leverage, and it is discussed in more detail later in the chapter.

Each of these factors is determined partly by the firm's industry characteristics, but each of them is also controllable to some extent by management. For example, most firms can, through their marketing policies, take actions to stabilize both unit sales and sales prices. However, this stabilization may require firms to spend a great deal on advertising and/or price concessions to get commitments from their customers to purchase fixed quantities at fixed prices in the future.

As noted above, business risk depends in part on the extent to which a firm builds fixed costs into its operations. If fixed costs are high, even a small decline in sales can lead to a large decline in ROE; so, other things held constant, the higher a firm's fixed costs, the greater its business risk. Higher fixed costs are generally associated with more highly technical, capital-intensive firms and industries. Thus, hospitals have higher fixed costs, relative to total costs, than do home healthcare agencies. Also, businesses, such as many healthcare providers, that employ highly skilled workers who must be retained and paid even during periods of low demand have a relatively high proportion of fixed costs.

If a high percentage of a firm's total costs are fixed, the firm is said to have a high degree of operating leverage. In physics, leverage implies the use of a lever to raise a heavy object with a small force. In politics, if people have leverage, their smallest word or action can accomplish a great deal. In business terminology, a high degree of operating leverage, other factors held constant, implies that a relatively small change in sales results in a large change in ROE, even when no debt financing is used.

To what extent can firms control their operating leverage? To a large extent, operating leverage is determined by industry characteristics. Companies such as drug manufacturers, hospitals, and ambulatory care clinics simply must have heavy investments in fixed assets; this results in high fixed costs and operating leverage. On the other hand, companies such as home health agencies generally have significantly lower fixed costs and hence lower operating leverage. Still, although industry factors exert a major influence, all firms do have some control over their operating leverage. For example, a hospital can expand its diagnostic imaging capability by either buying a new imaging device or by leasing it on a per-procedure basis. (Per-procedure leases are discussed in Chapter 11.) If the device is purchased, the hospital would incur fixed costs, but the device's per-procedure operating costs would be relatively low. If the device is leased, the hospital would have lower fixed costs, but the variable (per-procedure) costs for the device would be high. Thus, by its financing decisions (and also by its capital budgeting decisions), a firm can influence its operating leverage and hence its business risk.

The concept of operating leverage was, in fact, originally developed for use in capital investment decision making. Competing projects that involve alternative methods for producing a given product or service often have different degrees of operating leverage and thus different break-even points and different degrees of risk. Santa Fe and many other companies regularly undertake a type of break-even analysis (the sensitivity analyses discussed in Chapter 8) for each proposed project as a part of their regular capital budgeting process. Still, once a firm's operating leverage has been established, it exerts a major influence on the capital structure decision.

Financial Risk

Financial risk is the additional risk placed on the common stockholders as a result of the decision to use debt (or preferred stock) financing. Conceptually, a firm has a certain amount of risk inherent in its operations. This is its business risk, which is defined as the uncertainty inherent in projections of future ROE, assuming that the firm is all-equity financed. If a firm uses debt financing, or financial leverage, its business risk is concentrated on the common stockholders.

To illustrate, suppose four physicians decide to incorporate a group practice. There is a certain amount of business risk in the operation. If the firm is capitalized only with common equity and if each physician buys 25 percent of the stock, they share the business risk equally. However, suppose the firm is capitalized with 50 percent debt and 50 percent equity, with two of the physicians putting up their capital as debt and the other two putting up their capital as equity. In this case, those investors who put up the equity will have to bear all of the business risk, so the common stock will be twice as risky as it would have been had the firm been financed only with equity. (Remember the Super Health illustration in Table 10–2; the use of 50 percent debt doubled the riskiness to stockholders.) Since the return to debtholders is fixed by contract and is independent of fluctuations in the firm's revenues and costs, creditors do not bear any of the firm's business risk. Thus, the use of financial leverage concentrates the firm's business risk on its stockholders.

Business and financial risk can be easily measured. Refer again to Table 10–2. The standard deviation of ROE to Super Health if it used no debt financing, $\sigma_{ROE(U)}$ where U stands for unleveraged (no debt), is a measure of the business risk seen by stockholders. The standard deviation of ROE at any positive debt level, $\sigma_{ROE(L)}$ where L stands for leveraged (some debt), is a measure of the actual stand-alone risk borne by stockholders. Because the use of debt financing increases the risk to stockholders, $\sigma_{ROE(L)}$ is always greater than $\sigma_{ROE(U)}$ and the financial risk seen by stockholders is $\sigma_{ROE(L)} - \sigma_{ROE(U)}$. Applying these measures to Super Health, we see that the business risk to stockholders is $\sigma_{ROE(U)} =$

10.6%, but the actual stand-alone risk borne by stockholders under 50 percent debt financing is $\sigma_{ROE(L)} = 21.2\%$, so the financial risk to stockholders is $\sigma_{ROE(L)} - \sigma_{ROE(U)} = 21.2\% - 10.6\% = 10.6\%$.

Operating leverage and financial leverage normally work in the same way; they both increase expected ROE, but they also increase the risk borne by stockholders. Operating leverage affects the business risk seen by stockholders, while financial leverage affects the financial risk borne by stockholders.

CAPITAL STRUCTURE THEORY FOR INVESTOR-OWNED FIRMS

The previous discussion pointed out that the use of debt financing increases the expected rate of return to stockholders, but it also increases their risk. The obvious question at this point is whether the benefit of debt financing (increased expected return) exceeds the cost of debt financing (increased risk). Capital structure theory attempts to establish the relationship between the amount of debt financing and the firm's stock price, and thus its goal is to determine whether, on net, the use of financial leverage is beneficial. This section discusses the two major capital structure theories, which were developed for investor-owned firms. The next major section discusses whether or not these theories apply to not-for-profit businesses.

The Trade-Off Theory

There are two major competing theories of capital structure: (1) the trade-off theory and (2) the asymmetric information theory. The trade-off theory is the most widely accepted debt/equity choice theory in corporate finance. This theory is based on the premise that the use of financial leverage (debt financing in lieu of equity financing) involves a trade-off between the costs and benefits associated with debt financing. In this framework, the optimal capital structure occurs when the marginal costs of debt financing equal the marginal benefits. At this structure, the net benefit of debt financing is maximized.

Let's begin the discussion of the trade-off theory by looking at the benefit of debt financing. The primary benefit of debt financing to taxable firms is the tax deductibility of interest payments. (We will ignore a second benefit, the capital pass-through of interest payments by third-party payers, since this benefit is being phased out.) Federal and state governments subsidize the use of debt financing by allowing firms to deduct interest payments from taxable income. No such subsidy exists for equity financing because the return to stockholders—net income and ultimately dividends—comes from after-tax earnings.

Since debt financing is subsidized while equity financing is not, shouldn't firms use virtually all debt financing? Common sense tells us that very high debt levels are bad, and the trade-off theory tells us why: The use of debt financing brings with it indirect costs. Note that the direct cost of debt financing is the interest expense, while the direct cost of equity financing is dividend payments. In general, the direct cost of equity is higher than the direct cost of debt. For example, the cost of equity to Columbia/HCA Healthcare might be 14 percent, while the firm's cost of debt might be 8 percent. The direct cost differential between these capital sources stems from the fact that debt is a less risky security for investors than common stock is. (The payment of interest is a contractual obligation, while the payment of dividends is not.)

The riskiness of debt and equity to the firm is the mirror image of the riskiness to investors. Thus, a firm is willing to issue common stock, even though its direct cost is greater than the cost of debt capital, because equity capital is less risky from the firm's perspective. If the debt and equity markets are efficient, the direct costs of the two capital sources to firms are exactly commensurate with the risks inherent in each type of capital; so, there is no benefit to debt over equity financing, even though the direct cost of debt is less than the direct cost of equity. The benefit of debt arises because U.S. tax laws effectively reduce the cost of debt below the market-determined rate; thus, its direct cost to the firm is less than that commensurate with its riskiness.

Now that we understand the direct costs of debt and equity financing, what are the indirect costs associated with debt financing? Assuming a business is reasonably profitable, a small amount of debt financing exposes creditors to an almost imperceptible probability of default. Thus, rating agencies will give the debt a high rating, and investors will demand a relatively low coupon rate in the debt markets. However, as a firm uses more and more debt financing (in place of equity financing), the probability of default increases, rating agencies will lower the firm's bond rating, and debt investors will demand higher coupon rates. This increase in the cost of debt as the proportion of debt in a firm's capital structure increases is one of the indirect costs of debt financing.

The same concept regarding the indirect cost of debt holds for equity financing. That is, the greater the use of debt financing, the greater the risk to stockholders. Thus, the cost of equity, like the cost of debt, increases as the proportion of debt financing increases.

There is a second indirect cost to debt financing that affects stockholders. Higher debt levels increase a firm's probability of facing financial distress that, at the extreme, can lead to bankruptcy and closure. Furthermore, financial distress produces costs that must be borne by the firm's stockholders. For example, financial distress diverts managers' energies away from their primary jobs of running the firm's operations, and financial distress can also lead to managerial decisions that are suboptimal in the long run. Finally, financial distress may cause employees, customers, and suppliers to hold the firm in low regard, which can result in a loss of sales and an increase in operating costs, both of which have a negative impact on a firm's financial condition. Other costs of financial distress include the legal and administrative costs associated with bankruptcy, the loss of asset value that can occur during liquidation proceedings, and the costs to the community of losing local healthcare services.

Under the trade-off theory, the use of debt financing has a tax benefit that increases as more and more debt is used (more debt leads to higher interest deductions). On the down side, debt brings with it risk and financial distress costs that increase with financial leverage. The benefits increase at a more or less constant rate because each additional dollar of debt produces a similar marginal benefit. However, the indirect costs first increase at a relatively slow rate, but as the firm uses more and more debt financing, the rate of increase in indirect costs itself increases.

The optimal capital structure is that mix of debt and equity financing that balances the marginal costs and marginal benefits of debt financing. Figure 10–2 depicts the benefit–cost relationship. The benefit from tax deductibility increases linearly with each additional dollar of debt financing. (Again, remember that we are

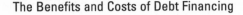

F I G U R E   10–2

The Benefits and Costs of Debt Financing

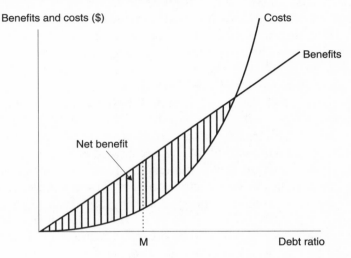

replacing one dollar of equity when we add a dollar of debt.) The indirect costs associated with debt financing are trivial for small amounts of debt but increase rapidly as more and more debt is added to a firm's capital structure. The net benefit of debt financing is the vertical distance between the two curves, and this benefit is maximized at point M. Any debt added beyond Point M has a marginal cost that exceeds the marginal benefit, so the net benefit of debt financing is reduced if the firm's capital structure is to the right of this point.

Unfortunately, the trade-off model is more of a conceptual framework than a true model that provides managers the means to determine a firm's optimal capital structure. That is, we cannot apply some formula to a particular firm and end up knowing that the firm's optimal capital structure is, say, 35 percent debt and 65 percent equity financing. However, the trade-off theory does provide some insights as to which firms should use more debt financing and which firms should use less.

    1. Firms with higher business risk, as measured by the variability of ROE if the firm used no debt financing, ought to borrow less than lower-risk firms, other things being equal. The greater the variability of earnings, the greater the probability of financial distress at any level of debt and hence the greater the expected costs of financial distress. Thus, firms with lower business risk can borrow more before the indirect costs outweigh the tax advantage of borrowing.

2. Firms that employ tangible assets such as real estate and standardized equipment should borrow more than firms whose value is derived either from intangible assets such as patents and goodwill or from growth opportunities. The costs of financial distress depend not only on the probability of incurring distress but also on what happens if distress occurs. Specialized assets, intangible assets, and growth opportunities are more likely to lose value if financial distress occurs than are standardized, tangible assets.

3. Firms that are currently paying taxes at the highest rate, and that are likely to continue to do so in the future, should carry more debt than firms with current and/or prospectively lower tax rates. High corporate tax rates lead to greater benefits from debt financing; hence, high-tax-rate firms can carry more debt, other factors held constant, before the tax benefit is offset by indirect costs.

According to the trade-off model, each firm should set its target capital structure such that its indirect costs and benefits of leverage are balanced at the margin because such a structure will maximize its value. Once a firm estimates its optimal capital structure, or at least an optimal range, it becomes the firm's target structure. Financing decisions should be consistent with the goal of keeping the firm's actual capital structure within the target range. This implies a balanced approach to financing, in which both debt and equity funding are used over time.

Asymmetric Information Theory

Many surveys have been conducted to find out how managers of for-profit firms make financing decisions. For the most part, these surveys reach the following conclusions:

1. Firms prefer to finance with internally generated funds, that is, with retained earnings and depreciation cash flow.

2. Firms set target dividend payout ratios on the basis of their expected future investment opportunities and their expected future cash flows. (The dividend payout ratio is dividends/net income or the percentage of net income paid out as dividends.) The target payout ratio is set at a level such that retentions plus depreciation cash flow will meet capital expenditure requirements under normal conditions.

3. Dividends are "sticky" in the short-run. Firms are reluctant to make major changes in the dollar dividend, and they are especially reluctant to cut the dividend. Thus, in any given year, depending on realized cash flows and actual investment opportunities, a firm may or may not have sufficient internally generated funds to cover its capital expenditures.

4. If the firm has more internal cash flow than is needed for capital investment, it will invest the excess in marketable securities (safe, temporary investments) or else use the funds to retire debt.

5. If the firm has insufficient internal cash flow to finance its capital investments, it will first draw down its marketable securities portfolio, then issue debt, then issue convertible bonds (bonds that can be exchanged for stock in the future), and only as a last resort, issue new common stock.

Thus, surveys indicate that managers follow a "pecking order" of financing, not the balanced approach that is called for by the trade-off theory. Until recently, there was no theory to explain this observed behavior of firms, so the survey results were not given much credence by academicians. Then, the asymmetric information theory of capital structure was developed. The theory is based on two assumptions: (1) managers know more about their firms' future prospects than investors do, and (2) managers are motivated to maximize the wealth of their firms' current shareholders.

If managers think their firm's stock is undervalued in the marketplace, they will be motivated to use debt financing; but if managers think their firm's stock is overvalued, they will be motivated to issue new common stock. However, investors are rational, and they recognize the bias for managers to issue new common stock only when it is overvalued. New common stock issues are treated by investors as "signals" that management considers the stock to be overvalued, and thus investors revise downward their expectations for the firm, and the stock price falls.

Since new stock issues have an adverse impact on stock price, managers are reluctant to issue new stock. If external financing is required, debt is the first choice, and new common stock would only be used in unusual circumstances. Thus, the asymmetric information theory leads managers to act in accordance with the pecking order indicated by surveys.

A Summary of Capital Structure Theory

The trade-off theory is summarized in Figures 10–3a and 10–3b. The first graph shows the relationships between the amount of debt financing as measured by the debt ratio (total debt divided by total assets) and the cost of debt, cost of equity, and the overall cost of capital, while the second graph shows the relationship between debt usage and stock price. Note one very important point: Debt usage is measured by the percentage of debt financing, say 30 percent or 50 percent or 75 percent, not the dollar amount. Large firms use a large dollar amount of debt financing, and small firms use a small dollar amount; the critical variable here is the debt/equity

FIGURE 10–3a

Capital Costs and Stock Price under the Trade-Off Theory

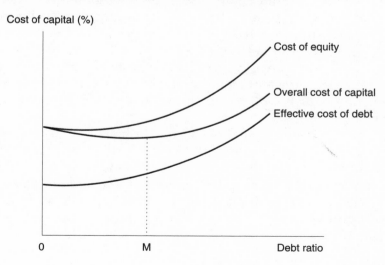

F I G U R E   10–3b

Stock Price

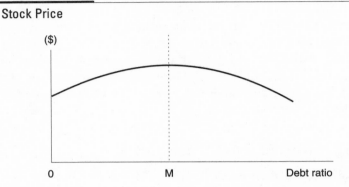

mix because we are trying to assess the effect of substituting debt financing for equity financing.

In Figure 10–3a, both the cost of debt and the cost of equity rise steadily with increases in leverage, but the rate of increase accelerates at higher debt levels, reflecting the increased probability of financial distress and its attendant costs. However, the cost of debt is effectively reduced by the tax subsidy, so the cost of debt curve is lower than it would be if interest expense were not tax deductible. The effective cost of debt to taxable firms plotted in Figure 10–3a is actually the before-tax cost multiplied by (1 − Tax rate).

The overall cost of capital is merely the weighted average of the costs of debt and equity. When the first amounts of debt are added to a firm's capital structure, the addition of the lower-cost debt causes the overall cost of capital to decline. However, as more and more debt is added, both the cost of equity and the cost of debt rise, and these increasing component costs eventually overcome the advantage inherent in adding more and more lower-cost debt. Thus, the overall cost of capital eventually hits a minimum and then begins to rise.

As shown in Figure 10–3b, the firm's stock price reacts to leverage similarly, but opposite, to the overall cost of capital. Stock price first rises, then reaches a maximum, and then falls. Note that the amount of debt that results in the lowest overall cost of capital also results in the highest stock price. This is shown as Point M in both figures. Thus, a firm's cost of capital is minimized, and its stock price is maximized at the same capital structure.

Unfortunately, it is extremely difficult for financial managers to actually quantify capital costs at different levels of debt, so it is virtually impossible to draw a real-world graph such as Figure 10–3b for a particular firm to pinpoint the capital structure that truly maximizes its stock price. Most experts believe such a structure exists for every taxable firm but that it changes substantially over time as tax laws, the nature of the firm, and the capital markets change. Most experts also believe that, as shown in Figure 10–3b, the relationship between stock price and financial leverage is relatively flat; thus, relatively large deviations from the optimum can occur without materially affecting stock price.

Now consider the asymmetric information theory. Because of asymmetric information, investors know less about a firm's prospects than its managers do. Furthermore, managers try to maximize value for current stockholders, not new ones; so if the firm has excellent prospects, management will not want to issue new shares, but if things look bleak, new stock may be sold. Therefore, investors take a stock offering to be a signal of bad news, so stock prices tend to decline when new issues are announced. As a result, new equity financing can be very expensive, and this fact must be incorporated into the capital structure decision. Its effect is to motivate firms to maintain a reserve borrowing capacity, which permits future investment opportunities to be financed by reasonably priced debt when internal funds are insufficient. Thus, asymmetric information creates the incentive for firms to operate at capital structures to the left of Point M in Figures 10–3a and 10–3b.

If the two theories are combined, this possible explanation for capital structure decisions of taxable firms results:

1. Debt financing provides benefits because of the tax deductibility of interest. Hence, firms should have some debt in their capital structures.

2. However, financial distress costs place limits on debt usage; beyond some point, these costs offset the tax advantage of debt.

3. Finally, because of asymmetric information, firms maintain a reserve borrowing capacity to take advantage of good investment opportunities and, at the same time, avoid having to issue stock at distressed prices.

APPLICATION OF CAPITAL STRUCTURE THEORY TO NOT-FOR-PROFIT FIRMS

So far, the discussion of capital structure theory has focused on investor-owned firms. Does the theory apply to not-for-profit firms? Although no rigorous research has been conducted into the optimal capital structures of not-for-profit firms, some loose analogies can be drawn. Not-for-profit firms do not receive a direct tax subsidy when debt financing is used, but they do have access to the tax-exempt debt markets, which provides an indirect tax subsidy because it permits them to borrow at below-market rates. Thus, not-for-profit firms receive about the same benefits from the use of debt financing as do investor-owned firms.

What about the costs associated with debt financing? As discussed in Chapter 6, a not-for-profit firm's fund capital has an opportunity cost that is roughly equivalent to the cost of equity of a similar investor-owned firm. Thus, we would expect the opportunity cost of fund capital to rise as more and more debt financing is used, just as for investor-owned firms, because more debt usage increases the riskiness to the noncreditor stakeholders. Furthermore, not-for-profit firms are subject to financial distress just like investor-owned firms, so these costs are equally applicable. Thus, we would expect the trade-off theory to be applicable to not-for-profit firms and hence for such firms to have optimal capital structures defined, at least in theory, as a trade-off between the costs and benefits of debt financing. Note, however, that the asymmetric information theory is not applicable to not-for-profit firms because such firms do not issue common stock.

Although the trade-off theory may be conceptually correct for not-for-profit firms, a problem arises when applying the theory. For-profit firms have more or less unlimited access to equity capital. Thus, if they have more capital investment opportunities than they can finance with retained earnings and debt financing, investor-owned firms can always raise the needed funds by a new stock issue. (According to the asymmetric information theory, managers may not want to issue new stock, but the opportunity still exists.) Furthermore, it is quite easy for investor-owned firms to alter their capital structures. If they are financially underleveraged (using too little debt), they can simply issue more debt and use the proceeds to repurchase stock. On the other hand, if they are financially overleveraged (using too much debt), they can issue additional shares and use the proceeds to retire debt. Not-for-profit firms do not have access to the equity markets. Their sole sources of "equity" capital are government grants, private contributions, and excess revenues (retained earnings).

Managers of not-for-profit organizations do not have the same degree of flexibility in either capital investment or capital structure decisions as do their proprietary counterparts. Thus, it is often necessary for not-for-profit firms to (1) delay new projects because of funding insufficiencies or (2) use more than the theoretically optimal amount of debt because that is the only way that needed services can be financed. Although these actions may be necessary, managers must recognize that such strategies are not ideal. Project delays mean that needed services are not being provided on a timely basis. Using more debt than optimal pushes the firm beyond the point of the greatest net benefit of debt financing; hence, aggregate capital costs are increased above the minimum. If forced into a situation where the firm is using more than the optimal amount of debt financing, its managers should plan to reduce the firm's level of debt as soon as the situation permits.

The ability of a not-for-profit firm to negotiate government payments, attract private contributions, and generate excess revenues plays an important role in establishing its competitive position. A firm that has an adequate amount of fund capital can operate at its optimal capital structure and thus minimize capital costs while at the same time funding all programs deemed worthwhile. If insufficient fund capital is available, too much financial leverage is often used, and the result is higher capital costs. Consider two not-for-profit hospitals that are similar in all respects except that one has more fund capital and can operate at its optimal structure, while the other has insufficient fund capital and thus must use more debt financing than the optimum. In effect, the hospital with insufficient fund capital must operate at an inefficient capital structure. The former has a significant competitive advantage because it can either offer more services at the same cost by using additional debt financing, or it can offer matching services at lower costs because its capital costs are lower. Thus, sufficient fund capital provides the flexibility to offer all the necessary services and still operate at the lowest cost structure.

Any firm that is forced to use more than the optimal amount of debt financing is operating inefficiently and hence has an economic incentive to obtain more fund capital. As in any competitive industry, not-for-profit healthcare managers have limited control over their firms' abilities to generate excess revenues. On the other hand, managers have much greater control over the amount of effort applied to public and private fund-raising. Thus, not-for-profit firms that require fund capital to operate efficiently must examine closely their fund-raising efforts. Years ago, public and private contributions were a critical source of funds for not-for-profit providers, but many firms deemphasized this source of capital during the cost-plus era of the 1970s and early 1980s. In the competitive healthcare market of the 1990s, fund-raising is again playing an important role in the capital acquisition process.

FACTORS THAT INFLUENCE THE CAPITAL STRUCTURE DECISION

Since it is impossible to determine precisely a firm's optimal capital structure, managers must apply judgment along with quantitative analysis. The judgmental analysis involves many different factors; in one situation a particular factor might have great importance, while the same factor might be relatively unimportant in another situation. This section discusses some of the more important judgmental factors that should be taken into account when setting a firm's target capital structure. Although some of the factors apply solely to investor-owned firms, most of the factors are applicable to all firms.

Long-Run Viability

Managers of large firms, especially those providing vital healthcare services, have a responsibility to ensure the long-run viability of the enterprise. In general, this means avoiding using financial leverage to the point where the firm's future financial condition is endangered.

Managerial Conservatism

Well-diversified investors have eliminated most, if not all, of the diversifiable risk from their portfolios. Therefore, the typical investor can tolerate some chance of financial distress because a loss on one stock will probably be offset by random gains on other stocks in his or her portfolio. However, managers often view financial distress with more concern. They are typically not well diversified in their careers, and thus the present value of their expected earnings can be seriously affected by the onset of financial distress. Thus, it is not difficult to imagine that managers of investor-owned firms might be more conservative in their use of financial leverage than the average stockholder would desire. If this is true, managers would set somewhat lower target capital structures than the ones that maximize firm value. The managers of a publicly owned firm would never admit this because, unless they owned voting control, they would quickly lose their jobs. However, in view of the uncertainties about what constitutes the optimal capital structure, management could always say that the structure employed is, in its judgment, optimal, and it would be difficult to prove otherwise.

For not-for-profit firms, one could argue that managerial conservatism is appropriate. Not-for-profit firms have no shareholders, and many of the stakeholders are typically not well diversified in regards to their relationships with the firm. Thus, these stakeholders have much more to lose if the firm fails than do well-diversified shareholders of investor-owned firms. However, the managers of not-for-profit firms can only adopt a conservative approach to capital structure if the firm is generating sufficient fund capital to meet the equity portion of its capital investment needs.

Lender and Rating Agency Attitudes

Regardless of a manager's own analysis of the proper leverage for his or her firm, there is no question but that lenders' and rating agencies' attitudes are frequently important determinants of financial structures. In the majority of situations, managers discuss the firm's financial structure with lenders, rating agencies, and investment bankers and give much weight to their advice. Also, if a particular firm's management is so confident of the future that it seeks to use leverage beyond the norms for its industry, its lenders may be unwilling to accept such debt increases or may do so only at a high price.

Reserve Borrowing Capacity

The discussion of the asymmetric information theory noted that it prescribes that firms should maintain a reserve borrowing capacity that preserves the ability to issue debt at favorable terms. For example, suppose Bristol-Myers Squibb (a pharmaceutical firm) had just successfully completed an R&D program on a new drug, and its internal projections forecast much higher earnings in the future.

However, the new earnings are not yet anticipated by investors and hence are not reflected in the price of its stock. The firm's managers would not want to issue stock at this time; they would prefer to finance with debt until the higher earnings materialized and were reflected in the stock price, at which time the firm could sell an issue of common stock, retire the debt, and return to its target capital structure. To maintain this borrowing capacity reserve, firms generally use less debt under "normal" conditions and hence present a stronger financial picture than they otherwise would. This is not necessarily suboptimal from a long-run standpoint, although it might appear so if viewed strictly on a short-run basis.

Industry Averages

Presumably, managers act rationally, so the capital structures of other firms in the industry (particularly the industry leaders) should provide insights as to the optimal structure. In general, there is no reason to believe that the managers of one firm are better than the managers of any other firm. Thus, if one firm has a capital structure that is significantly different from other firms in its industry, the managers of that firm should identify the unique circumstances that contribute to the anomaly. If unique circumstances cannot be identified, it is doubtful that the firm has identified the correct target structure.

Control of Investor-Owned Corporations

The effect of security issues on a management's control position may influence the capital structure decision. If a firm's management just barely has majority control (just over 50 percent of the stock), but it is not in a position to buy additional stock, debt may be the choice for new financings. On the other hand, a management group that is not concerned about voting control may decide to use equity rather than debt if the firm's financial situation is so weak that the use of debt might subject the company to serious risk of default.

Asset Structure

Firms whose assets are suitable as security for loans tend to use debt rather heavily. Thus, hospitals tend to be highly leveraged, but companies involved in technological research employ relatively little debt. Also, if the firm's assets carry high business risk, it will be less able to use financial leverage than a firm with low business risk. Accordingly, factors such as sales stability and operating leverage, which influence business risk, also influence a firm's optimal capital structure.

Growth Rate

Other factors being equal, faster-growing firms must rely more heavily on external capital. Slow growth can be financed with retained earnings, but rapid growth generally requires the use of external funds. As postulated in the information asymmetry theory, firms first turn to debt financing to meet external funding needs. Further, the flotation costs involved in selling common stock exceed those incurred when selling debt. Thus, rapidly growing firms tend to use more debt than do slower-growth companies.

Profitability

One often observes that firms with very high rates of return on investment use relatively little debt. This behavior is consistent with the asymmetric information theory. The practical reason seems to be that highly profitable firms simply do not need to do much debt financing; their high rates of return enable them to do most of their financing with retained earnings.

Taxes

Interest is a deductible expense, while dividends are not deductible, so the higher a firm's corporate tax rate, the greater the advantage of using corporate debt.

AN APPROACH TO SETTING THE TARGET CAPITAL STRUCTURE

Thus far in this chapter, two theories of capital structure and a host of factors that influence the capital structure decisions of most firms have been discussed. In this section, a pragmatic approach to setting the target capital structure that is used at the W. T. Mathews Teaching Hospital and Clinics is described. The approach requires judgmental assumptions, but it also allows the hospital's managers to see how alternative capital structures would affect future profitability, the firm's ability to meet its debt payments, and external financing requirements under a variety of assumptions.

The starting point for the analysis is the hospital's financial forecasting model, which also is set up to test the effects of capital structure changes. Basically, the model generates forecasted financial statements based on inputs supplied by the hospital's managers. Each data item can be fixed, or it can be allowed to vary from year to year. The required data include the most recent balance sheet and income statement, plus the following items, all of which represent either managerial expectations or policy variables:

1. Annual utilization and reimbursement rates.
2. Annual inflation rates for both revenues and costs.
3. Corporate tax rate (if investor owned).
4. Variable costs as a percentage of sales.
5. Fixed costs.
6. Interest rate on already outstanding (embedded) debt.
7. Marginal component costs of debt and equity.
8. Capital structure percentages.
9. Dividend growth rate (if investor owned).

The model uses the input data to forecast the hospital's balance sheets and income statements for five years. Further, the model calculates and displays other applicable financial information such as external financing requirements, return on equity (ROE), debt coverage ratios, and the overall cost of capital for projected future years.

To begin the process, the hospital's managers enter base-year values and data on expected utilization and reimbursement rates, expected inflation rates, and so on. These inputs are used by the model to forecast operating income and asset requirements that, in general, will not depend on financing decisions. Next, the managers must consider the financing mix. The model permits as inputs both the debt/equity mix and the debt-maturity mix. (By debt maturity, we mean the proportion of short-term versus long-term debt.) Further, the hospital's managers must estimate as best they can the effects of capital structure changes on the component costs of capital and then must enter these cost rate estimates. For example, a higher debt ratio (more debt in the capital structure) will lead to increases in the costs of all components and vice versa if less debt is used. With all inputs entered, the model then completes the forecasted financial statements.

Next, the model's output must be reviewed and analyzed. Since the focus here is on the capital structure decision, the hospital's managers would pay particular attention to forecasted earnings, debt coverage ratios, and external financing requirements. Finally, the model is used to analyze alternative scenarios. This analysis takes two forms: (1) changing the financing inputs to get some idea of how the financing mix affects the key outputs and (2) changing the operating inputs to see how the basic business risk of the hospital affects the key outputs under various financing strategies.

The model can generate the output "answers" quite easily, but it remains the responsibility of the hospital's managers to assign input values, to interpret the output, and finally, to set the target capital structure. The final decision maker must judge which factors are most relevant to his or her firm. Reaching a decision is not easy, but a capital structure forecasting model such as the one described here at least permits managers to analyze the effects of alternative courses of action, which is an essential element of good decision making. The managers of W. T. Mathews Teaching Hospital and Clinics identify the hospital's optimal capital structure by specifying the target range of debt. For example, their 1996 analysis indicated an optimal range of 30 to 35 percent debt financing, so future financings will be structured, if at all possible, to keep the hospital's capital structure within the target range.

THE DEBT-MATURITY DECISION

The second capital structure decision involves the choice between short-term and long-term debt: Given some target amount of debt financing, how much should be short-term debt and how much should be long-term debt? Most businesses, including healthcare firms, experience seasonal fluctuations in demand and hence revenues. Furthermore, almost all businesses are subject to cyclical swings in sales that result from local, regional, national, and global business cycles. In general, healthcare firms have relatively small seasonal and cyclical demand fluctuations compared to other industries. Nevertheless, predictable demand fluctuations do occur, and in areas where a large segment of the population is seasonal, such as the "snow bird" areas of Florida, seasonal demand variations at healthcare providers can be quite pronounced.

Seasonal and cyclical variations in demand for services affect a firm's asset levels. For simplicity, assume that a firm is not expanding or contracting. It would maintain sufficient fixed assets to meet its peak needs, so its level of fixed assets remains constant over time. The firm's current assets, on the other hand, fluctuate over time. During periods of peak activity, the firm's cash, receivables, and inventories are at high levels, but at seasonal or cyclical low periods, these assets decrease to some minimum level. The minimum level of total (fixed plus minimum current) assets constitutes the firm's permanent asset base. Thus, the firm's permanent assets represent the lowest level of assets required to support operations. During cyclical or seasonal operational peaks, the firm adds temporary assets, but these are later reduced when business declines.

There are three general approaches to the debt-maturity decision: (1) the aggressive approach, (2) the maturity-matching approach, and (3) the conservative approach. In the aggressive approach, some portion of the firm's permanent assets is financed with short-term debt as opposed to financing all permanent assets with permanent capital (equity, or fund, capital and long-term debt). For example, consider Suncoast Surgery, Inc., which operates six outpatient surgery centers in the Tampa Bay area. Its permanent level of assets is ten million dollars, but it must add two million dollars in temporary assets during the peak winter season. Its optimal capital structure calls for 50 percent debt and 50 percent equity, so it finances its ten million dollars in permanent assets with five million of debt and five million dollars of equity. However, its maturity structure for the five million dollars of debt financing consists of four million dollars of long-term debt and one million dollars of short-term debt. Thus, it is using one million dollars of short-term debt to finance its permanent assets. It then uses an additional two million dollars of short-term debt to finance its temporary peak assets, so it has one million dollars of short-term debt on the books during the slow summer season and three million dollars during the winter peak.

The aggressive approach calls for relatively large amounts of short-term debt, even during seasonal and cyclical lows. (Suncoast has one million dollars of short-term debt on the books during the slow season.) In general, the yield curve (which is a plot of interest rates versus term to maturity) is upward sloping, which indicates that interest rates on short-term debt are lower than rates on long-term debt. Since short-term debt is normally less costly than long-term debt, the aggressive approach, which uses the greatest amount of short-term debt, is generally the least-cost debt-maturity alternative.

However, short-term debt is also more risky to the issuer than long-term debt because (1) continuing use of short-term debt means that the firm's interest costs rise and fall with changing interest rates (rollover rate risk), and (2) temporary financial setbacks could result in lenders refusing to renew the loan (renewal risk). Long-term debt does not carry these risks because (1) the interest cost is fixed for a long period, and (2) loan renewal occurs only at lengthy intervals. Thus, Suncoast Surgery, with one million dollars of short-term debt as part of its permanent financing structure, continuously runs the risks of rising interest rates and loan renewal problems. Although the aggressive approach offers the potential for the lowest debt costs, the continuous dependence on short-term debt, even during seasonal and cyclical lows, brings with it substantial risk.

In the conservative approach, a firm makes maximum use of long-term debt and minimum use of short-term debt. For example, Suncoast Surgery could use six million dollars of equity and six million dollars of debt, all of which is long term. With this financing mix, the firm would carry two million dollars of marketable securities during the slow summer period, but these securities would be liquidated in the winter to buy supplies and carry receivables. The conservative approach potentially is the most costly of the three approaches because of its reliance on relatively costly long-term debt. On the other hand, the conservative approach, with its limited (or zero in our example) reliance on short-term debt exposes the firm to only a small amount of (or zero) rollover rate and renewal risk.

In the maturity-matching approach, a firm matches the maturities of the liabilities with the maturities of the assets being financed, where maturities are defined as permanent or temporary. The maturity-matching approach falls between the aggressive and conservative approaches. For example, Suncoast Surgery could use five million dollars of equity and five million dollars of long-term debt to finance it ten million dollars of permanent assets. Then, it would use two million dollars of short-term debt to finance its temporary winter needs. In effect, Suncoast is financing permanent assets with permanent capital and temporary assets with temporary capital. With a maturity mix in between those of the aggressive and conservative approaches, the maturity-matching approach exposes the firm to less rollover rate and renewal risk than the aggressive approach. At the same time, the maturity-matching approach uses more long-term debt and less short-term debt than the aggressive approach, so it is more costly.

The debt-maturity decision involves a choice between three levels of cost and risk. The aggressive approach promises the least cost but exposes the firm to the most risk. The maturity-matching approach offers a middle-of-the-road solution, while the conservative approach is the most costly but the least risky. Unfortunately, there is no clear-cut rule on which to base the choice among the three alternatives. Most firms use the maturity-matching approach, but some use the conservative approach. Few firms use the aggressive approach, presumably because managers tend to believe that the risk outweighs the reward. Note that the debt-maturity decision can be influenced by the capital structure decision since both decisions affect the riskiness of the firm's financial structure. If a firm assumes a great deal of risk in its capital structure (more debt and less equity), there is less room for that firm to assume maturity risk (a lot of short-term debt).

Finally, note that the maturity-matching approach does not call for financing current assets with current liabilities, which is sometimes also described as maturity matching. The latter type of maturity matching relies on accounting definitions, which do not recognize that some portion of a firm's current assets will always be carried and hence are permanent in nature. Maturity matching using accounting definitions is actually following the high-risk aggressive approach because the firm would be using short-term debt to finance its permanent level of current assets along with that portion that is temporary in nature.

After burning a lot of midnight oil, reading several books on healthcare financial management and turnaround situations, and with much support from the hospital's staff, Roberta was able to stem the tide and move the hospital in the right direction. Regarding the use of debt financing, she concluded that the large amount used by San Gabriel Memorial Hospital was not consistent with good managerial practices. With no unique factors, other than a recent lack of profitability, to indicate otherwise, Roberta concluded that San Gabriel's target debt ratio should be about 35 percent, the industry average.

The overuse of debt could not be corrected immediately; but by increasing profitability, she was able to use profit retentions to start reducing the amount of debt to a more reasonable level. After several years, she estimated that the hospital's debt level would be in line with the competition, which would give the hospital more flexibility, lower its risk, and help the bottom line.

SELF-ASSESSMENT EXERCISES

10–1 a. What is meant by a firm's capital structure decision?
   b. What is meant by a firm's debt-maturity decision?
   c. What are some common measures of debt utilization?

10–2 a. What is business risk? What factors influence a firm's business risk?
   b. What is financial risk?
   c. How is business risk measured? How is financial risk measured?

10–3 a. What is the goal of capital structure theory?
   b. What, in general, does the trade-off theory tell managers of for-profit firms about the use of debt financing? According to the theory, what factors influence a firm's decision to use more or less debt in its optimal capital structure?
   c. Briefly describe the asymmetric information theory of capital structure for investor-owned firms.
   d. What implications does capital structure theory have for not-for-profit firms?

10-4 What are the most important factors that firms consider when setting their optimal (target) capital structures?

10-5 Superior Care, Inc., is an investor-owned home health-care provider that is just being formed. Although Superior Care's first-year operating income (earnings before interest and taxes) is expected to be three million dollars, there is a great deal of uncertainty in the estimate, as indicated by the following probability distribution.

Probability	Operating Income
0.25	$1,000,000
0.50	3,000,000
0.25	5,000,000

Assume that Superior Care has only two financing alternatives: either an all-equity capital structure with $12,000,000 of stock or $6,000,000 of 12 percent debt plus $6,000,000 of equity. The firm's expected tax rate is 40 percent.

a. Construct partial income statements for each financing alternative at each operating income level. (Hint: Fill in the Xs in the following table through the net income line.)

	All Equity			50 Percent Debt		
Probability	0.25	0.50	0.25	0.25	0.50	0.25
Operating income	$1,000,000	$3,000,000	$5,000,000	$1,000,000	$3,000,000	$5,000,000
Interest	0	0	0	X	X	X
BT earnings	X	X	X	X	X	X
Taxes	X	X	X	X	X	X
Net income	X	X	X	X	X	X
ROE	X	X	X	X	X	X
Expected ROE		X			X	
Times interest earned	N/A	N/A	N/A	X	X	X
Standard deviation of ROE		X			X	

b. Now calculate the return on equity (ROE) and times-interest-earned (TIE) ratio for each financing alternative at each operating income level. (Hint: ROE = Net income/Total equity. Times interest earned is a measure of how well a firm's earnings cover its interest expense, and it is defined as TIE = Operating income/Interest. The higher the TIE, the greater the interest coverage and hence the less risky the debt usage.)

c. Finally, discuss the risk/return trade-offs under the two financing alternatives. (Hint: Use expected ROE as the return measure and the standard deviation of ROE as the risk measure.)

SELECTED REFERENCES

Boles, Keith E. "What Accounting Leaves Out of Hospital Financial Management." *Hospital & Health Services Administration*, March/April 1986, pp. 8–27.

Gapenski, Louis C. "Hospital Capital Structure Decisions: Theory and Practice." *Health Services Management Research*, November 1993, pp. 237–47.

Harris, John P. and Victor E. Schimmel. "Market Value: An Underused Financial Planning Tool." *Healthcare Financial Management*, April 1987, pp. 40–46.

McCue, Michael J. and Yazar A. Ozcan. "Determinants of Capital Structure." *Hospital & Health Services Administration*, Fall 1992, pp. 333–46.

Sterns, Jay B. and Todd K. Majidzadeh. "A Framework for Evaluating Capital Structure." *Journal of Health Care Finance*, Winter 1995, pp. 80-85.

Valvona, Joseph and Frank A. Sloan. "Hospital Profitability and Capital Structure: A Comparative Analysis." *Health Services Research*, August 1988, pp. 343–57.

Wedig, Gerald J., Frank A. Sloan, Mahmud Hassan, and Michael A. Morrisey. "Capital Structure, Ownership, and Capital Payment Policy: The Case of Hospitals." *Journal of Finance*, March 1988, pp. 21–40.

11

CHAPTER

Financing Decisions: Leasing

Sandy Gross, a neurologist on the staff of Seven Oaks Hospital, knew just what the hospital needed—a positron emission tomography (PET) unit—and he didn't hesitate to communicate his views to the hospital's CEO, Herb Cooper. Although Mr. Cooper was well aware of the diagnostic value of the unit, the high price tag, coupled with significant uncertainty associated with usage and reimbursement, put the risk of such an acquisition in the very high range. The board just didn't want to commit the scarce resources of the hospital to a project that might not come close to paying for itself. Of course, such arguments weren't enough for Dr. Gross, and he continued to push his views at every opportunity.

Then, a chance conversation between Dr. Gross and Mark Bedford, the chief of radiology, changed the entire situation. Dr. Bedford had just returned from Chicago, where he had attended the annual meeting of the Radiological Society of North America. At the meeting, one of the exhibitors, Pinnacle Credit Corporation, was promoting its new fee-per-scan financing. "It's really a kind of joint venture," Dr. Bedford had explained. "In most of the deals, providers pay a higher per-scan fee—say, four hundred dollars—for the first 75 to 100 scans performed in a month, *and a lower fee—say, two hundred dollars—after the threshold is reached. Best of all, there is no minimum payment, so Pinnacle would bear all of the usage uncertainty."*

When Mr. Cooper learned about the possibility of financing the PET unit with a per-procedure lease, his attitude towards the project changed. After you read this chapter, you will see why leasing an asset may be better than buying in certain situations. At the end of the chapter, you can read about Mr. Cooper's final decision on the PET project.

INTRODUCTION

Businesses generally own fixed assets, but it is the use of buildings and equipment that is important, not their ownership. One way to obtain the use of assets is to raise debt or equity capital and then use this capital to buy the assets. An alternative way to obtain the use of assets is to lease them. Prior to the 1950s, leasing was generally associated with real estate—land and buildings. Today, however, it is possible to lease virtually any type of fixed asset, and leasing is used extensively in the healthcare industry. In fact, about 40 percent of all new medical equipment acquired by providers is leased rather than purchased.

Healthcare managers need to understand that leasing represents a viable alternative to purchasing for many fixed-asset acquisitions. Furthermore, it is important that managers understand the reasons why leasing may be favorable under some circumstances but unfavorable under others. Finally, managers must be able to analyze lease terms to determine when leasing is the best financing choice. This chapter provides managers with the basic concepts and tools required to make better leasing decisions.

BASIC TERMINOLOGY

To begin, it is necessary to become familiar with the basic terminology used in lease transactions.

Lessee and Lessor

Lease transactions involve two parties, the owner of the asset and the user (operator) of the asset. The user of a leased asset is called the lessee, while the owner of the asset, usually the manufacturer or a leasing company, is called the lessor. Note that the term *lessee* is pronounced "less-ee," not "lease-ee," and *lessor* is pronounced "less-or."

Operating Leases

In operating leases, sometimes called service leases, the lessor generally provides both financing and maintenance. IBM was one of the pioneers of operating lease contracts, and computers and office copying machines, together with automobiles, trucks, and medical diagnostic equipment, are the primary types of equipment involved in operating leases. Ordinarily, operating leases require the lessor to maintain and service the leased equipment, and the cost of the maintenance is built into the lease payments.

Another important characteristic of operating leases is the fact that they are not fully amortized. This means that the payments required under the lease contract are not sufficient for the lessor to recover the full cost of the equipment. However, the lease contract is written for a period considerably less than the expected economic life of the leased asset, and the lessor expects to recover all costs either by subsequent lease renewal payments, by releasing the equipment to other lessees, or by sale of the equipment.

A final feature of operating leases is that they frequently contain a cancellation clause, which gives the lessee the right to cancel the lease and to return the equipment to the lessor before the expiration of the basic lease agreement. This is an important consideration to the lessee, for it means that the equipment can be returned if it is rendered obsolete by technological developments or if it is no longer needed because of a decline in the lessee's business.

Most operating leases require the lessee to make fixed payments, usually monthly but sometimes annually. However, a new type of lease contract becoming popular with healthcare providers is the per-procedure lease. Instead of fixed lease payments, the lessee pays the lessor a fixed amount per procedure performed on the equipment. Thus, if the equipment is used extensively, the lease payment will be relatively high, but if the equipment is barely used at all, the lease payment will be relatively low.

Another new feature that is being built into some operating leases is "future protection." Under such a provision, lessees pay an extra amount with each lease payment, which depends on the type and cost of the equipment. The lessor agrees to furnish to the lessee, at no additional cost, all upgrades affecting the capability of the leased equipment.

Financial Leases

Financial leases, which are often called capital leases, are differenti-ated from operating leases in that (1) they typically do not provide for maintenance service, (2) they typically are not cancelable, (3) they are generally for a period that approximates the economic life of the asset, and hence (4) they are fully amortized (that is, the lessor receives rental payments equal to the full cost of the leased asset plus a return on the capital employed). In a typical financial lease, the lessee selects the specific item it requires, and then it negotiates the price and delivery terms with the manufacturer. The lessee then arranges to have a leasing company (the lessor) buy the equipment from the manufacturer, and the using firm simultaneously executes an agreement to lease the equipment from the lessor.

The terms of the lease call for full amortization of the lessor's investment plus a rate of return on the unamortized balance that is close to the percentage rate the lessee would have paid on a secured term loan. For example, if a radiology group practice would have to pay 10 percent for a term loan to buy an X-ray machine, a rate of about 10 percent typically would be built into the lease contract by the lessor.

A sale and leaseback is a special type of financial lease that can be arranged by a user that currently owns some asset. Here, the user sells the asset to another party and simultaneously executes an agreement to lease the property back for a stated period under spe-cific terms. In a sale and leaseback, the lessee receives an immedi-ate cash payment from the sale in exchange for a series of future payments that must be made to rent the use of the asset sold.

The parallel to borrowing is obvious in a financial lease. Under a mortgage loan arrangement, the lender would normally receive a series of equal payments just sufficient to amortize the loan and to provide a specified rate of return on the outstanding loan balance. Under a financial lease, the lease payments are set up exactly the same way: The payments are just sufficient to return the full purchase price to the lessor plus a stated return on the lessor's investment.

In general, financial leases cannot be canceled unless the lessor is completely paid off. Also, the lessee generally pays the property taxes and insurance on the leased property. Since the lessor receives a return after, or net of, these payments, this type of lease is often called a net, net lease.

Although the distinction between operating and financial leases has historical significance, today many lessors offer leases under a wide variety of terms. Therefore, in practice, leases often do not fit exactly into the operating lease or financial lease category but, rather, combine some features of each. To illustrate, cancellation clauses are normally associated with operating leases, but many of today's financial leases also contain cancellation clauses. However, in financial leases, these clauses generally include provisions whereby the lessee must make penalty payments sufficient to enable the lessor to recover some or all of the remaining cost of the leased property.

TAX EFFECTS

Tax effects play an important role in the lease-versus-buy decision. In fact, as explained in a later section, tax differentials between the lessee and lessor are the driving force behind many lease contracts.

The full amount of the annual lease payment is a tax-deductible expense for investor-owned lessees provided that the Internal Revenue Service (IRS) agrees that a particular contract is a genuine lease, not simply an installment loan called a lease. This makes it important that a lease contract be written in a form acceptable to the IRS. A lease that complies with all of the IRS requirements is called a guideline, or tax-oriented, lease. In a guideline lease, ownership benefits (depreciation tax deductions) accrue to the lessor, but the lessee's lease (rental) payments are fully tax deductible.

A lease that does not meet the tax guidelines is called a non-tax-oriented lease. For this type of lease, only the interest portion implied in each lease payment is tax deductible to the lessee. However, the lessee is considered to be the owner of the leased equipment; thus, the lessee can take the tax depreciation.

To qualify as a lease under tax guidelines, a lease contract must meet the following provisions:

1. The lease term (including any extensions or renewals at a fixed rental rate) must not exceed 80 percent of the estimated useful life of the equipment at the commencement of the lease transaction. Thus, at the end of the lease, the equipment must have an estimated remaining useful life equal to at least 20 percent of its original life. Furthermore, the remaining useful life must not be less than one year. This requirement limits the maximum term of a lease to 80 percent of the asset's useful life.

2. The equipment's estimated value (in constant dollars without adjustment for inflation) at the expiration of the lease must equal at least 20 percent of its value at the start of the lease. Note that the estimated value of the asset at the end of the lease is called the residual value. This requirement also has the effect of limiting the maximum lease term.

3. Neither the lessee nor any related party can have the right to purchase the property from the lessor at a fixed price predetermined at the lease's inception. However, the lessee can be given a fair market value purchase option.

4. Neither the lessee nor any related party can pay or guarantee payment of any part of the price of the leased equipment. Simply put, the lessee cannot make any investment in the equipment, other than through the lease payments.

5. The leased equipment must not be "limited use" property, defined as equipment that can only be used by the lessee or a related party at the end of the lease.

The reason for the IRS's concern about lease terms is that, without restrictions, a taxable company could set up a "lease" transaction calling for very rapid lease payments, which would be tax deductions. The effect would be to depreciate the equipment over a much shorter period than the IRS allows in its depreciation guidelines. For example, suppose that Carolina Clinical Laboratories, Inc., an investor-owned company that owns clinical laboratories in North and South Carolina, planned to acquire a one million dollar automated clinical laboratory analysis system, which has a three-year tax depreciation (MACRS) class life. The annual depreciation allowances would be $330,000 in Year 1, $450,000 in Year 2, $150,000 in Year 3, and $70,000 in Year 4. If the firm were in the 40 percent federal-plus-state tax bracket, the depreciation would provide a tax savings of 0.40($330,000) = $132,000 in Year 1, $180,000 in Year 2, $60,000 in Year 3, and $28,000 in Year 4, for a total savings of $400,000. At a 6 percent discount rate, the present value of these tax savings would be $357,283.

Now suppose Carolina Clinical could acquire the equipment through a one-year lease arrangement with NationsBank for a payment of one million dollars, with a one-dollar purchase option. If the one million dollars payment were treated as a lease payment, it would be fully deductible, so it would provide a tax saving of 0.40($1,000,000) = $400,000 versus a present value of only $357,283 for the depreciation shelters associated with ownership. Thus, the lease payment and the depreciation would both provide the same total amount of tax savings (40 percent of one million dollars, or $400,000), but the savings would come in faster, and hence have a $400,000 − $357,283 = $42,717 higher present value, with the one-year lease. Therefore, if just any type of contract could be called a lease and given tax treatment as a lease, the timing of the tax shelters could be speeded up compared with ownership depreciation tax shelters. This speedup would benefit both lessees and lessors because the value could be shared, but it would be costly to the government. For this reason, the IRS has established the rules described above for defining a lease for tax purposes.

Even though leasing can be used only within limits to speed up the effective depreciation schedule, there are still times when very substantial tax benefits can be derived from a leasing arrangement. For example, if a taxable firm has a very large construction program that has generated so much depreciation that it has no current tax liabilities, depreciation shelters are not very useful. In this case, a leasing company set up by very profitable companies like General Electric can buy the equipment, receive the depreciation shelters, and then share these benefits with the lessee by charging lower lease payments. In fact, General Electric has a subsidiary, GE Capital Corporation, which is one of the largest lessors in the world. The subsidiary was originally set up to finance consumers' purchases of GE's durable goods such as refrigerators and washing machines, but it has become a major player in the commercial loan and leasing markets. The point to be made here is that if the lease parties are to obtain the normal tax benefits from leasing—deduction of the rental payments by the lessee and depreciation deductions by the lessor—the lease contract must be written in a manner that will qualify it as a true lease under IRS guidelines. If there is any question about the tax status of a lease contract, the firm's lawyers and accountants must check the latest IRS regulations.

FINANCIAL STATEMENT EFFECTS

Under certain conditions, neither the leased assets nor the liabilities imposed by the lease contract appear directly on the lessee's balance sheet. For this reason, leasing under these conditions is sometimes called off-balance-sheet financing. This point is illustrated in Table 11–1 by the balance sheets of two hypothetical firms, B (for buy) and L (for lease). Initially, assume the balance sheets of both firms are identical, and they both have debt ratios of debt/total assets = $50/$100 = 50%. Now, assume each firm decides to acquire a fixed asset costing one hundred dollars. Firm B borrows one hundred dollars and buys the asset, so both an asset

TABLE 11–1

Balance Sheet Effects of Leasing

Before Asset Increase, Firms B and L:			
Current assets	$ 50	Debt	$ 50
Fixed assets	50	Equity	50
Total assets	$100	Total claims	$100
Debt/assets ratio			50%
After $100 Asset Increase, Firm B, Which Buys the Asset:			
Current assets	$ 50	Debt	$150
Fixed assets	150	Equity	50
Total assets	$200	Total claims	$200
Debt/assets ratio			75%
After $100 Asset Increase, Firm L, Which Leases the Asset:			
Current assets	$ 50	Debt	$ 50
Fixed assets	50	Equity	50
Total assets	$100	Total claims	$100
Debt/assets ratio			50%

and a liability go on its balance sheet, and its debt ratio rises from 50 to 75 percent. Firm L leases the equipment. The lease may call for rental payments as high or even higher than the loan payments, and the obligations assumed under the lease may be equally or more dangerous from the standpoint of potential bankruptcy, but the firm's debt ratio remains at only 50 percent.

To correct the problem of firms acquiring assets and liabilities that do not appear on the balance sheet, accounting rules require firms that enter into capital leases to restate their balance sheets to report the leased asset as a fixed asset and the present value of the future lease payments as a liability. This process is called capitalizing the lease, and hence such a lease is called a capital lease. The net effect of capitalizing the lease is to cause Firms B and L to have similar balance sheets, both of which will, in essence, resemble the one shown for Firm B.

The logic behind the accounting rule is as follows. If a firm signs a capital lease contract, its obligation to make lease payments is just as binding as if it had signed a loan agreement—the failure to make lease payments has the potential to bankrupt a firm just as fast as the failure to make principal and interest payments on a loan. From a financial risk perspective, a capital lease is similar to a loan. This being the case, a capital lease agreement increases the firm's effective debt ratio. Therefore, if a firm has established its target capital structure, and if the firm is currently at that structure, then using lease financing requires additional equity support exactly like debt financing if the firm is to remain at its debt usage target.

If disclosure of the lease in our Table 11–1 example were not made, then Firm L's investors could be deceived into thinking that its financial position is stronger than it really is. Thus, even before accountants required that capital leases be included directly on the balance sheet, firms were required to disclose the existence of long-term leases in footnotes to their financial statements. At that time, it was debated whether or not investors fully recognized the impact of leases and, in effect, would see that Firms B and L were in essentially the same financial position. Some people argued that leases were not fully recognized, even by sophisticated investors. The question of whether investors were truly deceived was debated but never resolved. Those who believe strongly in efficient markets thought that investors were not deceived and that footnotes were sufficient, while those who questioned market efficiency thought that all leases should be capitalized. Current accounting standards represent a compromise between these two positions, though one that is tilted heavily toward those who favor capitalization.

Under accounting rules, a lease is classified as a capital lease, and thus capitalized and shown directly on the balance sheet, if one or more of the following conditions exist:

1. Under the terms of the lease, ownership of the property is effectively transferred from the lessor to the lessee.
2. The lessee can purchase the property at less than its true market value when the lease expires.
3. The lease runs for a period equal to or greater than 75 percent of the asset's life. Thus, if an asset has a 10-year life and the lease is written for eight years, the lease must be capitalized.
4. The present value of the lease payments is equal to or greater than 90 percent of the initial value of the asset. The discount rate used to calculate the present value of the lease payments must be the lower of (1) the rate used by the lessor to establish the lease payments (this rate is discussed later in the chapter) or (2) the rate of interest that the lessee would have to pay for new debt with a maturity equal to that of the lease. Also note that any maintenance payments embedded in the lease payment must be stripped out prior to checking this condition.

These rules, together with strong footnote disclosure rules for operating leases, are sufficient to insure that no one will be fooled by lease financing. In effect, a capital lease for a particular asset has the same economic consequences for the firm as does a loan in which the asset is pledged as collateral. Thus, leases are regarded as debt for capital structure purposes, and they have the same effects as debt on the financial condition of the firm.

In closing, note that the rules that accountants follow in making the decision whether or not to capitalize a lease are not identical to the rules that the IRS follows to decide whether or not the lease is a guideline lease. In most cases, however, leases that meet IRS guidelines are operating leases and will not be capitalized, while leases that do not meet IRS guidelines are financial leases and will be capitalized. Remember, however, that even operating (noncapitalized) leases must be disclosed in the footnotes to the firm's financial statements.

EVALUATION BY THE LESSEE

Leases are evaluated by both the lessee and the lessor. The lessee must determine whether leasing an asset is less costly (on a risk-adjusted basis) than obtaining equivalent alternative financing and buying the asset, and the lessor must decide what the lease payments must be to produce a rate of return consistent with the riskiness of the investment. This section focuses on the analysis by the lessee.

In the typical case, the events leading to a lease agreement follow the sequence described below:

1. The firm decides to acquire a particular building or piece of equipment; this decision is based on normal capital budgeting procedures, as discussed in Chapters 7 and 8. The decision to acquire the asset is not an issue in most lease analyses—this decision was made previously as part of the firm's capital budgeting process. In lease analysis, the concern is simply whether to obtain the use of the asset by lease or by purchase.

2. Once the firm has decided to acquire the asset, the next question is how to finance its acquisition. Most businesses do not have excess cash lying around, so capital to finance new assets must be obtained from some source.

3. Funds to purchase the asset could be obtained by borrowing, by retaining earnings, or if the firm is investor-owned, by selling new equity. (If the firm is not-for-profit, perhaps the funds could be raised by soliciting contributions for the project.) Alternatively, the asset could be leased. Because of the capitalization/disclosure provisions for leases, leasing has about the same impact on a firm's financial condition as debt financing (borrowing).

As indicated earlier, a lease is comparable to a loan in the sense that the firm is required to make a specified series of payments and that failure to meet these payments could result in bankruptcy. Thus, when making lease decisions, the most appropriate comparison is the cost of lease financing versus the cost of debt financing, *regardless of how the purchase would actually be financed.* Even if the asset, if purchased, would be paid for with excess cash, leasing has the same risk implications for the lessee as financing the acquisition with debt, so a lease analysis must compare leasing with debt financing.

To illustrate the basic elements of lease analysis by the lessee, consider this simplified example. Radiology Associates of Charleston (RAC), an investor-owned group practice, has made the decision to acquire a piece of diagnostic equipment that costs $100,000, and now it must choose between leasing and buying the asset. If the asset is purchased, the bank would lend RAC the $100,000 at a rate of 10 percent on a two-year, simple interest loan. Thus, the firm would have to pay the bank $10,000 in interest at the end of each year, plus return the $100,000 in principal at the end of Year 2. For simplicity, assume that RAC could depreciate the asset over two years for tax purposes by the straight-line method if it is purchased, resulting in tax depreciation of $50,000 in each year. Also for simplicity, assume the asset's value at the end of two years (its residual value) is estimated to be zero.

Alternatively, RAC could lease the asset under a guideline lease for two years for a payment of $55,000 at the end of each year. RAC's tax rate is 40 percent. The analysis for the lease-versus-buy decision consists of (1) estimating the cash flows associated with borrowing and buying the asset, that is, the flows associated with debt financing; (2) estimating the cash flows associated with leasing the asset; and (3) comparing the two financing methods to determine which has the lower cost. Below are the borrow-and-buy cash flows.

Cash Flows if RAC Buys	Year 0	Year 1	Year 2
Equipment cost	($100,000)		
Loan amount	100,000		
Interest expense		($10,000)	($ 10,000)
Interest tax savings		4,000	4,000
Principal repayment			(100,000)
Depreciation tax savings		20,000	20,000
Net cash flow	$ 0	$14,000	($ 86,000)

Note that the interest tax savings in Years 1 and 2 is T(Interest expense) = 0.40($10,000) = $4,000, while the depreciation tax savings in those same years is T(Depreciation expense) = 0.40($50,000) = $20,000. The net cash flow is zero in Year 0 because the cost of the equipment is offset by the loan, positive in Year 1, and negative in Year 2. Since the operating cash flows (the revenues and operating costs generated by the equipment) will be the same regardless of whether the equipment is leased or purchased, they can be ignored. Cash flows that are not impacted by the decision at hand are said to be "nonincremental" to the decision.

Below are the cash flows associated with the lease:

Cash Flows if RAC Leases	Year 0	Year 1	Year 2
Lease rental payment		($55,000)	($55,000)
Payment tax savings		22,000	22,000
Net cash flow	$ 0	($33,000)	($33,000)

Here, the payment tax savings is T(Rental payment) = 0.40($55,000) = $22,000. Note that the two sets of net cash flows (buying and leasing) reflect the tax savings associated with interest expense, depreciation, and lease payments, as appropriate. If the lease had not met IRS guidelines, ownership would effectively reside with the lessee, and RAC would depreciate the asset for tax purposes whether it was "leased" or purchased, and hence the depreciation tax savings would be nonincremental to the decision. Furthermore, only the implied interest portion of the lease payment would be tax deductible. Thus, the analysis for a nonguideline lease would consist of simply comparing the after-tax financing flows on the loan with the after-tax lease payment stream.

To compare the cost streams of buying and leasing, the two sets of cash flows must be expressed on a present-value basis. As explained later, the correct discount rate is the after-tax cost of debt, which for RAC is 10%(1 – T) = 10%(1 – 0.40) = 6.0%. Applying this rate, the present value cost of buying is found to be $63,332, and the present value cost of leasing to be $60,500. Since leasing has the lower present value of costs, it is the less costly financing alternative and RAC should lease the asset.

This simplified example shows the general approach used in lease analysis, and it also illustrates a concept that can simplify the cash flow estimation process. Look back at the loan-related cash flows if RAC buys the asset. The after-tax loan-related flows are –$6,000 in Year 1 and –$106,000 in Year 2. When these flows are discounted to Year 0 at the 6.0 percent after-tax cost rate, their present value is –$100,000, the negative of the loan amount shown in Year 0. This equality results because the cost of debt is first used to estimate the future financing flows, and then this same rate is used to discount the flows back to Year 0, all on an after-tax basis. In effect, the loan amount positive cash flow in Year 0 and the present values of the loan cost negative cash flows in Years 1 and 2 cancel one another out. Below, is the cash flow stream associated with buying the asset after the Year 0 loan amount and the related Year 1 and Year 2 financing flows have been removed.

Cash Flows if RAC Buys	Year 0	Year 1	Year 2
Cost of asset	($100,000)		
Depreciation tax savings		$ 20,000	$ 20,000
Net cash flow	($100,000)	$ 20,000	$ 20,000

The present value cost of buying here is of course $63,332, the same value obtained when all the financing flows were included in the analysis. This result will always occur regardless of the specific terms of the debt financing; as long as the discount rate is the after-tax cost of debt, the cash flows associated with the loan can be ignored.

To examine a more realistic example of lease analysis, consider the following lease-versus-buy decision facing Northside Medical Center, a for-profit hospital:

1. Northside plans to acquire a new computer system, which will automate its patient accounts records. The computer has an economic life of eight years and costs $200,000, delivered and installed. However, Northside plans to lease the equipment for only four years because it believes that computer technology is changing rapidly, and it wants the opportunity to reevaluate the situation at that time.

2. Northside could borrow the required $200,000 from its bank at a before-tax cost of 10 percent.

3. The computer's estimated scrap value is $10,000 after eight years of use, but its estimated residual value when the lease expires after four years of use is $40,000. Thus, if Northside buys the equipment, it would expect to receive $40,000 before taxes if the equipment is sold after four years.

4. Northside can lease the equipment for four years at a rental charge of $50,000, payable at the beginning of each year, but the lessor will own the equipment upon the expiration of the lease. (The lease payment schedule is established by the potential lessor, as described in the next major section, and Northside can accept it, reject it, or attempt to negotiate its terms.)

5. The lease contract stipulates that the lessor will maintain the computer at no additional charge to Northside. However, if Northside borrows and buys the computer, it will have to bear the cost of maintenance, which would be performed by the equipment manufacturer at a fixed contract rate of two thousand dollars per year, payable at the beginning of each year.

6. The computer falls into the MACRS five-year class life for tax depreciation, the hospital's marginal tax rate is 30 percent, and the lease qualifies as a guideline lease.

Dollar Cost Analysis

Table 11–2 shows the steps involved in a complete dollar cost analysis. Again, the approach here is to compare the cost of owning (borrowing and buying) the computer to the cost of leasing the computer. All else the same, the lower cost alternative is preferable. Part I of the table is devoted to the cost of borrowing and buying. Note that whenever an analyst sets up cash flows on a time line, the first decision that must be made is what time interval will be used—months, quarters, years, or some other period. As a starting point, analysts often assume that all cash flows occur at the end of each year. If, at some point later in the analysis, another interval appears to be better, the analysis can always be changed. Longer intervals, such as years, simplify the analysis but introduce some inaccuracies because all cash flows do not actually occur at year-end. For example, tax benefits occur quarterly because businesses pay taxes on a quarterly basis. On the other hand, shorter intervals, such as months, complicate the model and imply a degree of forecasting accuracy that often just does not exist.

Line 1 of Table 11–2 contains the equipment's cost and Line 2 shows the maintenance expense; both are cash costs, or outflows.

T A B L E   11–2

Lessee's Dollar Cost Analysis

I. Cost of Owning (Borrowing and Buying)					
	Year 0	**Year 1**	**Year 2**	**Year 3**	**Year 4**
1. Net purchase price	($200,000)				
2. Maintenance cost	(2,000)	($ 2,000)	($ 2,000)	($ 2,000)	
3. Maintenance tax savings	600	600	600	600	
4. Depreciation tax savings		12,000	19,200	11,400	$ 7,200
5. Residual value					40,000
6. Residual value tax					(1,800)
7. Net cash flow	($201,400)	$10,600	$17,800	$10,000	$45,400
8. PV cost of owning = ($133,148)					

II. Cost of Leasing					
	Year 0	**Year 1**	**Year 2**	**Year 3**	**Year 4**
9. Rental payment	($50,000)	($50,000)	($50,000)	($50,000)	
10. Payment tax savings	15,000	15,000	15,000	15,000	
11. Net cash flow	($35,000)	($35,000)	($35,000)	($35,000)	$0
12. PV cost of leasing = ($126,851)					

III. Cost Comparison

13. Net advantage to leasing (NAL) = PV cost of leasing - PV cost of owning
    = –$126,851 – (–$133,148) = $6,297

Notes:
a. The MACRS depreciation allowances are 0.20, 0.32, 0.19, and 0.12 in Years 1 through 4, respectively.
b. In practice, a lease analysis such as this would be done using a spreadsheet program.

Line 3 lists the maintenance tax savings; since the maintenance expense is tax deductible, Northside saves 0.30($2,000) = $600 in taxes by virtue of paying the maintenance fee. Line 4 contains the depreciation tax savings, which is the depreciation expense times the tax rate. To begin the calculation, it is necessary to know the MACRS allowances, which are 0.20 for Year 1, 0.32 for Year 2, 0.19 for Year 3, and 0.12 for Year 4. To illustrate the calculation, the Year 1 depreciation expense is 0.20($200,000) = $40,000, and the resulting tax savings is 0.30($40,000) = $12,000. The depreciation tax savings for the remaining years are calculated similarly.

Lines 5 and 6 contain the residual value cash flows: the residual value is estimated to be $40,000, but the tax book value after four years of depreciation is $200,000 − $40,000 − $64,000 − $38,000 - $24,000 = $34,000. Thus, Northside is forecasting that it will sell (or at least have the opportunity to sell) the computer for $40,000, when it has "told" the IRS that it is only worth $34,000. In effect, Northside has taken too much depreciation, so the IRS is going to "recapture" the excess depreciation. Northside will have to pay taxes on the difference between the estimated residual value and the tax book value of 0.30($40,000 − $34,000) = 0.30($6,000) = $1,800. This tax liability is shown on Line 6. Line 7, which sums the component cash flows, contains the net cash flows associated with borrowing and buying.

Part II of Table 11–2 contains an analysis of the cost of leasing. The rental payments, shown on Line 9, are $50,000 per year; this rate, which includes maintenance, was established by the prospective lessor and offered to Northside. If the hospital accepts the lease, the full amount will be a deductible expense, so the tax savings, shown on Line 10, is 0.30(Rental payment) = 0.30($50,000) = $15,000. The net cash flows associated with leasing are shown on Line 11.

The final step in the analysis is to compare the net cost of owning with the net cost of leasing. However, we must first put the annual cash flows associated with owning and leasing on a common basis. This requires converting them to present values, which brings up the question of the proper rate at which to discount the net cash flows. We know that the riskier the cash flows, the higher will be the discount rate used to find the present value. This principle, which was applied in security valuation and capital budgeting decisions, applies to all discounted cash flow analyses, including lease analysis. Just how risky are the cash flows under consideration here? Most of them are relatively certain, at least when compared with the types of cash flow estimates associated with stock investments or Northside's operating cash flows. For example, the loan payment schedule is set by contract, as is the lease payment schedule. Depreciation expenses are established by law and not subject to change, and the annual maintenance fee is fixed by contract as well. The tax savings are somewhat uncertain, but they will be as projected so long as Northside's marginal tax rate remains at 30 percent. The residual value is the least certain of the cash flows, but even here, Northside's management is fairly confident because the loss of value over time for computers has been relatively constant over the past 10 years.

Since the cash flows under both the lease and borrow-and-purchase alternatives are relatively certain, they should be discounted at a relatively low rate. Most analysts recommend that the company's cost of debt financing be used, and this rate seems reasonable in our example. However, Northside's cost of debt, 10 percent, must be adjusted to reflect the tax deductibility of interest payments, since this benefit of borrowing and buying is not accounted for in the cash flows. Thus, Northside's effective cost of debt becomes (Before-tax cost)(1 − Tax rate) = 10%(1 − 0.30) = 7.0%. Accordingly, the net cash flows shown in Lines 7 and 11 are discounted at a 7.0 percent rate. The resulting present values are \$133,148 for the cost of owning and \$126,851 for the cost of leasing, as shown on Lines 8 and 12. Leasing is the lower cost financing alternative, so Northside should lease, rather than buy, the computer.

The cost comparison can be formalized by defining the net advantage to leasing (NAL) as follows:

$$NAL = PV \text{ cost of leasing} - PV \text{ cost of owning}$$
$$= -\$126,851 - (-\$133,148) = \$6,297.$$

A positive NAL indicates that leasing is a lower-cost alternative to buying, so Northside should lease the equipment. Furthermore, the NAL shows that the value of Northside is increased by \$6,297 if the hospital leases, rather than buys, the computer.

Percentage Cost Analysis

The last section examined Northside Medical Center's lease decision on a dollar cost basis—does it cost fewer dollars to buy or to lease? Northside's lease-versus-buy decision can also be analyzed by looking at the effective cost rate on the lease and comparing it to the effective cost rate on a loan. Signing a lease is similar to signing a loan contract—the firm has the use of equipment, but it must make a series of payments under either type of contract. We know the cost rate built into the loan; it is 7 percent after taxes. If the after-tax cost rate inherent in the lease is less than 7 percent, there is an advantage to leasing.

Table 11–3 sets forth the cash flows needed to determine the percentage cost of the lease.

Here is an explanation of the table:

1. The first step is to calculate the leasing versus owning net cash flows. To do this, merely subtract the owning net cash flows, Line 7 from Table 11–2, from the leasing net cash flows, Line 11 from Table 11–2. The differences are the cash flows that Northside would obtain if it leases rather than buys the computer. In other words, these are the incremental cash flows of leasing as opposed to buying.

2. Note that Table 11–3 consolidates the analysis shown in Table 11–2 into a single set of cash flows. At this point, it is easy to discount the consolidated net cash flows shown on Line 3 of Table 11–3 by 7.0 percent to obtain the NAL, $6,297. In Table 11–2, the net cash flows associated with owning and leasing were discounted separately, and then the present values were subtracted to obtain the NAL. In Table 11–3, the net cash flows associated with buying and leasing were first subtracted to obtain a single set of incremental flows, and then the present value of the con-solidated flows was calculated. The end result (the NAL) is the same.

3. The incremental cash flows shown on Line 3 of Table 11–3 provide a good insight into the economics of leasing. If Northside leases the computer, it avoids the Year 0 cash outlay required to buy the equipment and hence saves

T A B L E 11–3

Lessee's Percentage Cost Analysis

	Year 0	Year 1	Year 2	Year 3	Year 4
1. Leasing cash flow	($ 35,000)	($35,000)	($35,000)	($35,000)	$ 0
2. Less: Owning cash flow	(201,400)	10,600	17,800	10,000	45,400
3. Leasing versus owning CF	$166,400	($45,600)	($52,800)	($45,000)	($45,400)
NAL = $6,297.					
IRR = 5.3%.					

$166,400, but the business is then obligated to a series of cash outflows in Years 1 through 4.

4. By entering the Table 11–3 leasing versus owning cash flows into the cash flow registers of a calculator and then pressing the IRR (internal rate of return) button, or by using a spreadsheet model, it is easy to find the cost rate inherent in the incremental cash flow stream; it is 5.3 percent. This is the equivalent after-tax cost rate implied in the lease contract. Since this cost rate is less than the 7 percent after-tax cost of a regular loan, leasing is cheaper than borrowing and buying. Thus, the percentage cost analysis confirms the NAL analysis.

Some Additional Points about the Lessee's Analysis

So far, the main features of a lessee's analysis has been discussed. However, it is worthwhile to note the following points before moving on:

1. The dollar cost and percentage cost approaches will always lead to the same decision. Thus, one method is as good as the other from a decision standpoint.

2. If the net residual value cash flow (residual value and tax effect) is considered to be much riskier than the other cash flows in the analysis, it is possible to account for this risk by applying a higher discount rate to this flow, which results in a lower present value. Since the net residual value flow is an inflow in the cost-of-owning analysis, a lower present value leads to a higher present value cost of owning. Thus, increasing residual value risk decreases the attractiveness of owning an asset and hence increases the attractiveness of leasing the asset.

To illustrate, assume that Northside's managers believe that the computer's residual value is much riskier than the other flows in Table 11–2. Furthermore, they believe that 10.0 percent, rather than 7.0 percent, is the appropriate discount rate to apply to the residual value flows. When the Table 11–2 analysis is modified to reflect this risk, the present value cost of owning increases to $136,199 versus $133,148, while the NAL increases from $6,297 to $9,348. The riskier the residual value, the more favorable leasing becomes because a lease contract passes the residual value risk to the lessor. Of course, the more risky the residual value, the more risky the lease contract becomes for the lessor and hence the higher the rental payment.

3. In Chapter 7, in the discussion of the basics of capital investment analysis, the concept of net present value (NPV) was introduced. Basically, NPV is the dollar present value of a project assuming that it is financed using debt and equity financing. In lease analysis, the NAL is the additional dollar present value of a project (the additional NPV) attributable to leasing rather than using conventional (debt) financing. Thus, as an approximation of the value of a leased asset to the firm, the project's NPV can be increased by the amount of NAL.

$$\text{Adjusted NPV} = \text{NPV} + \text{NAL}$$

The value added through leasing, in some cases, can turn unprofitable (negative NPV) projects into profitable (positive adjusted NPV) projects.

Lease Analysis by Not-for-Profit Firms

The example used to illustrate a lessee's analysis was based on a lease decision by Northside Medical Center, a for-profit hospital. If the analysis were being performed by a not-for-profit corporation, the approach would be identical to the example; that is, the cost of leasing the asset is compared with the cost of borrowing and buying the asset, on either a dollar cost or percentage cost basis. The only analytical differences attributable to ownership are (1) non-taxable businesses will not have tax implications associated with the decision, and (2) the cost of debt to not-for-profit firms will often be the cost of tax-exempt debt.

Looking back at Table 11–2, a not-for-profit lessee would not show Lines 3, 4, or 6 in Part I, nor Line 10 in Part II. When a zero tax rate, which is equivalent to tax-exempt status, is entered into the model used to conduct the analysis and the discount rate is left at 10 percent, the NAL drops from $6,297 to $5,311. The decrease in NAL occurs because, under these particular lease terms and tax rates, tax effects favor leasing over owning. That is, the tax shelters associated with leasing are greater, on a present value basis, than the tax shelters associated with owning.

However, if the tax-exempt firm doing the analysis had access to 7 percent tax-exempt (municipal) debt financing, the NAL drops to –$4,483. Thus, the access to lower-cost debt financing, coupled with the loss of the tax benefits associated with leasing, drives the decision to favor owning. In this example, the lessor would have to lower the rental payment to make the lease attractive to a not-for-profit lessee with access to 7 percent tax-exempt debt.

EVALUATION BY THE LESSOR

Thus far, the discussion has considered leasing only from the lessee's viewpoint. It is also useful to analyze the transaction as the lessor sees it: Is the lease a good investment for the party that writes the lease, that is, the party that must put up the money to buy the asset? The lessor will generally be a specialized leasing company, a bank or bank affiliate, or a manufacturer such as General Electric Medical Systems that uses leasing as a sales tool. It is important for healthcare managers to understand the viewpoint of the lessor because (1) this knowledge enables lessees to drive better lease bargains in situations where the lease terms are negotiated, and (2) lessees are better able to understand in what situations leasing is likely to make financial sense and in what situations it is not.

The lessor's analysis involves (1) determining the net cash outlay, which is usually the invoice price of the equipment to be leased less any rental payments made in advance; (2) determining the periodic cash inflows, which consist of the rental payments minus both income taxes and any maintenance expense the lessor must bear; (3) estimating the after-tax residual value of the property when the lease expires; and (4) determining whether the rate of return on the lease is adequate for the risk of the investment.

To illustrate a lessor's analysis, assume the same facts as for the Northside Medical Center lease analysis but with these modifications: (1) The potential lessor is CompuLease, Inc., a commercial leasing company that specializes in leasing computers to healthcare providers. CompuLease's marginal federal-plus-state tax rate, T, is 40 percent. (2) To provide maintenance to Northside, CompuLease, like Northside, must contract with the computer manufacturer, but CompuLease has a volume contract with the manufacturer that reduces the maintenance payment to one thousand dollars at the beginning of each year. (3) CompuLease has better access to the market for used medical computer systems, so it estimates the residual value at $50,000, $10,000 higher than Northside's estimate. (4) CompuLease views computer lease arrangements as relatively low-risk investments. There is, however, some small chance of default on the lease, so CompuLease typically assumes that a lease investment is about as risky as buying AA-rated corporate bonds. Since four-year AA-rated bonds are yielding about 9 percent, CompuLease could earn an after-tax yield of $(9.0\%)(1 - T) = (9.0\%)(0.6) = 5.4\%$ on such investments. This is the after-tax return that CompuLease can obtain on alternative investments of similar risk and hence its opportunity cost rate.

The lease analysis from the lessor's standpoint is developed in Table 11–4. Here we see that the nature of the cash flows to the lessor is similar to those for the lessee shown in Table 11–2. Line 1 of Table 11–4 contains the purchase price of the computer, $200,000. Line 2 contains the maintenance costs, while Line 3 lists the tax savings attributable to these costs. Line 4 contains the depreciation tax savings, or tax shields, that accrue to the owner of the computer. Line 5 shows the annual rental payment as an inflow, while the taxes that must be paid on the rental payments are shown in Line

TABLE 11–4

Lessor's Analysis

	Year 0	Year 1	Year 2	Year 3	Year 4
1. Net purchase price	($200,000)				
2. Maintenance cost	($1,000)	($1,000)	($1,000)	($1,000)	
3. Maintenance tax savings	400	400	400	400	
4. Depreciation tax savings		16,000	25,600	15,200	$ 9,600
5. Rental payment	50,000	50,000	50,000	50,000	
6. Tax on rental payment	(20,000)	(20,000)	(20,000)	(20,000)	
7. Residual value					50,000
8. Tax on residual value					(6,400)
9. Net cash flow	($170,600)	$45,400	$55,000	$44,600	$53,200
NPV = $3,180.					
IRR = 6.2%.					

6. Lines 7 and 8 contain the residual value and resulting taxes. Finally, the cash flows are summed in Line 9.

The value of the lease contract to CompuLease can be easily found by discounting the Line 9 net cash flows at the firm's after-tax opportunity cost of capital, 5.4 percent, and then summing the resultant present values. For CompuLease, the NPV of the lease investment is $3,180, which means that the firm is better off by that amount, on a present-value basis, if it writes the lease rather than invests in comparable-risk AA-rated bonds. Conversely, if the NPV of the lease were negative, CompuLease would be better off investing in the bonds. Since we saw earlier that the lease is also advantageous to Northside, the transaction is beneficial to both parties and hence should be completed.

We can also calculate CompuLease's expected percentage rate of return on the lease by finding the internal rate of return (IRR) of the net cash flows shown on Line 9 of Table 11–4. Simply use the IRR function on a financial calculator, or a spreadsheet's @IRR function. The answer is 6.2 percent. Thus, the lease provides a 6.2 after-tax rate of return to CompuLease, which exceeds the 5.4 percent after-tax return available on alternative investments of similar risk, AA-rated four-year bonds. So, both the dollar rate of return (NPV) method and the percentage rate of return (IRR) method indicate that the lease is a good investment for the lessor. In general, both methods will lead to the same conclusion about the financial attractiveness of a lease investment.

In closing, note that the lease investment is actually slightly more risky than the alternative bond investment because the residual value cash flow is less certain than the principal repayment on an AA-rated bond. Thus, the lessor would probably require a rate of return somewhat above the 5.4 percent promised on the bond investment; and the higher the residual value risk, the higher the required rate of return. To incorporate differential residual value risk into the analysis, a higher discount rate could be applied to the residual value cash flows. This would lower the NPV, and hence make the lease investment look less attractive vis-à-vis the bond investment. Of course, as demonstrated in the next section, CompuLease could always raise the rental payment to boost the risk-adjusted return on the lease.

Setting the Lease Payment

The Northside–CompuLease example assumed that the rental payment had already been specified. However, as a general rule, in large leases the parties will sit down and work out an agreement as to the size and timing of the rental payments, with these payments being set so as to provide the lessor with some minimum required rate of return. In situations where the lease terms are not negotiable, which is often the case for small leases, the lessor must still go through the same type of analysis, setting terms that provide a target rate of return, and then offering these terms to potential lessees on a take-it-or-leave-it basis. Note, however, that competition among leasing companies forces lessors to build market-related returns into their lease payment schedules.

To illustrate lease payment setting, suppose CompuLease, after examining other alternative investment opportunities, decides that the 6.2 percent after-tax return on the Northside lease is too low and that the lease should provide a 12.0 percent pretax return (7.2 percent after taxes). What lease payment would provide this return? To answer this question, note again that Table 11–4 contains the lessor's cash flow analysis. If the basic analysis is set up on a spreadsheet, it is very easy to change the lease payment until the lease's NPV is zero at a 7.2 percent discount rate or, equivalently, its IRR is 7.2 percent. In the example, CompuLease must set the lease payment at $51,800 to obtain an expected after-tax rate of return of 7.2 percent. At this rental level, Northside's NAL is $1,730, so the lease deal remains favorable to both parties.

LEASE ANALYSIS SYMMETRY

Stop for a moment and compare the cash flows in Tables 11–2 and 11–4. Note that every line that appears in the lessee's analysis in the costs of owning and leasing sections (Parts I and II) also appears in the lessor's analysis. Some of the numbers are different, but the nature of the entries is the same.

In the example, the lessee had an NAL of $6,297, while the lessor's NPV was $3,180, so the lease contract was favorable to both parties. However, if both Northside and CompuLease "saw" the same set of cash flows, it would not be possible to set a rental payment that was acceptable to both parties.

To illustrate, assume that both parties (1) had the same tax rate, 30 percent; (2) estimated the same residual value, $40,000; (3) had to pay the manufacturer the same amount for maintenance, $2,000 per year; and (4) used the same pretax discount rate, 10 percent. Under these assumptions, the cash flows would be the same to each party, but some would have opposite signs. For example, the rental payment is an outflow to the lessee but an inflow to the lessor. The end result is that the net cash flows to the lessee and the lessor would be equal but opposite in sign. With these symmetrical inputs, Northside's NAL is $6,297 (the original value), but CompuLease's NPV is now –$6,297. When there is symmetry between the lessor and the lessee (same tax rates, discount rates, estimated salvage values, and so on), leasing is a zero-sum game. That is, the NAL to the lessee and the NPV to the lessor are equal but opposite in sign. Under symmetrical conditions, it is impossible to structure lease terms that are acceptable to both the lessee and lessor.

MOTIVATIONS FOR LEASING

Since leasing cannot be attractive to both the lessee and lessor when the lease inputs are symmetrical, why is leasing so popular? The answer, of course, is that numerous situations arise in the real world in which the lease inputs to the lessee and lessor are not symmetrical. It is asymmetries between the lessee and lessor that create the incentives required to make leasing a viable alterative to conventional (debt) financing. Here are some of the more common motivations for leasing brought about by asymmetries between the lessee and lessor.

Taxes

One of the most common motivations for leasing is differential tax rates. When the lessee and lessor are taxed at different rates, it is often possible to structure lease terms that are favorable to both parties. If the lessor has the higher rate, and this certainly holds when the lessee is a not-for-profit business, leasing permits the lessor to gain more tax advantages of ownership than would be available to the lessee, and some of the tax savings can then be passed on to the lessee in the form of lower rental payments. (Of course, the availability of tax-exempt debt makes leasing less attractive.) Even when the lessee has the higher tax rate, it is possible to structure lease terms so that the tax benefits associated with leasing (the tax deductibility of rental payments) is greater than the tax benefits associated with owning (depreciation tax shields).

Another tax-related motivation for leasing is the alternative minimum tax (AMT). Taxable corporations are permitted to use accelerated depreciation and other tax shelters to reduce taxes paid but then to use straight-line depreciation for stockholder reporting and hence to report high profits. Thus, some companies have reported high earnings in many years yet have paid little or no federal income taxes. The AMT, which is roughly calculated as 20 percent of profits as reported to shareholders, is designed to force profitable companies to pay at least some taxes.

Many companies are exposed to heavy tax liabilities under the AMT, so they are looking for ways to reduce reported income. Leasing can be beneficial here: Use a relatively short period for the lease and consequently have a high annual payment, and the result will be lower reported profits and hence a lower AMT liability. Note that the lease payments do not even have to qualify as a deductible expense for regular tax purposes; all that is needed is that they reduce reported income as shown on a firm's income statement.

Residual Value

Leasing companies are often more experienced in reselling used assets than are the lessee users. Thus, lessors are often able to obtain higher net prices when selling assets that come off lease than can lessees. This differential access to the used-asset market means that lessors can often build higher residual values into their lease analyses than can lessees. Higher net residual values may stem from negotiating higher sales prices, but they may also arise when the lessor's transaction costs in selling the used asset are less than those of the lessee. Finally, the lessor may elect to re-lease the asset to another lessee, and the value of re-leasing may be greater than the value inherent in selling the asset.

Residual Value Risk

Leasing is an attractive financing alternative for many high-technology items that are subject to rapid and unpredictable technological obsolescence. For example, assume a small, rural hospital wants to acquire a magnetic resonance imaging (MRI) device. If it buys the MRI equipment, it is exposed to the risk of technological obsolescence. In a relatively short time, some new technology might be developed that makes the current system almost worthless, and this large economic loss could create a financial burden on the hospital. Since it does not use much equipment of this nature, the hospital would bear a great deal of risk if it bought the MRI device.

However, a lessor that specializes in state-of-the-art medical equipment might be exposed to significantly less risk. By purchasing and then leasing many different high-tech items, the lessor benefits from equipment portfolio diversification; over time, some items will probably lose more value then the lessor expected, but these losses will be offset by other items that retain more value than was expected. Since the lessor is better able to bear the risk of technological obsolescence than the hospital, it would be able to charge a premium for bearing this risk that is less than the premium inherent in ownership. By passing the residual value risk to a party (the lessor) that is better able to bear this risk, leasing can be made more attractive to the hospital than owning.

Operating Risk

Per-procedure leases were mentioned briefly at the beginning of the chapter. In this type of lease, instead of a fixed annual or monthly payment, the lessor charges the lessee a fixed amount for each procedure performed. For example, the lessor may charge the hospital three hundred dollars for every scan performed using a leased MRI device. Since the per-procedure lease changes the hospital's cash flows for the MRI from a fixed payment under conventional financing to a variable payment that is highly correlated with the revenue stream, the hospital's risk is reduced. Conversely, the payment stream to the lessor is converted from a fixed stream to an uncertain stream, so the lessor's risk increases.

This type of arrangement can be beneficial to both parties if the lessor is better able to bear the usage risk than the lessee. As with residual values, if the lessor has written a large number of per-procedure leases, some of the leases will be more profitable than expected at the time the lease is written and some will be less profitable than expected, but if the lessor's expectations are unbiased, the aggregate return on all the leases will be quite close to that expected. Thus, the lessor mitigates the riskiness inherent in per-procedure leases through portfolio diversification and hence has lower risk than that faced by any lessee under conventional financing.

Leasing can also be attractive when a firm is uncertain about how long an asset will be needed. Again, consider the hospital industry. Hospitals sometimes offer services that are dependent on a single staff member—for example, a physician who does liver transplants. To support the physician's practice, the hospital might have to invest millions of dollars in equipment that can be used only for this particular procedure. The hospital will charge for the use of the equipment, and if things go as expected, the investment will be profitable. However, if the physician leaves the hospital staff, and if no other qualified physician can be recruited to fill the void, the project is dead, and the equipment becomes useless to the hospital.

In this situation, the annual usage may be quite predictable as long as the equipment is needed, but the need for the asset could suddenly cease. A lease with a cancellation clause would permit the hospital to simply return the equipment. The lessor would charge something for the cancellation clause because such clauses increase the riskiness of the lease to the lessor. The increased lease cost would lower the expected profitability of the project, but it would provide the hospital with an option to abandon the equipment, and such an option could have a value that exceeds the incremental cost of the cancellation clause. The leasing company would be willing to write this option because it is in a better position to remarket the equipment, either by writing another lease or by selling it outright.

Provision of Services

Some companies find leasing attractive because the lessor is able to provide services on favorable terms. For example, MEDEVAC Services, Inc., a for-profit ambulance and medical transfer service that operates in Pennsylvania, recently leased 25 ambulances and transfer vans. The lease agreement, with a large leasing company that specializes in purchasing, maintaining, and then reselling automobiles and trucks, permitted the replacement of an aging fleet that MEDEVAC had built up over seven years. "We are pretty good at providing emergency services and moving patients from one facility to another, but we aren't very good at maintaining an automotive fleet," said MEDEVAC's CEO.

Access to Financing

Finally, leasing may be financially attractive for smaller firms that have limited access to debt markets. For example, a small, recently formed physician group practice may need to finance one or more diagnostic devices, such as an EKG machine. The group has no credit history, so it would be relatively difficult, and hence costly, for a bank to assess the group's credit risk. Some banks might think the loan is not even worth the effort, while others might be willing to make the loan, but the high cost of credit assessment will be built into the loan rate. On the other hand, Medical Equipment Leasing Company has a division that specializes in leasing to group practices. Their analysts have assigned credit ratings to hundreds of group practices, and it is relatively easy for them to make the credit judgment. Thus, a specialized leasing company might be more willing to provide the financing, and charge lower rates, than conventional lenders.

Note, however, that the advantage of access to financing applies only to businesses that have limited access to conventional financing. Larger businesses that can easily issue debt securities and obtain bank loans do not benefit from improved access to financing. In such situations, leasing is attractive only if there are other considerations that make leasing preferable to conventional financing.

SOME CLOSING REMARKS

There are many reasons that might influence a firm to lease an asset rather than buy it. Often these reasons are difficult to quantify, so they cannot be easily incorporated into a numerical analysis. Nevertheless, a sound lease analysis must begin with a quantitative analysis, and then qualitative factors can be considered before making the final lease-or-buy decision. As a starting point in the decision process, remember that leasing companies are in business to make money, so they have to build an opportunity cost rate of return into every lease they write. To make leasing attractive to a potential lessee, there has to be some underlying economic rationale that favors leasing over conventional financing.

Discussions with financial managers in the healthcare industry indicate that standard numerical analyses rarely result in leasing being favored over buying. However, such analyses are extremely important to get a feel for the relative cost of leasing versus the cost of borrowing and buying. Then, other factors, such as the transfer of residual value risk, can be considered. Sometimes these factors can be quantified. For example, if risk transfer through a cancellation clause makes leasing less risky than owning, then the leasing cash flows can be discounted at a different rate than the owning cash flows. Since the flows being discounted are cash outflows (see Part II of Table 11–2), lower risk for the cost of leasing cash flows would lead to a higher discount rate, which would lower the cost of leasing, make leasing less expensive relative to owning, and hence reflect a favorable risk bias toward leasing. The problem, of course, is that there is no good way to know how much the discount rate applied to the leasing flows should be increased, so it is probably better to apply judgment rather than quantitative analysis when making the final decision.

When Dr. Gross informed Mr. Cooper of the availability of a per-procedure lease for the PET unit, he immediately directed the hospital's CFO to look into the matter.

After conducting a thorough analysis, the CFO concluded that using a fee-for-scan lease would decrease the expected profitability of the PET scanner, but, at the same time, it would substantially reduce the risk inherent in the project. The overall profitability of the project would be reduced because, at the expected level of usage, the cost of the lease payments would be greater than the implied cost of debt financing. However, at low usage rates, the cost of the lease would be less than the implied cost of debt financing, and hence the losses incurred if things went poorly would be mitigated by the per-procedure lease payments. In effect, the hospital would be paying a little more if things went well to transfer some downside risk to the lessor.

Since the main objection to the project was its riskiness, the project quickly obtained additional supporters. Within a month, the hospital's board of trustees agreed that such financing made the PET acquisition feasible, and within three months Seven Oaks had one up and running.

SELF-EXAMINATION EXERCISES

11–1   Who are the two parties to a lease agreement?

11–2   What are the two general types of leases?

11–3   a. How are leases classified by the Internal Revenue
          Service?

       b. How are leases classified by accountants?

11–4   a. Briefly discuss this statement: Leasing is a zero-sum
          game.

       b. What are the primary motivations for leasing rather
          than buying?

11–5   Goodhealth Diagnostics, a for-profit firm, is negotiat-
       ing a lease for a new one-million-dollar MRI system
       with Medical Leasing International. The terms of the
       lease offered by Medical Leasing call for a payment of
       $205,000 at the beginning of each year of the five-year
       lease. As an alternative to leasing, Goodhealth could
       borrow the needed million dollars at a 10 percent
       interest rate and use the funds to buy the MRI system.
       The equipment falls into the MACRS five-year class
       and has an expected residual value of $100,000.
       Maintenance costs would be included in the lease. If
       the system is purchased, a maintenance contract
       would be obtained that costs $10,000 at the beginning
       of each year. Medical Leasing has a 40 percent federal-
       plus-state marginal tax rate, while Goodhealth, which
       has a large amount of tax credits, has a tax rate of only
       20 percent.

       a. What is Goodhealth's present value of the cost of
          owning?

       b. What is Goodhealth's present value of the cost of
          leasing?

       c. Should Goodhealth purchase or lease the MRI sys-
          tem?

       d. Assume that Medical Leasing's best alternative to
          writing the lease is to invest in a five-year certificate
          of deposit that pays 9 percent before taxes. Should
          the lessor write the lease?

SELECTED REFERENCES

Beggan, John F. and Lauren K. McNulty. "Restrictions on Depreciation Where Tax-Exempt Entities Are Involved." *Topics in Health Care Financing*, Fall 1991, pp. 62–69.

Berg, Ian J. and Alan N. Frankel. "Equipment Leasing: How, When, and If." *Health Progress*, November 15, 1988, pp. 22–26.

Conbeer, George P. "Leasing Can Add Flexibility to High-Tech Asset Management." *Healthcare Financial Management*, July 1990, pp. 26–34.

Dine, Deborah Denaro. "Equipment Leasing Firms Offer Deals to Hospitals." *Modern Healthcare*, November 18, 1988, pp. 50–51.

Gapenski, Louis C. and Barbara Langland-Orban. "Leasing Capital Assets and Durable Goods: Opinions and Practices in Florida Hospitals." *Health Care Management Review*, Summer 1991, pp. 73–81.

Grant, Larry and Diane O'Donnell. "Watch for Pitfalls When Analyzing Lease Options." *Healthcare Financial Management*, July 1990, pp. 36–43.

"Leasing: Three Experts Discuss the Advantages of Equipment Leasing." *HealthWeek*, November 1989, pp. 51–53.

Meyers, Stewart C., David A. Dill, and Alberto J. Bautista. "Valuation of Financial Lease Contracts." *Journal of Finance*, June 1976, pp. 799–819.

Rosenthal, Robert A. "Creative Leasing Strategies for Medical Office Buildings." *Healthcare Financial Management*, December 1992, pp. 30–34.

12

CHAPTER

Dealing with Capitation

*J*ohn Griffin, the CEO of Capital City Health System, a newly formed integrated delivery system, knew that he had his work cut out for him. After only a year of operation, the PHO (physician–hospital organization) had to respond to a proposal by an HMO that would give Capital City a single dollar amount per member per month to provide all of the in-area healthcare services (excluding pharmacy) required by its eight thousand local members.

To respond to this proposal, John, and the System's board of directors, had to allocate the monthly premium among physicians and the hospital as well as develop a risk-sharing plan that would ensure both financial responsibility and quality services. The job would not be easy, but the board was convinced that it could not afford to lose the revenues associated with this patient population. As you read this chapter, think about what you might propose if you were in John's shoes. At the end, you will see how Capital City responded.

INTRODUCTION

Thus far in the book, we have focused on financial analysis and decision making in what might be termed a conventional reimbursement environment. In such an environment, providers are reimbursed on the basis of each patient encounter. Thus, each hospital stay and each patient visit generates additional revenue. The basis for payment may be charges, discounted charges, prospective payment, per diem, or some other methodology, but the key feature of conventional reimbursement is that higher patient volume, whether inpatient or outpatient, leads to increased revenues. Further, in most conventional payment methodologies, the greater the intensity of service provided, and hence the higher the costs, the greater the reimbursement amount.

In recent years, a new reimbursement methodology called capitation has been introduced that completely changes providers' financial incentives. Under capitation, providers receive a fixed fee for each member (patient) enrolled, regardless of the amount or intensity of services provided. Clearly, capitation represents a reimbursement methodology that requires a different approach to financial analysis and decision making than that used under conventional reimbursement. The basic principles of finance, such as discounted cash flow analysis, risk and return, and opportunity costs, remain unchanged, but the manner in which these concepts are applied must recognize the unique features of capitation.

In this chapter, we first present some background information about capitation; then we discuss the mechanics of capitation and its implications for healthcare financial analysis and decision making.

AN OVERVIEW OF CAPITATION

Formally defined, capitation is a flat periodic payment per enrollee to a healthcare provider that is the sole reimbursement for providing defined services to a defined population. The word *capitation* is derived from the term *per capita*, which means per person. Generally, capitation payments are expressed as some dollar amount per member per month (PMPM), where the word *member* typically means enrollee in a managed care plan, usually a health maintenance organization (HMO). For example, a primary care physician may receive a capitated payment of $14 PMPM for attending to the healthcare needs of 250 HMO enrollees. Under this contract, the physician would receive $14(250)(12) = $42,000 in total capitation payments over the year, and this amount must cover all of the primary care services specified in the contract that are provided to the covered population. Capitated payments often are adjusted for age and gender, but no other adjustments are typically made.

The primary impetus for capitation is the structural change that is occurring in the healthcare industry. Although the U.S. healthcare system accomplishes miraculous feats in curing disease and saving the lives of individuals with life-threatening injuries, it falls far short in the areas of prevention and health promotion. Also, delivery of healthcare services has become so expensive that employers, who are the primary purchasers of health insurance, are seeking lower-cost alternatives to the current system.

In an attempt to control costs, employers are forming coalitions to gain more bargaining clout when purchasing healthcare services. To illustrate, in 1995 10 major employers, including American Express, IBM, Merrill Lynch, and Sears, banded together to purchase one billion dollars of healthcare services for 600,000 employees from HMOs in 27 locations across the United States. The coalition gives the companies more leverage in controlling costs and quality than they would have on their own, especially at locations where each employer doesn't have a sufficient number of employees to wield much influence. Merrill Lynch's 1994 experience with a smaller coalition indicated that HMO premium rates dropped 7 percent in coalition cities but only 1 percent in other markets. These results are preliminary evidence that market forces are affecting, and even deflating, costs to healthcare purchasers. Furthermore, Merrill Lynch estimated that buyer coalitions result in healthcare costs that are about 8 percent lower than when companies contract individually. The coalition invites bids from 200 HMOs, selecting two to four plans in each market, on the basis of both quality and costs, to help foster competition.

It appears, at least for now, that healthcare purchasers are dictating the increased use of managed care as a potential means of both controlling costs and increasing emphasis on disease prevention. Within managed care plans, the preferred choice of employers is the HMO, and within HMOs, capitation is a commonly used payment mechanism.

THE IMPACT OF CAPITATION ON PROVIDERS

Capitation has a dramatic impact on provider incentives and hence on provider behavior. To begin our discussion of these issues, we will discuss the impact of capitation on provider incentives. Then, we present some evidence on what has occurred in markets that are dominated by capitated payment systems.

Incentives Under Capitation

Consider Figure 12–1, which depicts revenues and costs to a provider under both fee-for-service and capitated payment. Regardless of the payment system, total costs (TC), which are merely the sum of fixed costs (FC) and variable costs (VC), are tied directly to volume, so the greater the volume of services delivered, the greater the amount of total costs. The difference between the two graphs is the revenue line and how profits and losses are realized. Under fee-for-service, the revenue line (Rev) is upward sloping, and it starts at the origin. At zero volume, the provider receives zero revenue, and the greater the volume, the higher the revenue. Under capitation, assuming a fixed number of enrollees, revenues are fixed independently of volume, and hence the revenue line is horizontal. On each graph, breakeven (BE) is shown at that volume where revenues equal total costs.

FIGURE 12–1

Revenue and Cost Structures Under Fee-for-Service and Capitation

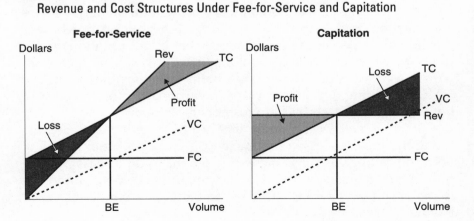

Although the graphs are somewhat similar in general appearance, there is a profound difference in how profits and losses occur. First, consider fee-for-service. All volumes to the left of breakeven produce a loss for the provider, while all volumes to the right of breakeven produce a profit. Thus, the incentive for providers is to increase utilization because increased volume leads to increased profits. Now look at the capitation graph. Here, all volumes to the left of breakeven produce a profit, whereas all volumes to the right of breakeven result in a loss. Under capitation, providers have the incentive to decrease utilization because decreased volume leads to increased profits. The only way to increase revenues under capitation is to increase the number of covered lives (enrollees).

Capitation completely reverses the actions that providers must take to assure financial success, and many providers will find it difficult to adjust to the new, perverse (by conventional reimbursement standards) incentive system. Under fee-for-service, the keys to success are to work harder, increase volume, and hence increase profits; while under capitation, the keys to profitability are to work smarter and decrease volume. Since the primary means to profitability with fee-for-service is increased volume, increased reimbursement rates, or both, the primary task of managers is to maximize utilization and reimbursement rates. Furthermore, any deficiencies in cost control often can be overcome by higher volume. Under capitation, the primary path to profitability is through cost control, so the key to success is lower volume and cost-effective treatment plans.

Although much has been written about the negatives of capitation, particularly the incentive to withhold needed services, it must also be recognized that there are positive aspects to capitation:

1. Providers receive a fixed payment regardless of whether services are actually rendered. Capitation revenues are predictable and timely, and thus are less risky than revenues from conventional payment methodologies, which are tied to volume.

2. Capitation payments are received before services are rendered so in effect, payers are extending credit to providers rather than vice versa, as under conventional reimbursement.

3. Capitation supports national healthcare goals, primarily increased emphasis on cost control as well as wellness and prevention.

4. Capitation may ease the reimbursement paperwork burden and hence reduce expenditures on administrative costs.

5. Capitation aligns the economic interests of physicians and hospitals because risk-sharing systems are typically established that allow all providers in a capitated system to benefit from reducing costs.

6. Similarly, capitation encourages utilization of lower-cost treatments, such as outpatient surgery and home healthcare, as opposed to higher-cost inpatient alternatives. Thus, capitation creates incentives to use those services that are typically preferred by patients when such alternatives are clinically appropriate.

Behavior under Capitation

In attempting to predict the future, it is interesting to examine the impact of capitation on provider behavior in those markets where managed care has the strongest presence. Several markets, such as Rochester, New York, and Madison, Wisconsin, now have HMOs controlling more than 50 percent of the healthcare market, but the managed care plans and integrated delivery systems in southern California have been particularly aggressive in gobbling up market share. For example, in Los Angeles, seven large integrated networks control 75 percent of the city's commercial healthcare market. Thus, southern California in general and Los Angeles in particular are often cited as examples where providers have already responded to the pressures of capitation and hence represent a view of what the entire country would resemble if capitation becomes the predominant reimbursement system.

Table 12–1 illustrates the impact of capitation on hospital utilization. Whereas current hospital utilization averages over 700 inpatient days annually per one thousand patient population, capitated systems that aggressively control inpatient stays have reduced utilization to only 238 inpatient days. When these data are converted to daily census, and allowing for 85 percent occupancy

TABLE 12-1

Impact of Capitation on Annual Hospital Utilization

Age	Number of Inpatient Days per 1,000 Covered Population		
	National Average	HMO Average	Capitated Target
Under 65	433	297	155
Over 65	2,676	1,691	850
Overall*	702	465	238

*Based on an age mix of 12 percent over age 65.

Source: Estimated by Jennings Ryan & Kolb on the basis of 1994 data from the National Center for Health Statistics, *Managed Care Digest* (Marion Merrill Dow, 1994), and the Advisory Board Government Committee.

as full capacity, only about 0.8 beds are required per one thousand population versus a current need of about 2.3 beds per thousand based on national average usage rates. The implication for hospitals is clear: If the capitated targets are realistic, and if the bulk of the U.S. population becomes covered by HMO plans, the hospital industry has significant overcapacity, and continued shrinkage is likely to occur. Even if the most aggressive utilization targets are not met, HMO penetration and capitation will surely increase the pace of hospital closings, consolidation, and downsizing already taking place.

Table 12–2 focuses on the impact of capitation on selected physician utilization. The key feature here is that managed care, with its emphasis on wellness and prevention as opposed to treatment, requires a different mix and fewer physicians than currently exists. Furthermore, managed care plans use more physician extenders, such as nurse practitioners and physician assistants, than are currently utilized.

Of course, not all predictions come true, and the structure of the healthcare industry may not change as drastically as these forecasts indicate. However, experience to date suggests two powerful trends: fewer hospital beds and a physician mix that contains a greater proportion of primary care physicians. Most importantly, the data tell us that historical utilization rates based on conventional reimbursement methodologies are not good predictors of future utilization when the payment system is capitation.

T A B L E   12–2

Impact of Capitation on Physician and Physician Extender Utilization

Specialty	FTEs per 100,000 Covered Population		Percent of Current Supply Needed Under Capitation
	1992 Supply	HMO Needs	
Family practice/ general medicine	29.3	11.7	39.9%
Internal medicine	23.3	23.8	102.1
Pediatrics	13.1	11.9	90.8
Total primary care	65.7	47.4	72.1%
Obstetrics/gynecology	11.4	10.1	86.0%
Medical specialties	17.8	12.7	71.3
Surgical specialties	32.5	21.2	65.2
Total specialists	61.7	44.0	71.3%
Total physicians	127.4	91.4	71.7%
Physician extenders	19.6	25.0	127.6%

Source: Adapted from Jonathan P. Weiner, "Forecasting the Effects of Healthcare Reform on U.S. Physician Workforce Requirements: Evidence from HMO Staffing Patterns," *Journal of the American Medical Association,* July 20, 1994.

FINANCIAL RISK UNDER CAPITATION

One of the key issues facing providers is the impact of capitation on financial risk. To examine this issue, we will first present a descriptive picture of financial risk, then examine the nature of financial risk, and finally present the results of an analysis that examined the financial risk inherent in capitation contracts.

Descriptive Risk

One way to assess the risk inherent in capitation versus other reimbursement contracts is to describe in words the nature of the risks incurred.

Table 12–3 lists the most common provider reimbursement methodologies and describes the financial risks inherent in each system. Fee-for-service is the least risky because the only risk facing providers is the risk that volume will be too low to cover total costs, including both variable and fixed costs. Note that regardless of the reimbursement method, providers bear the cost of service risk, in that costs can exceed revenues. However, a primary difference among the reimbursement types is the ability of the provider to influence the revenue/cost ratio. If providers set fees for each type of service provided, they can most easily ensure that revenues exceed costs. Furthermore, if providers have the power to set rates above those that would exist in a truly competitive market, fee-for-service becomes even less risky. Finally, providers can increase usage by churning—creating more visits, ordering more tests, extending inpatient stays, and so on—which in turn increases revenues and reduces

TABLE 12–3

Descriptive Risk under Various Reimbursement Methodologies

Contract Type	Provider Risks
Fee-for-service (charges)	Volume too low to cover total costs
Discounted fee-for-service (discounted charges)	Volume too low to cover total costs
Prospective payment	Volume too low to cover fixed costs Case intensity Length of stay
Per diem	Volume too low to cover fixed costs Case intensity Case mix Payer limited length of stay
Global pricing	Volume too low to cover fixed costs Case intensity Pre- and postoperative care Physician services
Capitation	Volume too high for payment amount Case intensity Case mix Utilization Actuarial accuracy

risks. Discounted fee-for-service may lower the profit potential of providers, but it does not alter the risks borne by providers.

Prospective payment, in which a fixed payment is made on the basis of each patient's diagnosis, adds a second dimension of risk to reimbursement contracts because the bundle of services needed to treat a particular patient may be more costly than that assumed in the payment. If, on average, patients require more intensive treatments and, for hospitals, a longer length of stay than assumed in the prospective payment amount, the provider must bear the added costs.

Per diem reimbursement, whereby providers are paid a preset amount per patient day, is often used for hospitals and long-term care facilities. In addition to a single all-inclusive per diem rate, stratified per diems are sometimes used whereby different rates are paid for dissimilar categories of care, such as general acute inpatient, obstetrical, and intensive care. Even under stratified per diems, one rate usually covers a large number of diagnoses, so providers bear case-mix risk along with intensity risk. In addition, providers bear the risk that the payer, through utilization reviews, will constrain lengths of stay and hence increase intensity during the days that a patient is hospitalized. Thus, under per diem, the "compression" of services and shortened lengths of stay can put significant pressure on providers' profitability.

Under global pricing, payers pay a single prospective payment that covers all services delivered in a single episode, whether the services are rendered by a single or by multiple providers. For example, a global fee may be set for all obstetric services associated with a pregnancy provided by a single physician, including all prenatal and postnatal visits, as well as the delivery itself. Or a global price may be paid for all physician and hospital services associated with a cardiac bypass operation.

From a payer's perspective, global pricing eliminates the potential for problems associated with unbundling and upcoding. Unbundling involves pricing the individual components of a service separately, rather than as a package. For example, a physician's treatment of a fracture could be bundled and hence billed as one episode, or it could be unbundled, with separate bills submitted for diagnosis, X-rays, setting the fracture, removing the cast, and so on. The rationale for unbundling is usually to provide more detailed records of treatments rendered, but often the result is higher total charges for the parts than would be charged for the entire package.

Upcoding is the practice of billing for a procedure that yields a higher prospective payment than the one actually performed. Clearly, the more services that must be rendered for a single payment, the more providers are at risk for intensity of services.

Finally, under capitation, providers receive a fixed payment per member per month to provide all covered services to some defined population. Now, providers assume utilization and actuarial risks along with the risks assumed under the other reimbursement methods.

When the risks under different reimbursement systems are outlined in this descriptive fashion, it is easy to jump to the conclusion that capitation is by far the riskiest to providers, while fee-for-service is the least risky. However, before finalizing our conclusions regarding the risk to providers under capitation contracts, we need to examine the issue a little more closely. We begin our more detailed examination with a discussion of the nature of financial risk.

The Nature of Financial Risk

As discussed in Chapters 2 and 8, financial risk stems from uncertainties inherent in expected cash flows. If all forecasted cash flows were known with certainty, there would be no financial risk. However, because of uncertainties, there is some probability that a reimbursement contract will be less profitable than expected, and the greater the probability of a realized profitability far below that expected, the greater the financial risk.

Note that financial risk and profitability are two separate and distinct attributes of a reimbursement contract. Under any reimbursement methodology, rates can be set too low to cover costs, resulting in losses to the provider. However, such losses do not necessarily imply financial risk because financial risk (as classically defined and used in this book) depends on the uncertainty of profitability, not its level. To illustrate, a hospital contract with a payer that promises a certain loss of $50,000 has no financial risk because there is no uncertainty regarding the contract's financial outcome. In many situations, payers offering capitated contracts have a great deal of bargaining power that can be used to negotiate payment terms that are unfavorable to hospitals. The resulting losses are not a result of the financial risk inherent in capitation contracts but, rather, stem from concessions made by the hospital, presumably due to the negotiating power of the payer.

A Quantitative Analysis

The financial risk associated with provider contracts stems from uncertainty in profitability, so both revenues and costs must be considered. We will use hospitals to analyze the financial risk inherent in prospective payment and capitation contracts, but the results apply to physicians and other healthcare providers. Under prospective payment, there is significant revenue risk since the amount of reimbursement depends on the number of admissions, with higher volume yielding greater revenues. However, under capitation, and assuming a fixed number of enrollees, there is virtually no revenue risk. The hospital will receive the contractually fixed amount per member per month regardless of patient volume.

On the cost side, the financial risks are identical under the two contracts. There are fixed costs inherent in providing the service that must be met regardless of volume, and variable costs that are incurred for each patient admission. Thus, total costs, the sum of fixed and variable components, are dependent on volume. If we assume, at least initially, that the number and nature of admissions are unaffected by the reimbursement contract, realized total costs are the same for a given population whether the payment method is prospective payment or capitation.

The financial risk facing hospitals is tied to uncertainty in profitability and hence stems from both uncertainties in the revenue stream and uncertainties in total costs. To examine the impact of these uncertainties, we will consider two hospitals: Hospital F, whose costs are all fixed, and Hospital V, whose costs are all variable. Clearly, no real-world hospital has all fixed or all variable costs, but by looking at these extremes we can gain a better appreciation of the factors that influence financial risk under prospective payment and capitation.

To keep the analysis manageable, assume a hypothetical situation in which the contract involves one thousand members; the annual capitation payment is three hundred dollars per member per year (PMPY); the expected number of inpatient stays is 0.1 PMPY, or one hundred admissions per year; and the prospective payment per admission is three thousand dollars. On the cost side, assume Hospital F has fixed costs of $300,000, and no variable costs, to treat the population served, while Hospital V has variable costs of three thousand dollars per inpatient stay, and no fixed costs.

Table 12–4 contains the annual cash flows to each hospital associated with the two contracts. Note that the initial values were chosen so that the revenues are the same under each contract type and that total costs are the same at both hospitals. Also, for ease, the values were chosen so that the net income under both contracts is zero.

Now, let's introduce risk into the analysis. Again, to keep the example manageable, assume that the only uncertainty in the contracts is patient volume. That is, the capitation payment, prospective payment per admission, fixed costs, and variable costs per inpatient stay are known with certainty at the beginning of the year (beginning of the contract period). What would happen to profitability if realized volume differed from expected volume? Table 12–5 answers this question.

Uncertain volume has no effect on Hospital F under capitation or on Hospital V under prospective payment. In each instance, revenues and costs move in step with one another. Hospital F has all fixed costs, and under capitation its revenues are fixed, so changes in volume have no impact on profitability. Under prospective pay-

TABLE 12–4

Annual Cash Flows

	Hospital F		Hospital V	
	Prospective Payment	Capitation	Prospective Payment	Capitation
Total revenues	$300,000	$300,000	$300,000	$300,000
Fixed costs	300,000	300,000	0	0
Variable costs	0	0	300,000	300,000
Net income	$ 0	$ 0	$ 0	$ 0

TABLE 12–5

Net Income at Different Volume Levels

	Hospital F		Hospital V	
Number of Inpatient Stays	Prospective Payment	Capitation	Prospective Payment	Capitation
80	($60,000)	$0	$0	$60,000
85	(45,000)	0	0	45,000
90	(30,000)	0	0	30,000
95	(15,000)	0	0	15,000
100	0	0	0	0
105	15,000	0	0	(15,000)
110	30,000	0	0	(30,000)
115	45,000	0	0	(45,000)
120	60,000	0	0	(60,000)

ment, revenues vary with volume, while costs are fixed, so higher volume leads to higher profitability. Thus, with prospective payment contracts, Hospital F has a financial incentive to increase volume because increased volume leads to higher profits.

The situation is reversed at Hospital V. When all costs are variable, profits are constant under prospective payment but variable under capitation. Increased volume leads to increased revenue under prospective payment, but the revenue increase is offset exactly by higher costs. Hospital V receives three thousand dollars for each admission, but its variable costs also equal three thousand dollars per admission, so additional admissions add nothing to the bottom line. Lower volume means lower costs regardless of the reimbursement method, but under capitation the revenue stream is fixed, so Hospital V has a financial incentive with capitation to decrease volume because lower volume leads to higher profits.

The analysis could be extended to include uncertainty in variable costs and prospective payment per admission, but the general results would remain the same. If all costs are fixed, there is less financial risk to capitation contracts than to prospective payment contracts. If all costs are variable, there is less financial risk to prospective payment contracts than to capitation contracts.

When assessing the relative financial risk of capitation contracts, the key question to providers is this: Are the costs at my organization predominantly fixed or predominantly variable? If the costs are mostly fixed, financial risk is actually reduced when moving from prospective payment to capitation because the fixed revenue stream better matches the fixed cost structure. On the other hand, if the cost structure is predominantly variable, moving to capitation will increase financial risk since the fixed revenue stream is a poor match for a cost structure that is highly correlated to volume.

Most healthcare providers, and hospitals in particular, have relatively high fixed-to-total-cost ratios. Thus, for most providers, capitation contracts can result in less financial risk than prospective payment contracts because financial risk is reduced by matching the uncertainties inherent in the revenue and cost streams. When organizations have a high percentage of fixed costs, a fixed revenue stream stabilizes profits and hence reduces financial risk.

If the quantitative analysis concludes that financial risk is reduced under capitation contracts, why did the descriptive analysis conclude that capitation is more risky than prospective payment? One reason, of course, is that the descriptive assessment did not consider in any systematic way the relationships between revenues and costs. More importantly, the quantitative analysis ignored some types of risk inherent in capitation contracts. The quantitative analysis assumed that providers know their cost structures and population characteristics well enough to be confident of the revenue and cost estimates. Under these conditions, capitation contracts are clearly less risky to providers with a high percentage of fixed costs.

However, to limit the financial risk of capitation contracts to that shown in the quantitative analysis, it is necessary that providers be able to forecast accurately costs and volumes for a large number of diagnoses. For example, assume a hospital signs a capitation contract to provide all common inpatient services to a patient population of 100,000. If the hospital is to limit its financial risk, it must know with some confidence the expected volume by diagnosis, as well as the costs for treating those diagnoses. Thus, the hospital needs relatively sophisticated actuarial and cost data.

Even if a contract has substantial underlying financial risk, its effective riskiness is lessened if management can take actions to counter unexpected adverse trends as they develop. Suppose a hospital enters into a capitation contract without good estimates of volume and costs. If six months into the contract, realized total costs exceed estimates, the contract will likely be less profitable than expected, and if the volume and cost estimates were very inaccurate, the results could prove disastrous. The only means available to turn the bad contract into a good one is to decrease volume, lower costs, or both.

In the past, hospitals with profitability problems solved such problems by raising charges and increasing volume. Under capitation, however, the prescription for increased profit requires actions—decreasing volume or lowering costs and increasing enrollment—with which providers have limited experience and hence are more difficult to implement than previous prescriptions. Furthermore, when a high proportion of costs is fixed, cost reduction efforts are extremely challenging because they can be achieved only by selling off plant and equipment and shrinking the labor force. Under capitation contracts, providers are less able to influence the profitability of a contract once it goes into force, so they are less able to cope with the given amount of financial risk faced.

Another risk that providers face under capitation is the impact of outliers. The costs associated with a single patient, especially to a hospital, can fall well beyond normal bounds, and hence one or just a few outliers can result in financial losses well beyond those estimated at the time a contract is signed. In general, prospective payment contracts have outlier provisions, so providers are somewhat protected against the risks associated with high-cost outliers. If capitation contracts do not contain such provisions, the risk of outliers increases the financial risk inherent in such contracts. Furthermore, to increase the probability that realized volume, and hence cash flows, will be close to that forecasted, providers must have a relatively large number of covered lives under capitation contracts.

Finally, we have ignored inter-contract-year risks. Most DRG and per diem contracts are awarded by payers to multiple providers within a given service area. Here, the variation of utilization from year to year on a given contract due to patients using alternative providers is relatively small. Conversely, capitation contracts are typically awarded to a single provider (or single panel) in a given service area. If a payer awards the contract currently held by one provider to a competing provider, the negative utilization, and hence profitability, consequences for the former can be severe. Additionally, the negotiating power of payers using single-provider capitation contracts is obviously greater than payers using multiple-provider contracts with other reimbursement methodologies.

Our quantitative analysis leads to two primary conclusions about the relative risk of capitation contracts. First, the pure quantitative financial risk inherent in capitation contracts is not as high as most people think. Providers with a high percentage of fixed costs can actually stabilize earnings under capitation, and hence reduce financial risk. Second, the overall financial risk of capitation contracts can be very high if providers (1) do not have the actuarial and cost data available to make sound capitation pricing decisions and (2) do not have the capability to reduce volume and cut costs, if necessary, to react to any adverse trends that might develop.

Taken together, these conclusions have several implications for healthcare providers. To prosper in a healthcare system moving rapidly towards capitation, providers must be able to estimate accurately not only their own costs but also the diagnoses and patient volumes that would result from a particular contract. This means that many providers will need better costing systems than they currently have and also that providers will need to acquire actuarial expertise, a domain historically left to insurers. Without these data, it will be impossible to enter into capitation contracts without bearing a high degree of subjective financial risk.

One efficient way for providers to acquire actuarial data is to enter into integrated networks that possess such data, so the trend towards networks can reduce the riskiness inherent in capitation contracts. Also, providers will have to break with traditional paradigms. Financial problems can no longer be solved by raising charges and increasing volume. Under capitation, raising charges (having a high bid on a contract proposal) will mean fewer patients for the provider, which will have an adverse impact both on revenues and on achieving a capitated population sufficiently large to realize actuarial predictions. Furthermore, the key to success once the contract has been signed is to lower costs and volume. This requires nontraditional strategies, so today's healthcare managers must exhibit flexibility and adaptability to successfully manage the transition to capitation.

Finally, providers that are less efficient than their local counterparts confront very difficult issues when negotiating managed care contracts. Capitation contracts are usually set at rates that assume the efficient delivery of services in order to control unnecessary services and costs. Less efficient providers will experience more challenges under capitation since they must choose between accepting rates that may not cover costs, at least in the short run, or losing market share that they may not be able to regain. The difficulties inefficient providers face do not result from financial risk differentials but, rather, from prior management practices that did not sufficiently stress the efficient delivery of services.

ALLOCATION OF PREMIUM DOLLARS

Organizations such as HMOs collect premium dollars from employers and, in return, provide healthcare services to covered employees. The premium dollars collected must be sufficient to (1) pay for the medical services consumed, (2) cover the HMO's administrative expenses, and (3) provide for profits.

To better understand this process, consider Table 12–6, which shows how a typical premium dollar is spent. First, HMOs have the same types of management and marketing expenses as any other business, and the premium dollar must cover such costs. Also, it is necessary for HMOs to earn profits, both to create reserves for contingencies and for distribution to stockholders if investor-owned. About 16 percent of the premium dollar goes for administration and profit, while the remaining 84 percent is paid out to providers. The biggest provider expense typically is for physicians, with approximately 12 percent of the premium dollar going to primary care physicians and 32 percent to specialists that are part of the HMO's provider panel.

The next major item is payments for hospital and other institutional care provided within the system (within the HMO's provider panel), which totals 36 percent of the premium dollar. Finally, HMO members sometimes require services from providers that are out of the HMO's system, either because there are no in-system providers for that service or the services were required outside the geographic area served by the HMO. Payments to out-of-system providers, including both physicians and hospitals/institutions, average 4 percent of the premium dollar.

TABLE 12–6

Typical Allocation of the HMO Premium Dollar

Total premium dollar	100%
Administration and profit	16%
Paid to within-system physicians:	
Primary care	12%
Specialists	32%
Total to within-system physicians	44%
Paid to within-system hospitals/institutions	36%
Paid to out-of-system providers	4%

Source: Jennings Ryan & Kolb.

Note that the Table 12–6 percentages are averages; there are wide variations among HMOs as to how the premium dollar is allocated. Healthcare purchasers want a high percentage of the premium dollar going to providers to encourage them to provide needed services in a timely manner. Conversely, HMOs have an incentive to lower the amount paid to providers, both to increase profits and to ensure competitive pricing to buyers in an increasingly hostile marketplace.

RISK-SHARING ARRANGEMENTS

In an integrated delivery system, or within the provider panel of a managed care plan, different providers are brought together in some type of formal or informal arrangement to provide healthcare services to a defined population. Often, provider participants are paid under different reimbursement methods, and different reimbursement systems clearly create different incentives. To illustrate, assume that an integrated delivery system uses capitation for primary care physicians, discounted fee-for-service for specialists, and per diem for institutional providers. In such a system, primary care physicians have the incentive to shift care to specialists and institutions because primary care physicians are capitated and hence not rewarded for higher utilization. On the other hand, specialists and institutions would welcome the added volume because they are being paid on the basis of the amount of services provided. Overall, this differential in reimbursement creates incentives that increase total system costs and hence costs to insurers and purchasers.

If both primary care and specialist physicians are capitated, primary care physicians would still have the incentive to make unnecessary referrals, but such referrals would no longer be welcome by specialists. If the institutions also are capitated, no provider wants increased volume, so conflicts are bound to occur between primary care physicians and specialists and between physicians and institutions.

In such situations, risk-sharing arrangements are often implemented to create incentives that encourage providers to act in the best interest of the system rather than in their own self-interest. Generally, proper incentives are created within integrated systems by establishing withholds, or risk pools, which are pools of money that are initially withheld and then distributed to providers only if preestablished goals are met.

Risk-Sharing Basics

Risk pools can be used with any type of reimbursement system, such as the use of withholds in a per diem system, whereby the hospital is rewarded if utilization is less than expected and, in effect, is penalized by not getting some portion or all of the amount withheld if utilization exceeds targets. In effect, risk pools are designed to reward those providers that are most able to control costs through better utilization management, better cost control, or both. Risk-sharing arrangements can occur among physicians only, among physicians and institutions, or among all providers. Furthermore, risk pools can be established to promote only financial goals or some combination of financial and nonfinancial goals.

Note that if a system is fully integrated and all subsidiary providers are owned by, and hence directly responsible to, the same parent, there is only one bottom line (and only one boss), so there is no need for risk-sharing arrangements. Proper incentives are created by managerial control. However, in most systems today, providers are loosely affiliated in some way rather than part of the same corporation, and hence risk-sharing arrangements are needed to align the incentives of the diverse parties involved.

Typically, risk-sharing arrangements allocate 10 to 20 percent of each reimbursement dollar to one or more risk pools, often for primary care, specialty (referral) care, and institutional care. Then, throughout the year, expenses are charged against the applicable pools, and at year-end, each pool's expenses are reconciled, that is, compared with those budgeted. Any surpluses are distributed to the participating providers on the basis of a prearranged formula. Any deficits are typically funded from network reserves, which, as we will discuss later, are established specifically to cover system cost overruns.

The best way to grasp the basics of risk sharing is through an example. Here, we illustrate a risk pool arrangement for primary care physicians (PCPs) used by Healthy HMO. The HMO pays its PCPs by capitation, but a percentage of the total capitated amount is held in reserve and distributed to individual physicians if certain financial goals are met. In general, PCP goals are based on specialty care and hospital costs. Of course, the goal is to lower the overall cost of providing care, but cost reduction goals should not reduce the quality of care afforded to patients.

Assume that Healthy HMO's capitation payment to PCPs is $15 PMPM, but that 20 percent of this amount is placed into the PCP risk pool. The budgeted amount for specialty and hospital costs is $45 PMPM. Of course, the purpose of the pool is to encourage PCPs to take actions that result in realized specialty and hospital costs that are less than those budgeted. For simplicity assume that there are only three PCPs in the plan: Physician L (for low-cost), Physician M (for medium-cost), and Physician H (for high-cost). Furthermore, assume that each physician has one thousand patients under the plan, so there are three thousand patients in total.

Table 12–7 contains the risk pool distributions under two different outcome scenarios. Line 1 gives each PCP's initial annual capitation payment: $15 PMPM(12 months)(1,000 members) = $180,000. Thus, 3($180,000) = $540,000 in total is allocated for PCP payments. However, 20 percent of the capitated amount is placed into the risk pool, so each PCP's annual capitated payment is reduced by 0.20($180,000) = $36,000. This reduction and the resulting $144,000 actual payment are shown on Lines 2 and 3. Note that each of the members served by the three PCPs is allocated $45 for specialty and hospital costs, so the budgeted goal for these costs is 1,000($45)(12) = $540,000 per PCP, or $1,620,000 in total, as shown

TABLE 12-7

Primary Care Physician (PCP) Risk Pool
(annual amounts)

	Physician L	Physician M	Physician H
1. Allocated amount	$180,000	$180,000	$180,000
2. Withhold (20 percent)	(36,000)	(36,000)	(36,000)
3. Initial payment	$144,000	$144,000	$144,000
4. Budgeted referral costs	$540,000	$540,000	$540,000
Scenario 1: Distribution Based on Aggregate PCP Performance			
5. Actual referral costs	500,000	560,000	680,000
6. Referral gain (loss)	40,000	(20,000)	(140,000)
7. Withhold returned	0	0	0
8. Total compensation	$144,000	$144,000	$144,000
Scenario 2: Distribution Based on Individual PCP Performance			
9. Actual referral costs	500,000	560,000	600,000
10. Referral gain (loss)	40,000	(20,000)	(140,000)
11. Withhold returned	36,000	16,000	0
12. Total compensation	$180,000	$160,000	$144,000

on Line 4. Also, note that the total amount in the PCP risk pool is
3($36,000) = $108,000.

Now consider Scenario 1, contained in Lines 5, 6, 7, and 8.
Here, we assume that no PCP will receive any funds from the pool
if it is empty at year end. The actual referral costs for each PCP are
the amounts shown on Line 5. The referral gain (loss) for each PCP
is shown on Line 6, and the total gain (loss) for all three PCPs is
$40,000 – $20,000 – $140,000 = –$120,000. This exceeds the $108,000
in the risk pool, so no funds remain for distribution. In fact,
Healthy HMO will have to fund the $108,000 – $120,000 = –$12,000
shortfall from its own reserves. Since no funds remain in the pool
for distribution, each PCP's realized compensation would be his or
her initial capitation payment, $144,000.

Clearly, there is a problem with the way the risk pool is allocated. Since no funds remained in the pool, all three PCPs were
equally penalized, even though Physician L did an excellent job of

controlling costs and Physician M came in only $20,000 over budget. The real cause of the failure to meet the overall referral budget was Physician H, who was a whopping $140,000 over budget. Is it fair to penalize L and M because of H's actions? If, over time, it appears to Physicians L and M that the risk pool will always be exhausted due to actions beyond their control, they will have no motivation to continue to practice as efficiently as they do now. Also, it is important to know whether Physician H's failure to meet the risk pool budget was a result of practice patterns or having an extraordinary number of high-cost patients. If the patient mix is not equal across PCPs, obvious problems will arise, so Healthy HMO must be careful in assigning patients to ensure (to the extent possible) that the usage and intensity mix is evenly spread across PCPs or that adjustments are made to account for such differences.

Scenario 2 in Table 12–7 is similar to Scenario 1, except that payments are made from the withhold to individual physicians regardless of the aggregate position of the pool. In this situation, the aggregate pool is really an artificiality; what counts is each physician's pool because Healthy HMO will reward individual PCPs that come in at or under budget regardless of aggregate performance. Thus, as shown on Line 11, Physician L, because he or she came in below budget, would receive the entire withhold amount from his or her pool, which results in total compensation of $144,000 + $36,000 = $180,000. Physician M would receive $36,000 – $20,000 = $16,000 from his or her pool, for total compensation of $160,000, while Physician H would receive nothing from his or her pool, for a total compensation of $144,000. This type of arrangement creates better incentives for PCPs, but Healthy HMO has to bear the total cost of the pool payments, $52,000, because the actions of Physician H depleted the pool. The key here is to modify the behavior of Physician H so that funds remain in the pool to make the incentive payments. Perhaps, after one year, Physician H will be motivated to follow lower-cost practice patterns because of the potential monetary rewards.

Note that there is an almost infinite number of ways in which a PCP risk pool can be distributed. Another alternative to Scenario 2 would be this: If the aggregate risk pool is depleted, payments to individual physicians will be cut in half. If this were the situation in Scenario 2 in Table 12–7, Physician L would get only $18,000 from the pool on Line 12, while Physician M would be paid $8,000. Now, the actions of Physician H have a direct bearing on the payments to L and M, so it is in the best interests of L, M, and the system to encourage H to lower costs. Also, with this distribution system, the HMO does not replace the full amount of the pool if it is depleted.

Performance-Based Pools

Often, risk pools are designed to control utilization and costs, but such pools can be structured to influence other types of behavior. To illustrate, primary care as well as specialty physicians may participate in a performance-based pool, wherein the pool is distributed on the basis of both financial and nonfinancial performance. Here is how a performance-based pool might work for primary care physicians. Some percentage, say, 20, of the total capitation payment is withheld. At the end of the year, the pool is distributed to physicians based on performance in four areas: (1) quality of care, (2) quality of service, (3) cost control, and (4) organizational participation. Thirty percent of the pool is allocated to each of the first three areas, and 10 percent is allocated to organizational participation. Physicians are "graded" in each area. For example, quality of care could be based on chart reviews, continuing medical education hours, and number of liability claims; quality of service could be based on patient satisfaction surveys, as well as visit waiting times and the ease with which patients can make appointments; cost control could depend on cost of referrals and other resource utilization; and organizational participation could be based on number of staff meetings attended and committee posts held.

At the end of the year, the pool distribution would reward those physicians who scored highest in each area and penalize those physicians who scored lowest. For example, assume that $10,000 remained in a pool for three physicians, so $0.30(\$10,000) = \$3,000$ is available for distribution based on quality-of-care performance. Furthermore, the physicians' quality-of-care performance scores are 55 for Physician X, 44 for Physician Y, and 33 for Physician Z. Note that these scores have no absolute meaning, but they do tell us how well the physicians have performed relative to one another on the quality-of-care dimension. Since the scores total 132, Physician X would receive $55/132 = 0.42$ of the $3,000 pool, or

$1,260; Physician Y would receive 44/132 = 0.33 of the pool, or $990; and Physician Z would receive the remaining $750. Of course, some minimum score could be established, so that physicians would receive nothing from the pool if the minimum level of performance were not met. It is clear that the type of risk pool described in this section creates incentives for physicians to perform well along both financial and nonfinancial dimensions.

FINANCIAL RISK MANAGEMENT

As discussed earlier, capitated payments expose providers to financial risks that differ from those associated with conventional reimbursement systems. As with all financial risks, there are actions that can be taken to reduce the impact of capitation-induced risks. We discuss two in this section: (1) the establishment of reserves and (2) stop-loss provisions (reinsurance).

Reserves

The first line of defense against financial risk by any organization is the maintenance of adequate reserves. Any provider that assumes the financial risk for covered lives without having adequate reserves could easily end up, so to speak, as roadkill along the capitation highway. When healthcare providers accept capitated rates, they agree to provide whatever services are required for a fixed monthly fee. If all goes well, that is, if utilization and costs are controlled, the provider will end the year with a profit. But, if realized utilization and costs exceed estimates, the losses have to be covered in some way, and hence the need for reserves becomes apparent. There are several classifications of reserves. We will cover the two most important types: required reserves and reserves for incurred but not reported costs.

Required Reserves

Required reserves are those reserves necessary to cover costs that exceed capitation revenues. The term *required reserves* stems from the fact that insurance companies—and HMOs are considered insurance companies in most states—are required by state regulators to maintain reserves. Typically, such regulations specify a minimum fixed dollar amount of reserves, some percentage of premium income, or even some dollar amount per individual insured. It is interesting to note that some state insurance regulators are now examining the risk positions of providers to ascertain whether it would be appropriate to require licensure and reserves.

At the provider level, where reserves are not currently required by law, its makes good business sense to have sufficient cash and marketable securities on hand (in reserve) to cover losses that have a reasonable likelihood of occurring.

In Chapter 9, we discussed the use of sensitivity and scenario analyses to assess a project's riskiness. The same techniques can be applied to the firm as a whole. A firm's cash inflows and outflows are not known with certainty, so in any period, say, a month, cash outflows could exceed inflows, and a reserve cash balance should be established to cover the potential shortfall. The concept is exactly the same for capitation reserves, but here it is applied to a particular contract. By applying scenario analysis (or Monte Carlo simulation) to utilization and costs, it is possible to estimate the sizes and probabilities of occurrence of potential contract losses. Then, based on the risk aversion of the organization's managers, a reserve can be established to cover all but the most unlikely loss scenarios.

To illustrate the concept, consider a capitation contract that OceanView Memorial Hospital has with a local HMO to serve 50,000 enrollees. The capitation rate is $27.50 PMPM, resulting in $16.50 million in total revenue. Table 12–8 contains OceanView's best estimate for the cost distribution of enrollees along with the resulting profit distribution. These distributions were developed on the basis of estimates of enrollees' admission rates, average length of stay, and average per diem cost. The expected total contract cost is $15.78 million, resulting in an expected profit of $720,000, which gives OceanView a profit margin of 4.4 percent.

Focusing solely on this one contract, it is clear that OceanView's profit is not guaranteed. There is a 60 percent chance that the profit realized will be greater than the $720,000 estimate. That's the good news. The bad news is that there is a 40 percent chance that the profit will be less than expected, and a 10 percent chance that the contract will lose money. How can OceanView protect itself against the possibility that losses on this contract will push the hospital into financial distress? Of course, the answer is to

TABLE 12–8

OceanView Memorial Hospital: Contract Cost and Profit Distribution
(millions of dollars)

Probability	Contract Cost	Contract Profit or Loss
0.10	$14.00	$2.50
0.20	15.00	1.50
0.30	15.50	1.00
0.20	16.00	0.50
0.10	16.50	0.00
0.05	17.50	(1.00)
0.03	19.00	(2.50)
0.02	21.50	(5.00)
1.00		
Expected value =	$15.78	$0.72

Note: Contract revenues total $16.50 million.

have sufficient reserves. On the basis of the Table 12–8 distributions, OceanView could fund a five million dollar reserve that would totally protect the hospital (assuming that the probability distribution itself is correct). But this very conservative approach to reserves would, assuming a opportunity cost rate of 10 percent, cost OceanView $500,000 in annual carrying costs and hence almost wipe out the contract's expected profit.

As an alternative, OceanView might conclude that a 2 percent probability of occurrence represents a very unlikely event and hence does not warrant reserve protection. If this were the case, OceanView would set a reserve for the contract of less than $5,000,000, say, $1,000,000 or $2,500,000. The choice is a risk/return trade-off, with more risk protection requiring a larger reserve, which in turn leads to lower contract profits. In general, the larger the contract, and the greater the uncertainty in contract costs, the higher the reserve must be to offer realistic protection against negative outcomes.

In most situations, the reserve requirement is not as clear-cut as discussed here. First, it is not easy to estimate utilization and cost distributions, so it is very difficult to have much confidence in the Table 12–8 values. Second, most providers have a large number of contracts with numerous payers, and what is most relevant is the chance of an overall loss rather than the probability of a loss on a particular contract. If the loss distributions on the individual contracts are not perfectly positively correlated, portfolio effects will mitigate somewhat the risks inherent in each contract.

Note that financial withholds are, in effect, a type of reserve. If certain financial goals are met, the withhold is distributed to providers. However, if goals are not met, the withhold is used to cover the excess costs incurred. Also, note that of all the providers, physicians are particularly vulnerable when entering capitation contracts because historically they have not used reserves. In most cases, physician group practices do everything they can to clear their books at year-end. Instead of posting profits that would be taxable, the tendency has been to spend any surplus on salaries and equipment. With this type of behavior as the norm, it is especially difficult to think in terms of establishing reserves.

Reserves for Incurred but Not Reported (IBNR) Costs

Another type of reserve is that held to cover incurred but not reported (IBNR) costs. To illustrate these reserves, consider Healthy HMO. At the end of every accounting period—for our purposes, assume a year—it must close its books and reconcile its established risk pools. Healthy HMO uses capitation to pay for primary care services, but it uses fee-for-service reimbursement to pay for specialist services. When it closes its books at the end of the year, Healthy HMO might not realize that specialist services have been provided that have not yet been billed. Indeed, some referrals likely have been made that have not yet occurred, so there are specialist services, and hence costs, that are still pending.

If a provider is capitated yet has referral responsibility for services that it does not provide, there is a strong likelihood that at the end of the year there will be payment obligations for costs that have been incurred but not reported. Obviously, such costs must be planned for and covered, and the impact of such costs on risk-pool distributions must be taken into account. There are relatively sophisticated methods available for establishing IBNR reserves, as well as some rather ad hoc methods such as setting two or three months worth of historical IBNR dollar claims aside as a reserve. It is not important for you to know the details of setting up IBNR reserves—we will leave that to the accountants—but it is important for you to recognize that such reserves are required whenever providers are responsible for payments for other services.

Stop-Loss Provisions (Reinsurance)

Rather than establishing reserves to cover every conceivable cost situation, many providers elect to "reinsure" the risk. Such insurance, which is now offered by dozens of insurance companies, is called reinsurance or medical stop-loss insurance. (The term *reinsurance* has traditionally been used to mean insurance bought by insurance companies from other insurance companies to limit the risk assumed by the first insurer in covering potential losses. However, the term is now being used in the healthcare industry when a provider seeks insurance to limit capitation risk.)

Providers have several options for handling stop-loss insurance. One option is to have the HMO withhold a portion of the capitation rate for the sole purpose of buying insurance. However, if the HMO elects to self-insure and then fails to establish adequate reserves, the provider remains at risk. Another option is for the provider to receive the full capitation payment and then purchase stop-loss insurance directly from a company that specializes in such insurance. Of course, the option always exists for the provider to self-insure.

Stop-loss insurance is written to protect providers from losses on individual patients rather than from aggregate losses on a contract. The idea is to insure the provider against catastrophic "budget buster" patients, not to guarantee a certain level of overall profitability. For example, a hospital might purchase stop-loss insurance with a deductible, or threshold, of $100,000 per patient. The insurer might agree to pay 80 percent of billed charges in excess of this threshold amount. Of course, the lower the threshold and the higher the percentage of any excess paid by the insurer, the higher the stop-loss insurance premium.

John's first task was to allocate each premium dollar to the system's providers. As a guide, he used data similar to that contained in Table 12–3 but developed from currently available information. Then he devised a risk-sharing plan that combined both financial and nonfinancial factors to reward both physicians—including primary care and specialists—and the hospital if certain goals were met. Finally, he made sure that Capital City used some of the premium dollars to refine its information system so that it would have real-time data on patients' utilization patterns and costs.

Getting everyone on board was not easy, and the first year was rough. However, some minor changes were made on the basis of experience, and the second year was a resounding success for the system. In fact, with experience in operating under capitation, and having the systems in place to support close and continuous monitoring of utilization, Capital City now prefers capitation to other forms of reimbursement.

SELF-ASSESSMENT EXERCISES

12–1 a. What is capitation reimbursement?
      b. How does capitation differ from conventional reimbursement in regard to the relationship between utilization and profitability?

12–2 Based on experience in the California market, what impact does capitation have on the need for hospital and physician providers?

12–3 Explain the relationship between financial risk under capitation and provider's fixed-cost ratios.

12–4 a. What are risk pools?
      b. How can risk pools be used to align incentives within managed care plan (or integrated delivery system) panels?

12–5 What risk management techniques can providers use to reduce capitation risk?

SELECTED REFERENCES

Baker, Judith J. "Activity-Based Costing for Integrated Delivery Systems." *Journal of Health Care Finance,* Winter 1995, pp. 57–61.

Bond, Michael T. and Brenda Stevenson Marshall. "Offsetting Unexpected Healthcare Costs with Futures Contracts." *Healthcare Financial Management,* December 1994, pp. 54–58.

Bond, Michael T. and Brenda Stevenson Marshall. "Managing Financial Risk with Options on Futures." *Healthcare Financial Management,* May 1995, pp. 50–56.

Cave, Douglas G. "Vertical Integration Models to Prepare Health Systems for Capitation." *Health Care Management Review,* Winter 1995, pp. 26–39.

Coyne, Joseph S. and Stuart D. Simon. "Is Your Organization Ready to Share Financial Risk with HMOs?" *Healthcare Financial Management,* August 1994, pp. 30–34.

Davidson, Daniel M. and John Wester. "Addressing Integrated Systems' Tax-Exemption Problems." *Healthcare Financial Management,* January 1995, pp. 46–50.

Finkler, Steven A. "Capitated Hospital Contracts." *Health Care Management Review,* Summer 1995, pp. 88–91.

Keegan, Arthur J. "Hospitals Become Cost Centers in Managed Care Scenario." *Healthcare Financial Management,* August 1994, pp. 36–39.

Kolb, Deborah S. and Judith L. Horowitz. "Managing the Transition to Capitation." *Healthcare Financial Management,* February 1995, pp. 65– 69.

Herrle, Gregory N. and William M. Pollock. "Multispecialty Medical Groups: Adapting to Capitation." *Journal of Health Care Finance,* Spring 1995, pp. 37–43.

Pallarito, Karen. "Gatekeepers of Capitation." *Modern Health Care,* June 27, 1994, pp. 93–100.

Peregrine, Michael W. and D. Louis Glaser. "Choosing Medical Practice Acquisition Models." *Healthcare Financial Management,* March 1995, pp. 58–64.

Ryan, J. Bruce and Scott B. Clay. "How to Determine Financial Reserves for Capitated Contracts." *Healthcare Financial Management,* March 1995, p. 18.

Seaver, Douglass J. and Stephen H. Kramer. "Direct Contracting: The Future of Managed Care." *Healthcare Financial Management,* August 1994, pp. 21–27.

Shortell, Stephen M. "The Future of Integrated Systems." *Healthcare Financial Management,* January 1995, pp. 24–30.

Schultz, Donald V. "The Importance of Primary Care Providers in Integrated Systems." *Healthcare Financial Management,* January 1995, pp. 58–63.

Teske, Jeffrey M. "Second-Generation Legal Issues in Integrated Delivery Systems." *Healthcare Financial Management,* January 1995, pp. 54–57.

Toso, Mark E. and Anne Farmer. "Using Cost Accounting Data to Develop Capitation Rates." *Topics in Health Care Financing,* Fall 1994, pp. 1–12.

Witek, J. Edward and Heather Davidson. "Assessing Organizational Readiness for Capitation and Risk Sharing." *Healthcare Financial Management,* August 1994, pp. 18–19.

Solutions to Self-Assessment Exercises

Each chapter contains a set of self-assessment exercises that allows you to test your understanding of the most important material in that chapter. In addition to providing a check on comprehension, the exercises reinforce the key concepts and hence contribute to long-term retention. This appendix contains the solutions to the self-assessment exercises. I strongly recommend that you work the exercises and then use the solutions provided here to check your answers.

Chapter 1

1–1   a. The three forms of business organization are (1) sole proprietorship, (2) partnership, and (3) corporation.

        b. The sole proprietorship form of organization has three important advantages: (1) It is easily and inexpensively formed. (2) It is subject to few governmental regulations. (3) The business pays no corporate income taxes—all earnings of the business, whether they are reinvested in the business or withdrawn by the owner, are taxed as personal income to the proprietor.

          The sole proprietorship form of organization has three important limitations: (1) Unless the proprietor is very wealthy, it is difficult to obtain large sums of capital. (2) The proprietor has unlimited personal liability for the debts of the business. (3) The life of the business is limited to the life of the proprietor. The major advantages and disadvantages of a partnership are similar to those for a sole proprietorship.

          A corporation has three primary advantages: (1) A corporation has unlimited life. (2) It is easy to transfer ownership in an investor-owned corporation because ownership is divided into shares of stock and hence can be easily sold. (3) Owners of a corporation have limited liability. These three factors make it much easier for corporations to raise money in the capital markets than for sole proprietorships or partnerships.

The corporate form of organization does have two primary disadvantages: (1) Corporate earnings of taxable entities are subject to double taxation; once at the corporate level and then again at the personal level when dividends are paid to stock-holders. (2) Setting up a corporation and then filing the required periodic state and federal reports is more costly and time-consuming than for a sole pro-prietorship or partnership.

1–2   a. The stockholders (shareholders) are the owners of investor-owned companies, and they exercise con-trol by voting for the firm's board of directors.

The shareholders have a claim to the residual earnings of an investor-owned firm. Management may elect to retain some of the earnings in the firm rather than pay them out to the shareholders as divi-dends, but this is presumably done with the owners' blessing since the funds belong to the shareholders.

b. Legally, a not-for-profit firm has no owners. Not-for-profit firms are controlled by a board of trustees. Since board members are not responsible to a single set of outside constituents (shareholders in investor-owned firms), there is no outside monitoring of trustees, and hence managers, of not-for-profit firms.

Since not-for-profit firms have no shareholders, there is no single body of individuals with owner-ship rights to the firm's residual earnings. Since no well-defined clientele has a claim against residual earnings, managers of not-for-profit firms may not have the same incentive for profit making as do managers of investor-owned firms.

c. Tax-exempt status is granted to organizations that meet the Internal Revenue Service (IRS) definition of a charitable organization. In addition to a charitable purpose, a not-for-profit corporation must be organized and operated so that (1) it operates exclusively for the public, rather than private, interest, (2) none of the profits are used for private gain, (3) no political activity is conducted, and (4) if liquidation occurs, the assets will continue to be used for a charitable purpose.

d. Investor-owned firms are fully taxable by all levels of government; whereas, not-for-profit corporations are generally exempt from taxation, including both property and income taxes. Additionally, not-for-profit firms have the right to issue tax-exempt debt through municipal healthcare financing authorities. Finally, individual contributions to not-for-profit organizations can be deducted from taxable income by the donor, so not-for-profit firms have access to contribution capital.

1–3 a. The primary goal of investor-owned firms is shareholder wealth maximization, which translates to stock price maximization. Investor-owned firms do, of course, have other objectives. Managers, who make the actual decisions, are interested in their own welfare, in their employees' welfare, and in the good of the community and of society at large. Still, the goal of stock price maximization is a reasonable operating objective upon which to build financial decision rules.

b. In many situations, conflicts exist between the interests of managers and the interests of stockholders. When conflicts exist, managers will often favor self-interest over the interests of others. The divergence of interests between principals (owners) and agents (managers) is called the agency problem.

Many factors influence managers of investor-owned firms to act in the best interests of their shareholders, including (1) incentive compensation plans such as stock options and performance shares, (2) the threat of firing by stockholders, and (3) the threat of takeover by another firm.

c. A firm's stakeholders include all parties that have an interest (often financial but not necessarily so) in the firm. The typical list of stakeholders includes the board of directors (trustees), managers, employees, suppliers, shareholders, creditors, customers, and even the communities in which firms operate. Both investor-owned and not-for-profit firms have stakeholders, the only difference being that stockholders are absent in not-for-profit firms.

d. Typically, the goal of not-for-profit firms is stated in terms of some mission. For example, a not-for-profit hospital might have the goal to be a recognized, innovative healthcare leader dedicated to meeting the needs of the community.

The financial management goal of a not-for-profit firm is usually to maintain financial viability. Although stated differently, the financial goals of most investor-owned and not-for-profit firms are essentially the same.

1–4   a. The after-tax yield on any investment is the rate of return available to investors after taxes have been paid. Since T-bond interest is fully taxable, the investor must pay 28 percent taxes on the $80 annual interest received; consequently,

Tax on bond interest = 0.28($80) = $22.40
Interest available to investor = $80 − $22.40 = $57.60
After-tax yield on bond = $57.60/$1,000 = 0.0576 = 5.76%

A more efficient way to determine the after-tax yield is to recognize that the following relationship holds:

After-tax yield = Pre-tax yield(1 − Tax rate)
After-tax yield = 8.0%(1 − 0.28) = 8.0%(0.72) = 5.76%

b. Since municipal bonds are tax exempt, their pretax and after-tax yields are the same. For a T-bond to have the same $70/$1,000 = 0.070 = 7.0 percent after-tax yield, its pretax yield would have to be 9.72 percent:

After-tax yield = Pretax yield(1 − Tax rate) = 7.0%

$$\text{Pretax yield} = \frac{\text{After-tax yield}}{(1-\text{Tax rate})} = \frac{7.0\%}{(1-0.28)} = \frac{7.0\%}{0.72} = 9.72\%$$

1–5   a. The interest paid by a taxable corporation is tax deductible (deducted from operating income to obtain taxable income), while dividends are not deductible (they must be paid from after-tax income). Therefore, a firm in the 34 percent tax bracket needs only $1 of pretax earnings to pay $1 of interest expense, but it needs $1.52 of pretax earnings to pay $1 in dividends

$$\text{Dollars of pretax income} = \frac{\text{Dividend}}{(1-\text{Tax rate})} = \frac{\$1}{0.66} = \$1.52$$

because it must pay 0.34($1.52) = $0.52 in taxes on $1.52 of income.

The fact that interest is a tax deductible expense—while dividends are not—has a profound impact on the way businesses are financed. In effect, the government subsidizes debt financing; whereas, it does not subsidize equity financing. So the U.S. tax system favors debt financing over equity financing.

b. Interest income received by a taxable corporation is taxed as ordinary income at regular tax rates. However, 70 percent of the dividends received by one corporation from another can be excluded from taxable income, while the remaining 30 percent is taxed at the firm's ordinary tax rate. Thus, a corporation with a 34 percent marginal tax rate would have an effective tax rate of only 0.30(0.34) = 0.102 = 10.2% on any dividends it receives from another corporation. If a taxable corporation has surplus funds that can be temporarily invested in securities, the tax laws favor investment in stocks (including preferred stock), which pay dividends, rather than bonds, which pay interest. (Of course, other considerations may cause firms to favor bond investments over stock investments.)

c. Rate of Return to a Taxable Corporation

Bonds:

After-tax yield = Pretax yield $(1 - T)$
$= 10\%(1 - 0.34) = 10\%(0.66)$
$= 6.6\%$

Preferred Stock:

After-tax yield = Pretax yield $(1 - \text{Effective } T)$
$= 9\%(1 - [0.30][0.34])$
$= 9\%(1 - 0.102) = 9\%(0.898)$
$= 8.082\%$

Rate of Return to an Individual Investor
Bonds:

After-tax yield = Pretax yield $(1 - T)$
$= 10\%(1 - 0.28) = 10\%(0.72)$
$= 7.2\%$

Preferred Stock:

After-tax yield = Pretax yield $(1 - T)$
$= 9\%(1 - 0.28) = 9\%(0.72)$
$= 6.48\%$

Since individual investors can typically get higher yields from less risky bonds as compared to more risky preferred stocks, individual investors typically do not buy preferred stocks unless they are convertible into common stocks. Most nonconvertible preferred is owned by other corporations to take advantage of the corporate tax benefit of stock ownership.

1–6 a. A firm's true financial condition is a function of the amount of cash that flows into and out of the business. Thus, financial decisions must focus on cash flows, not profits as defined by accountants.

b. A dollar received today is more valuable that one to be received in the future because the dollar received today can be invested and earn interest. Any financial analysis that involves cash flows occurring at different points in time must incorporate time value differences.

c. Because of risk aversion, higher risk investments must offer higher expected rates of return. Thus, all financial decisions must not only consider returns but risk.

d. The use of a resource, including money, for any purpose deprives the organization of the use of that resource for any other purpose. This imposes an opportunity cost that must be considered in the decision process.

e. It is less risky to own portfolios (groups of assets) than it is to own a single asset. Thus, rational investors will own many assets, and the relevant measures of risk and return are related to the portfolio rather than to the individual assets.

1–7 a. An income statement reports an organization's revenues and expenses over some period of time. Its purpose is to report net income, which is an accounting measure of the firm's dollar earnings.

b. A balance sheet reports an organization's assets and liabilities at some point in time. Its purpose is to report the accounting value of the business's assets, and the claims against those assets, or how those assets were financed.

c. (1) The total margin (net income divided by net revenues) indicates the proportion of each dollar of net revenue that flows to total earnings.

(2) The operating margin (net operating income divided by net revenues) indicates how much operating income is generated per dollar of net revenue.

(3) Return on assets (net income divided by total assets) indicates how many dollars of net income is generated per dollar of total assets.

(4) Return on equity (net income divided by total equity) indicates how many dollars of net income are generated per dollar of equity investment.

(5) The debt ratio (total debt divided by total assets) reports the proportion of overall financing attributable to debt.

Chapter 2

2–1   a. Dollar Return:

Dollar return = Amount received – Amount invested
= $11,500 – $10,000
= $1,500

Rate of Return:

$$\text{Rate of return} = \frac{\text{Amount received} - \text{Amount invested}}{\text{Amount invested}}$$
$$= \frac{\$11,500 - \$10,000}{\$10,000} = \frac{\$1,500}{\$10,000} = 0.15 = 15\%$$

b. Dollar Return:

Dollar return = Amount received – Amount invested
= $9,500 – $10,000
= –$500

Rate of Return:

$$\text{Rate of return} = \frac{\text{Amount received} - \text{Amount invested}}{\text{Amount invested}}$$
$$= \frac{\$9,500 - \$10,000}{\$10,000} = \frac{-\$500}{\$10,000} = -0.05 = -5\%$$

2–2   a. Financial risk is associated with realizing a return that is less than the return expected. The higher the probability of a return far less than expected, the greater the financial risk. A simple example is a hospital's potential investment in a gamma knife unit. A financial analysis might indicate that the expected rate of return on the investment is 25 percent, but if usage is low, the hospital could lose 10 percent on the investment. Because the hospital could earn a return less than the expected 25 percent, the gamma knife investment is risky.

b. Risk aversion means that given the choice of two investments with the same expected rate of return but different risks, investors would choose the lower-risk investment. In other words, investors dislike risk. Risk aversion is important because it means that investments with higher risk must offer higher expected rates of return to induce investors to purchase those assets.

2–3   a. Expected Rate of Return:

Expected rate of return
= Probability of Return 1 × Return 1
+ Probability of Return 2 × Return 2
+ and so on
= 0.10(–10%) + 0.20(0%) + 0.40(10%)
+ 0.20(20%) + 0.10(30%) = 10.0%

b. Standard Deviation of Returns:

$$\text{Variance} = 0.10(-10\% - 10\%)^2 + 0.20(0\% - 10\%)^2$$
$$+ 0.40(10\% - 10\%)^2 + 0.20(20\% - 10\%)^2$$
$$+ 0.10(30\% - 10\%)^2 = 120.00$$

$$\text{Standard deviation} = \sigma = \sqrt{\text{Variance}}$$
$$= \sqrt{120.00} = 10.95\% \approx 11\%$$

c. Coefficient of Variation of Returns:

$$CV = \frac{\sigma}{E(\text{Value})} = 11\% / 10\% = 1.1$$

d. The standard deviation and coefficient of variation of returns measure variability about the mean, which is a measure of stand-alone risk.

e. Stand-alone risk is only relevant when the investment being evaluated is held in isolation; that is, the investment is not part of a portfolio of investments.

2–4   a. By holding portfolios of investments, investors can reduce the riskiness inherent in individual investments because returns less than expected on one investment may be offset by returns greater than expected on another investment. That is, the riskiness of the portfolio may be less than the riskiness inherent in each investment.

b. (1) The expected rate of return on the portfolio is simply the weighted average of the expected rates of return on the two investments.

(2) For the portfolio to have lower risk, the returns on
the two investments must be less than perfectly
positively correlated. In other words, the two sets
of returns cannot move together in perfect syn-
chronization as the state of the economy changes.

c. Portfolio risk is the risk inherent in a single investment that remains when the investment is held as
part of a well-diversified portfolio. Diversifiable risk
is the risk that is eliminated by portfolio effects.

d. There are two major implications: (1) Investors
should hold portfolios of investments rather than
individual investments. (2) Stand-alone risk is not
relevant to investments held in portfolios.

2–5   a. Portfolio risk occurs when (1) businesses hold portfolios of assets and (2) when individual investors
hold portfolios of stocks, which amount to very
large portfolios of individual corporate assets.

b. (1) Corporate risk is the contribution of a corporate
asset, such as an MRI unit, to the overall riskiness of the business.

(2) Corporate risk is measured by an asset's corporate beta, which is the slope of the asset's corporate characteristic line.

(3) Corporate $b_P = (\sigma_P / \sigma_F) r_{PF}$
where P stands for project, F stands for firm,
and r is the correlation coefficient.

(4) The larger the asset's standard deviation of
returns (σ_P) relative to the standard deviation of
the firm's returns (σ_F), and the higher the correlation between the two (r_{PF}), the greater an
asset's corporate risk.

c. (1) Market risk is the contribution of a corporate
asset, such as an MRI unit, to the overall riskiness of an individual investor's stock portfolio.

(2) Market risk is measured by an asset's market
beta, which is the slope of the asset's market
characteristic line.

(3) Market $b_P = (\sigma_P / \sigma_M) r_{PM}$
where M stands for the market.

(4) The larger the asset's standard deviation of returns (σ_P) relative to the standard deviation of a well-diversified stock portfolio (σ_M), and the higher the correlation between the two sets of returns (r_{PM}), the greater an asset's market risk.

d. Stand-alone risk is relevant only when the asset is operated in isolation, which is almost never the case. Corporate risk is relevant when the asset is owned by a not-for-profit corporation with a large portfolio of individual projects. Market risk is relevant when the asset is owned by an investor-owned company with stockholders holding well-diversified portfolios of stocks.

Chapter 3

3–1   a. (1) A term loan is a contract under which a borrower agrees to make a series of interest and principal payments, on specified dates, to a lender. Investment bankers are generally not involved: Term loans are negotiated directly between the borrowing firm and a financial institution.

(2) A bond is a long-term contract under which a borrower agrees to make payments of interest and principal, on specific dates, to the holder of the bond. Although bonds are similar to term loans, a bond issue is generally registered with the Securities and Exchange Commission, advertised, offered to the public through investment bankers, and actually sold to many different investors.

(3) With a mortgage bond, the issuer pledges certain real assets as security (collateral) for the bond.

(4) Often, firms have several types of debt outstanding at any one time. Debt that has a priori-

ty claim on earnings and bankruptcy liquidation proceeds is called senior debt, while debt that has an inferior claim is called junior debt. Thus, first mortgage bonds are senior debt, while second mortgage bonds are junior to the first mortgage bonds.

(5) A debenture is an unsecured bond, and, as such, has no lien against specific property as security for the obligation. Debenture holders are, therefore, general creditors whose claims are protected by property not otherwise pledged.

(6) Subordinated debt has a claim on assets in the event of bankruptcy only after senior debt has been paid off. Debentures may be subordinated either to designated notes payable—usually bank loans—or to all other debt. In the event of liquidation, holders of subordinated debentures cannot be paid until senior debt, as named in the debenture, has been paid.

(7) Municipal bonds are long-term debt obligations issued by states and their political subdivisions, such as counties, cities, and healthcare authorities. The key feature of most municipal bonds is that they are tax exempt.

b. (1) An indenture is a legal document, which may be several hundred pages long, that spells out the rights of both bondholders and the issuing corporation.

(2) Indentures usually include a set of restrictive covenants that cover such points as the conditions under which the issuer can pay off the bonds prior to maturity, the financial condition that the company must maintain to issue additional debt, and restrictions against the payment of dividends unless earnings meet certain specifications.

(3) A trustee is an official (usually of a bank) who represents the bondholders and makes sure that the terms of the indenture are being carried out.

(4) A call provision gives the issuer the right to call a bond for redemption, that is, the right to pay off the bondholders in entirety and retire the issue.

(5) A sinking fund is a provision that provides for the systematic retirement of a bond issue. Typically, a sinking fund provision requires the issuer to retire a portion of its bonds each year.

3–2 a. The two major rating agencies are Moody's Investors Service (Moody's) and Standard & Poor's Corporation (S&P), which rate both corporate and municipal bonds with regard to their probability of default.

Bonds are rated from triple A for the highest quality to C (or D for Standard & Poor's) for bonds in or near default. Bonds with a BBB and higher rating are called investment grade, and they are the lowest-rated bonds that many banks and other institutional investors are permitted by law to hold. Double B and lower bonds are called junk bonds, and many financial institutions are prohibited from buying them.

b. Bond ratings are important both to firms and to investors. Most importantly, a bond's rating is an indicator of its default risk, so the rating has a direct, measurable influence on the bond's interest rate and hence on investors' returns and on the firm's cost of debt capital.

c. Credit enhancement, or bond insurance, is a relatively recent development for upgrading a municipal bond's rating to AAA. Credit enhancement is offered by several credit insurers, including the Municipal Bond Investors Assurance (MBIA) Corporation and AMBAC Indemnity Corporation.

3–3 a. (1) *Productive opportunities.* The ability of businesses to pay for borrowed capital depends on the investment opportunities within the economy. The greater the productive opportunities, the greater the return on business investment, and the more firms can offer to pay potential lenders for use of their savings.

(2) *Time preferences for consumption.* Individuals who have met their basic current consumption needs and who are concerned about saving for retirement might be willing to loan funds at relatively low rates because their preferences are for future consumption. Such individuals have a low time preference for consumption. Other individuals, however, might have a high need for current consumption and hence be willing to forgo consumption (lend) only if the interest rate is very high. Such investors have a high time preference for consumption.

(3) *Risk.* The risk inherent in the business environment affects the ability of borrowers to repay loans and hence affects the return investors will require: The higher the perceived risk, the higher the required rate of return.

(4) *Inflation.* Since the value of money in the future is affected by inflation, the higher the expected rate of inflation, the higher the interest rate demanded by savers.

b. k^* = the real risk-free rate of interest, which is the rate that would exist on a riskless security if zero inflation were expected. The real risk-free rate of interest cannot be measured directly, but it is thought to be in the range of 2 to 4 percent.

IP = inflation premium. IP is equal to the average expected inflation rate over the life of the security. As inflation expectations increase, so does the required rate of return on all securities.

DRP = default risk premium. This premium reflects the possibility that the issuer will not pay interest or principal on a security at the stated time and in the stated amount. The greater the probability of default, the greater the risk to investors and hence the higher the default risk premium.

LP = liquidity premium. This is a premium charged by lenders to reflect the fact that some securities cannot be converted to cash on short notice at a "fair market" price. The less liquid the security, the higher the liquidity premium, and hence the higher the required interest rate.

PRP = price risk premium. Longer-term bonds are exposed to a significant risk of price declines if interest rates rise in the economy, and a price risk premium is charged by lenders to reflect this risk. The longer the maturity on a debt security, the greater the price risk, the greater the price risk premium, and hence the higher the required interest rate.

3–4   a. The relationship between long- and short-term rates is known as the term structure of interest rates, and the yield curve is the plot of interest rates versus maturity for a given type of debt security, such as Treasury securities.

Since an upward-sloping yield curve is most prevalent, people often call this shape a normal yield curve. Conversely, a yield curve that slopes downward is called an inverted, or abnormal, yield curve.

b. The yield curve is important both to healthcare managers, who must decide whether to borrow by issuing long- or short-term debt, and to investors, who must decide whether to buy long- or short-term debt. Firms reduce risk by borrowing long term to finance assets that have long economic lives, but long-term rates are usually higher than short-term rates. Thus, managers must decide whether the risk reduction is worth the added cost. Financing decisions would be easy if managers could develop accurate forecasts of future interest rates, but forecasting interest rates is very difficult, if not impossible.

3–5   a. The Security Market Line is

$$k_i = k_{RF} + (k_M - k_{RF})b_i$$

where

k_i = required rate of return on Stock i.

k_{RF} = risk-free rate of return, in this context generally measured by the return on long-term U.S. Treasury bonds.

b_i = market beta coefficient of Stock i. The beta of an average stock is $b_A = 1.0$.

k_M = required rate of return on a portfolio consisting of all stocks, which is the market portfolio.

RP_M = market risk premium = $(k_M - k_{RF})$. This is the additional return over the risk-free rate required to compensate an investor for assuming average ($b_A = 1.0$) risk.

RP_i = risk premium on Stock i = $(k_M - k_{RF})b_i$.

The SML is an important tool in financial management because it expresses the relationship between market risk as measured by beta and required rate of return.

b. (1) The market risk premium is $(k_M - k_{RF})$
   = 12.4% − 7.4% = 5 percentage points.

   (2) Using the SML,

$$k_{Beverly} = k_{RF} + (k_M - k_{RF})b_{Beverly}$$
$$= 7.4\% + (12.4\% - 7.4\%)1.25$$
$$= 7.4\% + (5\%)1.25$$
$$= 7.4\% + 6.25\% = 13.65\%.$$

   (3) $k_{Beverly} = 8.5\% + (5\%)1.25 = 8.5\% + 6.25\% = 14.75\%$.
   (4) $k_{Beverly} = 7.4\% + (5\%)1.10 = 7.4\% + 5.5\% = 12.9\%$.

Chapter 4

4–1   a. $FV_n = PV(1 + i)^n = \$1,000(1.08)^6 = \$1,000(1.58687) = \$1,586.87$

With a financial calculator,

Inputs	6	8	−1,000		
	n	i	PV	PMT	FV
Output					= 1,586.87

b. $FV_n = PV(1 + i)^n = \$1{,}000(1.04)^{12} = \$1{,}000(1.60103)$
$= \$1{,}601.03$

With a financial calculator,

Inputs   12   4   −1,000

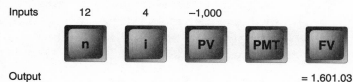

Output   = 1,601.03

4–2   a. $FV_n = PV(1 + i)^n$; $\$600 = \$500(1 + i)^2$; $i = 9.54\%$

With a financial calculator,

Inputs   2   −500   600

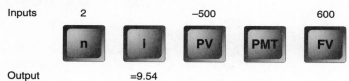

Output   =9.54

b. Assume any value for the present value and double it for the future value. For example, we used \$100 for the present value:

$FV_n = PV(1 + i)^n$; $\$200 = \$100(1 + i)^5$; $i = 14.87\%$

With a financial calculator,

Inputs   5   −100   200

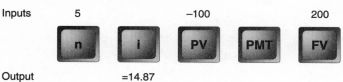

Output   =14.87

4–3   a. Calculator solution = \$5,637.09.

Inputs   5   6   −1,000

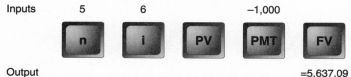

Output   =5,637.09

b. If the \$1,000 payments occur at the beginning of each year, the future value of the ordinary (regular) annuity from 4–3a is compounded for one more year. Thus,

FVA_n (Annuity due) $= FVA_n(1 + i) = \$5{,}637.09(1.06)$
$= \$5{,}975.32$ (or \$5,975.33)

Note that most financial calculators have a switch or key marked DUE or BEG that permits you to change the setting from end-of-period payments (ordinary annuity) to beginning-of-period payments (annuity due). When this mode is activated, the display will normally show the word *BEGIN*. Thus, as an alternative solution, press the BEG key and proceed as before.

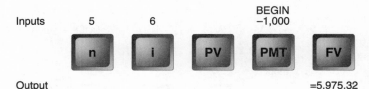

Since most problems will deal with end-of-period cash flows, don't forget to switch your calculator back to the END mode.

c. Calculator solution = $5,731.94.

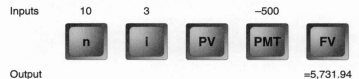

Note that to use the calculator in the normal way to solve these types of problems, the compounding period and payment period must be the same; in this case both are semiannual. If this is not the situation, each cash flow must be treated individually or an effective periodic rate must be calculated and then applied as above.

4-4   a.
$$PV = \frac{FV_n}{(1+i)^n} = \frac{\$1,000}{(1.07)^8} = \$582.01$$

With a financial calculator,

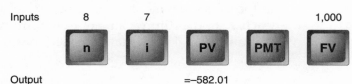

Note that annual compounding is assumed if not otherwise specified.

b. Calculator solution = $4,060.55.

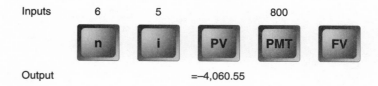

Inputs   6   5   800

Output   =–4,060.55

c. An opportunity cost arises whenever a resource is committed to a particular purpose. In discounted cash flow analysis, the commitment of funds to a particular investment deprives the investor of using those funds for any other purpose. Thus, an opportunity cost is incurred. This cost is the return foregone on alternative investments of similar risk, and this cost rate is used as the discount rate in time value of money problems.

4–5   a. One solution would be to sum the present values of each cash flow:

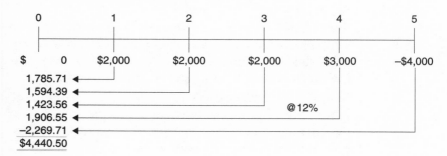

Alternatively, you could use the net present value function on your calculator. Enter the cash flows in the calculator's cash flow registers, then enter i = 12, and finally use the NPV function to obtain the present value, $4,440.51.

Note that the Year 5 cash flow is negative (an outflow). This sign carries over to its present value. Moving to the right (compounding) or to the left (discounting) on a time line changes the value of the cash flow, but the sign of the cash flow is unaffected.

b. Effective annual rate:

$$\left(1+\frac{i_{Nom}}{m}\right)^{m} - 1.0 = \left(1+\frac{0.12}{12}\right)^{m} - 1.0$$

$$= (1.01)^{12} - 1.0$$
$$= 1.1268 - 1.0 = 0.1268 = 12.68\%$$

Chapter 5

5–1   a. Financial assets are all valued in the same way, by finding the present value of the asset's expected cash flow stream. Note that the discount rate used in the valuation process is the opportunity cost rate, which is the rate of return available on alternative investments of similar risk.

b. Interest rates go up and down over time, and, as rates change, so do the values of outstanding bonds. When interest rates rise, the value of outstanding bonds will fall. Thus, bond investors are exposed to the risk of loss of value from rising interest rates, which is called price risk. An investor's exposure to price risk depends on the maturity of the bonds; the longer the maturity, the greater the price risk.

c. Reinvestment rate risk is the risk that an investment will be rolled over, or reinvested, at a rate less than the current rate on the security. For example, if your holding period is five years, investment in a one-year bond means that you would have to reinvest the principal and interest at the end of the first year. If interest rates fall, the return that you will earn during the second year is less than the return earned during the first year.

5–2   a. PV of a 4-year, $70 payment annuity at 14 percent = $203.96
PV of a $1,000 lump sum discounted 4 years = 592.08
Value of bond = $796.04

The value of the bond can also be found using most financial calculators.

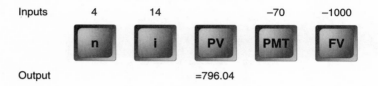

Inputs	4	14		−70	−1000
	n	i	PV	PMT	FV
Output			=796.04		

b. PV of an 8-period, $35 payment annuity at 7 percent = $209.00

PV of a $1,000 lump sum discounted 8 periods = 582.01

Value of bond = $791.01

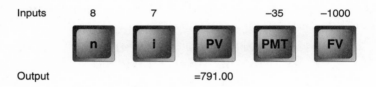

Inputs	8	7		−35	−1000
	n	i	PV	PMT	FV
Output			=791.00		

c. PV of a 40-period, $35 payment annuity at 7 percent = $466.61

PV of a $1,000 lump sum discounted 40 periods = 66.78

Value of bond = $533.39

Inputs	40	7		−35	−1000
	n	i	PV	PMT	FV
Output			=533.39		

5–3

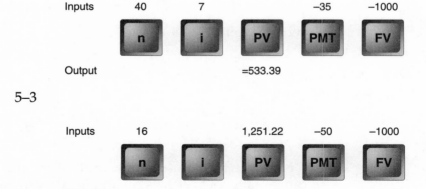

Inputs	16		1,251.22	−50	−1000
	n	i	PV	PMT	FV
Output		=3.00			

Note that the value for i, 3.00 percent, is the semiannual YTM, so it is necessary to multiply it by 2 to get the annual YTM, which is 2(3.00%) = 6.00%.

5–4   a. This is a zero-growth stock, or perpetuity.

$$E(P_0) = \frac{D_0[1+E(g)]}{k_s - E(g)} = \frac{\$4.00[1+0]}{0.12 - 0.00} = \frac{\$4.00}{0.12} = \$33.33$$

b.

$$E(P_0) = \frac{D_0[1+E(g)]}{k_s - E(g)} = \frac{\$2.00[1+0.10]}{0.20 - 0.10} = \frac{\$2.20}{0.10} = \$22.00$$

Since the stock is currently selling at $25.00, it is overvalued by $3.00, and you should not buy it.

c.

Expected rate of return	=	Expected dividend yield	+	Expected growth rate, or capital gains yield
E(R)	=	$\dfrac{E(D_1)}{P_0}$	+	E(g)

Expected Dividend Yield:

$$\frac{E(D_1)}{P_0} = \frac{D_0[1+E(g)]}{P_0} = \frac{\$1.50(1.05)}{\$15.75} = 0.10 = 10\%$$

Expected Capital Gains Yield:

$$\frac{\text{Capital gain}}{\text{Beginning price}} = \frac{E(P_1) - P_0}{P_0} = \frac{P_0[1+E(g)] - P_0}{P_0}$$

$$= \frac{\$15.75(1.05) - \$15.75}{\$15.75} = \frac{\$0.79}{\$15.75} = 0.05 = 5\%$$

Note that, for a constant growth stock, the expected capital gains yield always equals E(g), the expected dividend growth rate, which in this case is 5 percent.

5–5   a.

$$E(P_0) = \frac{D_0\left[1 + E(g)\right]}{k_s - E(g)} = \frac{\$2.00[1 - 0.05]}{0.15 - (-0.05)} = \frac{\$2.00(0.95)}{0.15 + 0.05} = \frac{\$1.90}{0.20} = \$9.50$$

For a constant growth stock, stock price is expected to grow each year at the expected dividend growth rate, E(g), so

$E(P)_3 = E(P_0)[1 + E(g)]^3 = \$9.50(1 - 0.05)^3$
$= \$9.50(0.95)^3 = \$8.15$

b. The value of a stock that is never expected to pay a dividend is zero because its value is the present value of its expected dividend (cash return to investors) stream. Now, some of you may say that the stock is worth something because it will grow in price, and hence value will stem from capital gains. However, sooner or later, investors will recognize that no cash will be forthcoming from the firm, so no one will be willing to buy the stock.

Chapter 6

6–1   a. Long-term debt, preferred stock (if used), and common stock (or fund capital for not-for-profit organizations) are the primary sources of long-term capital for most firms, so they are the components that are routinely included in a firm's overall cost of capital estimate.

b. Here is the generic formula for the cost of capital:

Cost of capital = $w_d k_d (1 - T) + w_s(k_s$ or $k_f)$

where w_d and w_s are the target weights for debt and common equity, respectively; k_d is the before-tax cost of debt; T is the firm's tax rate; k_s is the cost of equity; and k_f is the cost of fund capital.

c. Yes. For investor-owned firms, the tax benefit associated with debt financing can be incorporated either in the cash flows of the project being ana-

lyzed or in the cost-of-capital estimate. It is generally easier to incorporate the tax benefit of debt
financing into the cost-of-capital estimate.

d. Our primary purpose in developing a firm's cost of
capital is to use it in making capital investment
decisions, which involve future asset acquisitions
and future capital financing. Thus, for cost-of-capital purposes, the relevant costs are the marginal
costs of new funds to be raised in the future (normally during some planning period, say, a year) and
not the cost of funds raised in the past.

6–2   a. Perhaps the easiest way to estimate a firm's cost of
debt is to talk to the firm's investment banker.
Investment bankers are constantly bringing new
issues to the market, and since the firm's banker
will be familiar with the firm's credit rating, the
banker will be able to easily provide an estimate of
the firm's current cost of debt.

If the firm has publicly held debt outstanding
that is frequently traded, the firm's current cost of
debt can be approximated by the yield to maturity
(YTM) on existing debt.

Another method of estimating a firm's cost of
debt is to use the coupon rate on recent new issues
by firms similar to the firm in question.

b. Flotation costs are the administrative costs associated with issuing new debt (principally bonds). The
costs consist of accounting costs, legal fees, printing
costs, and the fees paid to governmental entities and
investment bankers. Flotation costs increase the
effective cost of a new debt issue but typically only
by a small amount, so it is common practice to
ignore flotation costs when estimating a firm's cost
of debt.

6–3   a. The residual earnings of a firm, its net income,
belong to the stockholders and serve to "pay the
rent" on stockholder supplied capital. If part of the
earnings are retained, an opportunity cost is

incurred: Stockholders could have received these earnings as dividends and then earned a return on the earnings by investing the dividends in stock, bonds, real estate, commodity futures, and so on.

b. The two primary methods used to estimate the cost of equity are the capital asset pricing model (CAPM) and the discounted cash flow (DCF) model.

c. Within the CAPM, the equation that relates risk to return is called the security market line (SML).

$$k_s = \text{Risk-free rate} + \text{Risk premium}$$
$$= k_{RF} + (k_M - k_{RF})b$$

Here,

k_s = estimated cost of equity.

k_{RF} = risk-free rate, the required rate of return on riskless securities.

k_M = required rate of return on the market.

b = beta coefficient of the stock in question.

$(k_M - k_{RF})$ = market-risk premium, the premium above the risk-free rate that investors require to buy a stock with average risk.

$(k_M - k_{RF})b$ = stock risk premium; the premium above the risk-free rate that investors require to buy the stock in question.

Typically, the rate of return on long-term Treasury securities (T-bonds) is used as the proxy for the risk-free rate. The required rate of return on the market is most often obtained from investment banking houses. Alternatively, the historical average market risk premium $(k_M - k_{RF})$ as reported by Ibbotson Associates can be used in the SML. Beta coefficient estimates are provided by many investment banking houses, as well as by investor advisory services such as Value Line.

d. If the firm is a constant-growth firm, the following form of the DCF model can be used to estimate k_s:

$$k_s = \frac{E(D_1)}{P_0} + E(g)$$

$E(D_1)$, the dividend expected over the next year, can be estimated from the current dividend. Also, most investment banking house analysts, as well as investor advisory services firms, give estimates of $E(D_1)$ for many companies.

The current stock price, P_0, can be obtained from many publications, including *The Wall Street Journal*. The most difficult parameter to estimate is the expected dividend growth rate, $E(g)$. Future dividend growth can be extrapolated from historical growth rates. Also, many stock analysts provide dividend growth rate estimates. Additionally, several investment advisory services compile individual analyst's forecasts and provide median dividend growth forecasts.

6–4   a. Not-for-profit firms raise equity, or fund, capital in two ways: by receiving contributions or government grants and by earning an excess of revenues over expenses (by retained earnings).

In recent years, there has been considerable controversy over the "cost" of this capital to not-for-profit firms. At least four positions can be taken on this question. (1) Fund capital has zero cost. (2) Fund capital has some cost, but it is not very high. (3) Not-for-profits must earn a return on equity sufficient to fund inflation and real asset growth. (4) Fund capital to not-for-profit firms has about the same cost as the cost of retained earnings to similar investor-owned firms.

Which of the four positions is most correct? By using fund capital to invest in real healthcare assets, the firm is deprived of the opportunity to use this capital for other purposes, so an opportunity cost must be assigned. Investment in real assets should return at least as much as the return available on securities investments of similar risk, or the return expected from investing in the stock of a similar investor-owned company.

b. This is Hamada's equation:

$$b_{Stock} = b_{Stock \text{ with no debt}}[1 + (1 - T)(D/S)]$$

Here b_{Stock} is the beta coefficient of the stock of the firm, assuming that the firm uses some debt financing, $b_{Stock\ with\ no\ debt}$ is the inherent beta of the stock if the firm used no debt financing, T is the tax rate, D is the market value of the firm's debt, and S is the market value of the firm's equity.

Hamada's equation is useful because it permits us to convert the market-determined beta of an investor-owned firm to the beta of a not-for-profit firm in the same line of business but having a different (zero) tax rate and a different debt/equity mix.

c. The very first increment of internal funds used to finance any year's investments in new assets is depreciation-generated funds. Since depreciation is a return *of* capital rather than a return *on* capital, depreciation cash flow "belongs" to the original capital suppliers, which includes both stockholders and debtholders. Thus, depreciation-generated funds have the same cost as the firm's overall cost of capital.

d. To interpret the cost of capital, first note that the component cost estimates that make up a firm's cost of capital are based on the returns that investors require to supply capital to the firm. These required rates of return are based on investors' perceptions regarding the riskiness of their expected cash flow streams, which, in turn, are based on the inherent riskiness of the business and the amount of debt financing used. Thus, the firm's inherent business risk and capital structure are embedded in the cost-of-capital estimate. The firm can always earn its cost of capital by investing in similar risk stocks and bonds, so it should not invest in real assets unless it can earn at least as much. Remember, though, that the cost of capital has embedded in it the risk and capital structure of the firm's average project. Thus, the firm's cost of capital can be applied without modification only to those projects under consideration that have average risk and average debt capacity, where *average* is defined as that applicable to the firm's currently held assets in the aggregate.

6–5   a. The yield to maturity on NEHC's currently out-
         standing annual coupon bonds can be used as a
         proxy for the firm's pretax cost of debt. Using a
         financial calculator, enter PMT = 100, n = 20,
         FV = 1000, and PV = –789.26. Then, press i to
         obtain k_d = 13.00%.

Inputs   20   –789.26   100   1000

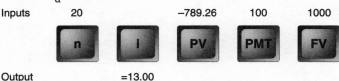

Output   =13.00

Note that the bond has annual coupon payments, so
it is not necessary to multiply the answer by two to
get the annual YTM. Since the firm's tax rate is 40
percent, its after-tax cost of debt is

$$k_d(1 - T) = 13\%(0.6) = 7.8\%$$

b. CAPM: $k_s = k_{RF} + (k_M - k_{RF})b$
              $= 10\% + (15\% - 10\%)1.2$
              $= 16.0\%$

   DCF: $k_s = E(D_1)/P_0 + g$
        $= \$2.00/\$20.00 + 5\% = 15.0\%$

Now judgment must be applied. Since the two
results are reasonably consistent, we could use a
weighted average of the two methods, and conclude
that the cost of equity, k_s, is 15.5%.

c. Cost of capital $= w_d k_d(1 - T) + w_s k_s$
              $= 0.4(13.0\%)(0.6) + 0.6(15.5\%)$
              $= 12.42\% \approx 12.4\%$

Chapter 7

7–1   a. Capital investments are business investments in
         long-term assets, and capital investment decision
         making is the process of choosing which capital
         investment proposals to accept and which to reject.
              Capital investment decisions are probably the
         most important decisions that managers make

because (1) the firm's strategic direction is defined by its capital investment decisions, and (2) the impact of capital investment decisions typically lasts a long time.

b. Within the healthcare industry, where goals other than shareholder wealth maximization are important, capital investment decisions should consider factors other than the financial impact of the project, such as medical staff preferences and the needs of the community. Note, however, that a firm is constrained in its ability to accept unprofitable projects by the necessity of maintaining financial soundness.

c. Here are the five steps of capital investment analysis:

   (1) First, the capital outlay, or cost, of the project must be estimated.

   (2) Second, the operating cash flows of the project (including termination cash flows) must be forecasted. Steps 1 and 2 constitute the cash flow estimation phase.

   (3) Next, the riskiness of the estimated cash flows must be assessed.

   (4) Then, given the riskiness of the cash flows, the project's cost of capital is estimated.

   (5) Finally, the profitability of the project is assessed, usually in terms of the project's net present value (NPV) or internal rate of return (IRR).

d. (1) Accounting income is profit as defined by generally accepted accounting principles; whereas, cash flow is the actual net dollars that flow into or out of the firm.

   (2) Incremental cash flow is defined as the difference in the firm's cash flows in each period if the project is undertaken versus the firm's cash flows if the project is not undertaken.

   (3) Project life is the estimated life of the project. Often, project life for analysis purposes is less than the true project life because it is very diffi-

cult, if not impossible, to estimate a project's cash flows 10, 20, or more years into the future.

(4) A sunk cost is an outlay that has already occurred (or has been irrevocably committed), so it is an outlay that is unaffected by the accept/reject decision under consideration.

(5) An opportunity cost is the value of an opportunity foregone by virtue of taking some action. For example, if a hospital is analyzing the building of a ambulatory care clinic on a piece of land it already owns, the net market value of that land must be charged as an opportunity cost against the project because using the land deprives the hospital of the opportunity to use the land for other purposes. To value the opportunity cost, it is generally best to use the net proceeds that would be received if the land were sold.

(6) Normally, expansion projects require additional inventories, and expanded sales also lead to additional accounts receivable. However, accounts payable and accruals will probably also increase as a result of the expansion, and these current liability funds will reduce the net cash needed to finance the increase in inventories and receivables. The difference between the increase in current assets and the increase in current liabilities that result from a new project must be charged against the project since it is just as much a cost as the cost of the new fixed assets.

(7) There are strong indications that project cash flow forecasts are not unbiased; rather, managers tend to be overly optimistic in their forecasts, and as a result, revenues tend to be overstated and costs tend to be understated. The end result is an upward bias in estimated profitability.

(8) Strategic value is the value of future investment opportunities that can be undertaken only if the project currently under consideration is accept-

ed. Failure to recognize a project's strategic value may cause a project's profitability to be understated.

(9) Because inflation is a fact of life, and because inflation effects can have a considerable influence on a project's profitability, inflation must be considered in capital budgeting analyses. Since inflation effects are already imbedded in the firm's cost of capital, and since the cost of capital will be used to discount the cash flows in our profitability measures, it is necessary to insure that inflation effects are also built into the project's estimated cash flows. The most effective way to deal with inflation is to build inflation effects into each cash flow element, using the best available information about how each element will be affected.

(10) Salvage value is the estimated value of a project at the end of its useful (economic) life. If the project's economic life corresponds to its analysis life, the salvage value may be low or even negative. However, if the project will be operated many years beyond the analysis life, the value at project termination (the terminal value) may be very large.

7–2   a. Volume (or unit sales) breakeven occurs when the number of procedures performed (or number of units sold) are just sufficent for the project to break even, or not lose any money. It is often useful to know how many procedures must be performed during some time period (week, month, or year) to create cash inflows that just match the operating cash outflows associated with the project. This type of breakeven focuses on operating cash flows.

b. A second type of breakeven measures how long it will take a project to generate the operating cash flow necessary to repay the initial investment in the project. This type of breakeven, which is an indicator of the project's risk and liquidity, measures the time it takes to break even and is called the payback, or payback period.

c. Net present value (NPV) is a profitability measure that uses discounted cash flow (DCF) techniques, so it is often referred to as a DCF measure. Simply put, NPV is the sum of the present values of all the project's cash flows.

   The interpretation of NPV is straightforward. An NPV of zero signifies that the project's cash inflows are just sufficient to (1) return the capital invested in the project and (2) provide the required rate of return on that invested capital. If a project has a positive NPV, it is generating excess cash flows. These excess cash flows are available to management to reinvest in the firm and, for investor-owned firms, to pay dividends. If a project has a negative NPV, its cash inflows are insufficient to compensate the firm for the capital invested, so the project is unprofitable and acceptance would cause the financial condition of the firm to deteriorate.

d. Whereas NPV measures a project's dollar profitability, internal rate of return (IRR) measures a project's percentage profitability, or its percentage rate of return. Mathematically, the IRR is defined as that discount rate which equates the present value of the project's expected cash inflows to the present value of the project's expected cash outflows, so the IRR is simply that discount rate which forces the NPV of the project to equal zero.

   A project's IRR is its expected rate of return. If the IRR exceeds the project's cost of capital, a surplus remains after paying for the capital. On the other hand, if the IRR is less than the project's cost of capital, taking on the project will have a negative impact on the firm's financial condition.

7–3   Except for the objective or subjective inclusion of strategic value, financial analysis techniques generally focus exclusively on the cash flow implications of a proposed project. Since healthcare firms, particularly not-for-profit firms, have the goal of producing social services along with commercial services, the proper analysis of proposed projects must systematically consider the social value of a project along with its pure financial, or cash flow, value.

When social value is considered, the total net present value (TNPV) of a project can be expressed as follows:

$$TNPV = NPV + NPSV$$

Here, NPV represents the standard NPV of the project's cash flow stream, and NPSV is the net present social value of the project. The addition of NPSV to the NPV method clearly differentiates capital budgeting in not-for-profit firms from that in investor-owned firms. NPSV represents managers' assessment of the social value of the project as opposed to the pure financial value measured by NPV.

7–4   a. To begin, consider Project X. Its NPV is $967 (or, using a financial calculator, $966.01). Here is the time line:

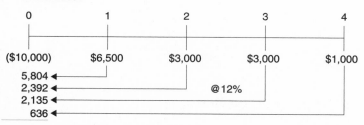

To find the payback, note that $9,500 is recovered in the first two years of operation, and $12,500 is recovered after three years of operation. Thus, the initial $10,000 investment is fully recovered after three years. Since only $500 remains to be recovered at the end of Year 2, if we assume that cash flows occur evenly throughout the year, payback occurs at

$$2 = \frac{\$500}{\$3,000} = 2.17 \text{ years.}$$

Project X's IRR, using a financial calculator, is 18.0%.

Here is a recap of the break-even and profitability measures for Project X, along with the values for Project Y:

	Project X	Project Y
Payback (years)	2.17	3.33
NPV	$966.01	–$887.95
IRR	18.0%	7.7%

b. From a purely financial basis, Project X is acceptable (profitable), while Project Y is unacceptable (unprofitable). The key here is that Project X has a positive NPV, while Project Y has a negative NPV. Also, Project X's IRR is greater than its 12 percent cost of capital, while Project Y's IRR is less than its 12 percent cost of capital.

7–5 a. Here are the depreciation schedule and cash flow statements for the project:

Depreciation Schedule:

Year	MACRS Factor	Depreciation Expense	End of Year Book Value
1	0.20	$120,000	$480,000
2	0.32	192,000	288,000
3	0.19	114,000	174,000
4	0.12	72,000	102,000
5	0.11	66,000	36,000
6	0.06	36,000	0
		$600,000	

Cash Flow Statements:

			Year			
	0	1	2	3	4	5
Equipment cost	($600,000)					
Net revenues		$300,000	$315,000	$330,750	$347,288	$364,652
Less: Labor/maint costs		100,000	105,000	110,250	115,763	121,551
Utilities costs		10,000	10,500	11,025	11,576	12,155
Supplies		18,750	19,688	20,672	21,705	22,791
Incremental overhead		5,000	5,250	5,513	5,788	6,078
Depreciation		120,000	192,000	114,000	72,000	66,000
Income before taxes		$ 46,250	($ 17,438)	$ 69,291	$120,455	$136,078
Taxes		18,500	(6,975)	27,716	48,182	54,431
Project net income		$ 27,750	($ 10,463)	$ 41,574	$ 72,273	$ 81,647
Plus: Depreciation		120,000	192,000	114,000	72,000	66,000
Plus: Equip salvage value						134,000
Net cash flow	($600,000)	$147,750	$181,538	$155,574	$144,273	$282,047

b. Net present value @ 10% (NPV) = $74,904
   Internal rate of return (IRR) = 14.4%

c. Since the project has a positive NPV (and an IRR
   that is greater than its cost of capital), its acceptance
   would be a positive contribution to Diagnostic
   Services' financial condition.

Chapter 8

8–1 a. One of the key principles of finance is that invest-
       ments of higher risk require higher rates of return.
       This principle is important not only to individual
       investors making decisions concerning securities
       purchases but also to corporate investors making
       capital investment decisions.

     b. Three separate and distinct types of project risk can
       be defined: (1) stand-alone risk, which views the
       risk of a project as if it were held in isolation; (2)
       corporate risk, which views the risk of a project
       within the context of the firm's portfolio of projects;
       and (3) market risk, which views a project's risk
       from the perspective of a shareholder who holds a
       well-diversified portfolio of stocks.

       Conceptually, stand-alone risk is only relevant
       in one situation: when a not-for-profit firm (that has
       no shareholders) is evaluating its first project. Firms
       usually offer a myriad of different products or ser-
       vices and thus can be thought of as having a large
       number (hundreds or even thousands) of individual
       projects. Thus, the relevant risk of a new project to a
       not-for-profit firm is its corporate risk, which is the
       contribution of the project to the firm's overall risk.
       Market risk is generally viewed as the relevant risk
       for investor-owned firms.

     c. By far, the easiest type of risk to measure in practice
       is stand-alone risk; hence, this type of risk, which is
       rarely the relevant risk, becomes important to deci-
       sion makers.

     d. In general, new projects are in the same line of busi-
       ness as the firm's other projects, so the returns on

new assets are usually highly correlated with
returns on existing assets. With highly correlated
returns, a project's stand-alone risk becomes a good
proxy for its corporate risk. Furthermore, the
returns on most projects, whether new or existing,
are highly correlated with the national economy, so
a project's stand-alone risk is also generally a good
proxy for its market risk.

Correlation among types of risk is important
because it is normally possible to measure only a
project's stand-alone risk. Thus, stand-alone risk
must be used as a basis for estimating the project's
corporate risk and, for investor-owned firms, the
project's market risk.

8–2 a. Sensitivity analysis is a technique that indicates
exactly how much a project's profitability (NPV or
IRR) will change in response to a given change in a
single input variable, other things held constant.

The primary strength of sensitivity analysis is
that it is relatively easy to perform and doesn't
require any information about the uncertainty inherent in the input variables. Unfortunately, it has
severe limitations. In general, a project's stand-alone
risk depends on both the sensitivity of its profitability to changes in key variables and the ranges of likely values of these variables. Because sensitivity
analysis considers only the first factor, it can give
misleading results. Furthermore, sensitivity analysis
does not consider any interactions among the uncertain variables—it considers each variable independent of the others.

b. Scenario analysis is a stand-alone risk measurement
technique that considers (1) the sensitivity of NPV
to changes in key variables, (2) the likely range of
variable values, and (3) the interactions among variables. To conduct a scenario analysis, managers generally pick a "worst-case" set of circumstances (low
utilization, low reimbursement levels, low salvage
value, and so on); an average, or "most-likely-case"

set; and a "best-case" set. The resulting input value estimates, along with their probabilities, are then used to create a probability distribution of NPV. Then, the probability distribution of NPV can be used to estimate the project's expected NPV, standard deviation of NPV, and coefficient of variation of NPV, which permits managers to quantitatively assess the project's stand-alone risk.

While scenario analysis is relatively easy to perform and provides useful information about a project's stand-alone risk, it is limited in that it only considers a few discrete outcomes (NPVs) for the project, although in reality there is an almost infinite number of possibilities. Additionally, it forces all best and worst input values to occur together, which may not reflect the actual situation. Finally, it is often very difficult to estimate what the worst- and best-case values are for the uncertain variables and the probabilities of occurrence.

c. Monte Carlo simulation is a sophisticated technique for measuring a project's stand-alone risk. In essence, uncertain variables are entered as continuous distributions (for example, a normal distribution), and the software picks values from these distributions to create many scenarios. The end result is an NPV probability distribution based on, say, five thousand individual "scenarios," which encompasses all of the likely financial outcomes.

Although Monte Carlo simulation provides the most information about a project's risk and return, it requires specialized software. More important, it is generally very difficult to specify (1) the uncertainty inherent in each variable (its distribution), (2) how this uncertainty varies over time, and (3) how the uncertainties in individual variables correlate to one another.

8–3 a. The most common method for incorporating risk into the capital budgeting process is to adjust the discount rate. The starting point is the firm's overall cost of capital, which reflects the aggregate riskiness of the firm (the riskiness of the firm's average project). If a project under consideration is judged to have above-average (high) risk, the cost of capital is increased to account for the project's differential risk (as compared to the firm's average project), while if the project has below-average (low) risk, the firm's cost of capital is decreased. One problem with the process is that there is no good way of estimating how large the adjustment should be, so many firms have standard adjustment procedures that, say, reduce the cost of capital by three percentage points for low-risk projects and increase the cost of capital by four percentage points for high-risk projects.

b. Most projects have one or more outflows followed by a series of inflows; hence, raising the discount rate (as would be done for a high-risk project) penalizes (reduces) the project's profitability. However, raising the discount rate on a cash outflow reduces its present value, which lowers the cost and hence makes the project look better. Thus, risk adjustments applied to cash outflows must be the reverse of those applied to normal projects: A cash outflow with above-average risk must be evaluated using a lower-than-average cost of capital, while a cash outflow with below-average risk requires a higher-than-average cost of capital.

8–4   Differences in the amount of debt financing applicable to a project should also be taken into account in the capital budgeting process. Some projects are able to support more debt financing than others and hence would be financed with a higher proportion of debt. When there are significant differences in debt capacity, the overall cost of capital weights should be adjusted to reflect the debt capacity of the project, rather than the overall debt capacity of the firm.

8–5   a. Here are the tabular results of a sensitivity analysis on procedures per day. Figure A–1 contains a graph of the results.

FIGURE A–1

Sensitivity Analysis

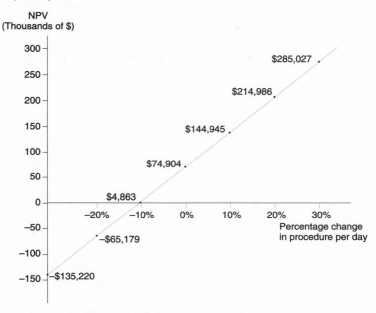

Percentage Change from Expected Value	Input Value	NPV
−30.0%	10.5	($135,220)
−20.0	12.0	(65,179)
−10.0	13.5	4,863
0.0	15.0	74,904
10.0	16.5	144,945
20.0	18.0	214,986
30.0	19.5	285,027

b. Here are the results of the scenario analysis:

Scenario	Average Probability	Number of Procedures	Collection	Equipment Salvage Value	NPV
Worst	0.25	10	$ 60	$100,000	($320,340)
Most likely	0.50	15	80	200,000	74,904
Best	0.25	20	100	300,000	594,665

Expected NPV	$106,033
Standard deviation of NPV	$324,998
Coefficient of variation of NPV	3.1

A scenario analysis provides quantitative information about a project's stand-alone risk and hence can be used to judge whether a project has below-average, average, or above-average risk.

c. (1) If the project had a coefficient of variation (CV) of NPV of 3.1, while the firm's average project had a CV in the range of 1.0–2.0, the project would be classified as a high-risk project.

(2) Since the project is judged to have high risk, the three percentage point risk adjustment would be added to the firm's 10 percent cost of capital, so the project's differential risk-adjusted cost of capital is 13 percent. If we recalculate the project's NPV using a 13 percent discount rate, we find the differential risk-adjusted NPV to be $22,313, so the project remains profitable even after adjustment for its high risk. However, it is not really necessary to recalculate the NPV because the project's 14.4 percent IRR indicates that the project is profitable even when the cost of capital is increased from 10 percent to 13 percent.

d. The risk being measured is the project's stand-alone risk, but the relevant risk in a not-for-profit hospital setting is the project's corporate risk. The hospital's managers must now determine whether the project's stand-alone risk is a good proxy for its corporate risk. Since the new project (diagnostic equipment) is in the same basic line of business as the hospital's other projects, it is likely that the new project's returns are highly correlated with the returns on the hospital's other projects; hence, that high stand-alone risk translates into high corporate risk. However, if the returns on the project under consideration were not highly correlated with the returns on the hospital's other projects, the stand-alone risk assessment would overstate the corporate risk of the project.

Chapter 9

9-1   There are a variety of motives behind mergers, some valid and some questionable. Here is brief discussion of the primary motives.

Synergy. From an economic perspective, the best motivation for mergers is to increase the value of the combined enterprise. If Companies A and B merge to form Company C, and if C's value exceeds that of A and B taken separately, then synergy is said to exist. When synergy drives a merger, value is created, and hence society benefits. Furthermore, such a merger can be beneficial to both A's and B's stockholders if the companies are investor-owned.

Availability of excess cash. Mergers are an easy, perhaps too easy, way for firms to get rid of excess cash. If a firm has a shortage of internal investment opportunities compared with its cash flow, it could (1) increase its dividend or repurchase stock if investor-owned, (2) invest in marketable securities, or (3) purchase another firm. Marketable securities often provide a good temporary parking place for money, but generally the rate of return on such securities is less than the return on real asset investments. Although there is nothing inherently wrong with using excess cash to buy other companies, the acquisition must create value to be economically worthwhile. Just making a company larger may benefit managers, but it does not necessarily benefit stockholders, patients, or society at large.

Purchase of assets at below replacement cost. Sometimes a firm will be touted as a possible acquisition candidate because the cost of replacing its assets is considerably higher than its market value. However, the true value of any business depends on its earning power, which sets the economic value of its assets. The real question, then, is not whether a business can be acquired for less than its replacement cost but, rather, whether it can be acquired for less than its economic value, which is a function of the cash flows that it is expected to produce in the future.

Diversification. Managers often claim that diversification into other lines of business is a reason for mergers. They contend that diversification helps to stabilize the firm's earnings stream, and thus benefits its owners. Stabilization of earnings is certainly beneficial to managers, employees, suppliers, customers, and other stakeholders, but its value is less certain from the standpoint of stockholders. If a stockholder is worried about the variability of a firm's earnings, he or she could diversify more easily by portfolio actions than could the firm.

Of course, there are some situations where mergers for diversification do make sense from a stockholder's perspective. For example, if you were the owner-manager of a closely held firm, it might be nearly impossible for you to sell part of your stock to diversify because this would dilute your ownership and perhaps also generate a large capital gains tax liability. In this case, a diversification merger might well be the best way to achieve personal diversification. Also, diversification mergers that better position firms to deal with future events are worthwhile, because such mergers can create operating synergies.

Even though diversification, without synergy, does not benefit shareholders directly, it clearly benefits a firm's other stakeholders. Thus, diversification-motivated mergers can be beneficial to not-for-profit firms. Furthermore, stockholders can obtain indirect benefits from diversification because making the firm less risky to managers, creditors, suppliers, customers, and the like could have positive implications for shareholders' wealth.

Personal incentives. Economists like to think that business decisions are based only on economic considerations. However, there can be no question that some business decisions are based more on managers' personal motivations than on economic analyses. Many people, business leaders included, like power, and more power is attached to running a larger corporation than a smaller one. Obviously, no executive would ever admit that his or her ego was the primary reason behind a merger, but knowledgeable observers are convinced that egos do play a prominent role in many mergers. It has also been observed that executive salaries, prestige, and perquisites are highly correlated with company size—the bigger the company, the higher these executive benefits. This could also play a role in the aggressive acquisition programs of some corporations. Of course, there is nothing wrong with executives feeling good about increasing the size of their firms or with their getting a better compensation package as a result of growth through mergers, provided the mergers make economic sense.

9-2   a. In a friendly merger, the boards of directors (trustees) of both firms agree to the merger. In a hostile merger, which can only occur between investor-owned firms, the acquiring company appeals directly to the target's shareholders, over the objections of the target firm's management. If more than half of the target's stockholders tender their shares, a hostile takeover occurs.

       b. No. As explained above, hostile takeovers involve a direct appeal to shareholders.

9-3   a. Merger regulation falls into the following two broad categories: (1) regulation concerning the procedures acquiring companies must follow in making hostile bids and (2) antitrust regulation to ensure that mergers do not lead to monopoly power.

       b. Prior to any merger regulation, raiders could put a great deal of pressure on target stockholders to tender their shares, even before a target's management could respond to the threat. This situation was thought to be unfair, and as a result, Congress passed the Williams Act in 1968. This law had two main objectives: (1) to regulate the way in which acquiring firms can structure takeover offers and (2) to force acquiring firms to disclose more information about their offers. Basically, Congress wanted to put target managements in a better position to defend against hostile offers. Additionally, Congress believed that shareholders needed easy access to information about tender offers—including information on any securities that might be offered in lieu of cash—in order to make a rational decision.

c. Antitrust laws are intended to ensure that no organization attains enough market power to act as a monopoly. Such laws are based on the assumption that vigorous competition is the most effective way to ensure that consumers receive the best possible goods and services at the lowest cost.

d. The two federal agencies that are charged with enforcing antitrust laws are the Federal Trade Commission (FTC) and the Justice Department (JD). The FTC and JD classify potential antitrust violations into two categories: per se and rule of reason. Per se violations are those so unlikely to produce redeeming consumer benefits that they are immediately presumed to be illegal. Examples would be two hospitals agreeing to fix prices for certain procedures or agreeing to allocate specific markets.

Actions that are not considered per se violations are evaluated using rule-of-reason analysis. Under rule-of-reason analysis, the FTC or JD must first determine whether a merger (or other combination) will enable a firm to exercise market power in an anticompetitive manner. If so, the agency must then analyze whether the activity produces economic efficiencies that outweigh the anticompetitive effects. If the benefits outweigh the anticompetitive consequences, the merger is allowed to take place. Mergers within the healthcare industry generally fall into the rule-of-reason category, so the regulators face a dilemma in deciding to what extent consolidation in a particular market leads to lower costs as opposed to market dominance.

9-4   The discounted cash flow (DCF) approach to valuing a business involves the application of classical capital investment analysis to an entire firm rather than to a single project. To apply this method, two key items are needed: (1) a set of pro forma statements that develop the incremental cash flows expected to result from the merger and (2) a discount rate, or cost of capital, to apply to these projected cash flows.

In market multiple analysis, a market-determined multiple is applied to some measure of the target's earnings such as net income or earnings per share. Like the DCF valuation method, the basic premise is that the value of any business depends on the earnings that the business produces. The DCF method applies this rationale to forecasted cash flows, while market multiple analysis uses comparative data to value earnings.

9-5   a. Hamada's equation can be used to approximate the effects of the leverage and tax rate change on beta. First, obtain the unlevered beta of Brandon Memorial Hospital, that is, the beta of the hospital assuming that it is financed entirely with equity:

$$b_{Assets} = \frac{b_{Firm}}{1+(1-T)(D/E)} = \frac{1.20}{1+(1-0.30)(0.10/0.90)} = \frac{1.20}{1.08} = 1.11$$

Next, relever Brandon's asset beta to reflect the 50 percent debt ratio and 40 percent tax rate that would be used in the acquisition.

$$b_{Firm} = b_{Assets}[1 + (1 - T)(D/E)]$$
$$= 1.11[1 + (1 - 0.40)(0.50/0.50)] = 1.11(1.6) = 1.78$$

Then, use the Security Market Line to estimate the postmerger cost of equity for the Brandon Memorial Hospital subsidiary. If the risk-free rate is 7 percent and the market-risk premium is six percentage points, then the cost of equity of the Brandon subsidiary, and hence the discount rate to apply to the forecasted net cash flows, would be about 17.7 percent:

$$\text{Cost of equity} = k_{RF} + (k_M - k_{RF})b$$
$$= 7\% + (6\%)1.78 = 17.7\%$$

b. Applying a 17.7 percent discount rate to the given cash flows, the value of Brandon to Continental is about $262 million.

c. In general, the merger of two not-for-profit firms does not require special consideration, but the acquisition of a not-for-profit firm by an investor-owned acquirer presents two significant problems. The first problem involves the charitable trust doctrine. This doctrine, which was first developed in English common law and has been adopted by most states, holds that assets used for charitable purposes must be held in trust. This doctrine shaped the state incorporation laws for not-for-profit firms, which require that assets being used for charitable purposes must be used for such purposes in perpetuity (forever). The end result is that the proceeds from the sale of a not-for-profit corporation to an investor-owned business must be held in trust and continue to be used for charitable purposes. These laws place two requirements on the board of trustees of a not-for-profit firm about to be acquired by an investor-owned firm. First, the trustees must ensure that the acquisition price reflects the full fair market value of the assets being acquired. Second, the trustees must establish a charitable foundation to administer the proceeds from the sale for a charitable purpose. The usual vehicle for continuing the charitable purpose of the not-for-profit corporation is the tax-exempt foundation.

The second major problem in the acquisition of a not-for-profit provider by an investor-owned company involves the tax-exempt, or municipal, debt that is often outstanding. Typically, such debt is issued for the sole purpose of funding plant and equipment owned by not-for-profit corporations. Furthermore, such debt usually has covenants that constrain the provider from merger activity that would lower the creditworthiness of the bonds or negatively affect the bonds' tax-exempt status.

However, the issuer normally has the right to refund that debt when transactions of this nature occur. The end result is that, in most situations, the entire amount of outstanding tax-exempt debt has to be refunded coincident with the acquisition of a not-for-profit provider by a for-profit firm.

Chapter 10

10–1 a. The capital structure decision sets the firm's optimal, or target, capital structure. In other words, the capital structure decision sets the optimal mix of debt and equity financing.

   b. Given the optimal amount of debt as set by the capital structure decision, a firm's managers must determine the optimal mix of debt maturities (short-term versus long-term debt).

   c. Three commonly used measures of debt usage are the debt ratio, debt-to-equity ratio, and the times-interest-earned (TIE) ratio.

$$\text{Debt ratio} = \frac{\text{Total debt}}{\text{Total assets}}$$

$$\text{Debt/equity ratio} = \frac{\text{Total debt}}{\text{Total equity}}$$

$$\text{TIE ratio} = \frac{\text{Operating income}}{\text{Interest expense}}$$

10–2 a. Business risk is the risk inherent in a firm's business operations. Thus, it is the riskiness of a firm if it uses no debt financing.

   Business risk depends on a large number of factors, including the following:

   (1) Competition.

   (2) Demand variability.

   (3) Input cost variability.

   (4) Ability to adjust output prices when input costs rise.

(5) Need to develop new products.

(6) Liability exposure.

(7) The extent to which costs are fixed: operating leverage.

b. Financial risk is the additional risk placed on stock-holders when a firm uses debt financing.

c. Business risk is measured by the standard deviation (variability) of a firm's return on equity (ROE = Net income/Total equity) assuming no debt financing.

If a firm uses debt financing, its standard deviation of ROE is higher than if it uses no debt financing. Further, the greater the debt/equity mix, the higher the standard deviation of ROE, and hence the greater the risk to the firm's stockholders. Financial risk is measured by the difference between the standard deviation of ROE with debt financing and the standard deviation of ROE assuming no debt financing.

10–3 a. The goal of capital structure theory is to define the relationship between the use of debt financing and firm value (stock price). If this relationship is known, managers can identify the capital structure that maximizes their firm's stock price.

b. The trade-off model indicates that the optimal capital structure is found, at least conceptually, by balancing the tax-shield benefits of leverage against the financial distress costs of leverage, so the costs and benefits are "traded off" against one another.

The trade-off model is not capable of specifying precise optimal capital structures, but it does point out three factors that influence debt usage:

(1) Higher-business-risk firms, as measured by the variability of returns on the firm's assets, ought to borrow less than lower-business-risk firms, other things being equal.

(2) Firms that employ tangible assets, such as real estate and standardized equipment, should borrow more than firms whose value is derived

either from intangible assets such as patents and goodwill, or from growth opportunities.

(3) Firms that are currently paying taxes at the highest rate, and that are likely to continue to do so in the future, should carry more debt than firms with current and/or prospectively lower tax rates.

c. The asymmetric information theory is based on two assumptions: (1) managers know more about their firms' future prospects than do investors, and (2) managers are motivated to maximize the wealth of their firms' current shareholders. If managers think that their firm's stock is undervalued, they will be motivated to use debt financing because selling stock at a "bargain" is detrimental to the firm's existing shareholders. However, if managers think that their firm's stock is overvalued, they will be motivated to issue new common stock. But, investors are rational, so they treat new common stock issues as "signals" that management considers the stock to be overvalued. Thus, investors revise downward their expectations for the firm, and the stock price falls. Since new stock issues have an adverse impact on stock price, managers are reluctant to issue new stock. If external financing is required, debt is the first choice, and new common stock would only be used in unusual circumstances.

d. Although no rigorous research has been conducted into the optimal capital structures of not-for-profit firms, some loose analogies can be drawn. Not-for-profit firms do not receive a direct tax subsidy when debt financing is used, but they do have access to the tax-exempt debt markets, which provides an indirect tax subsidy. Thus, not-for-profit firms receive about the same benefits from the use of debt financing as do investor-owned firms. Furthermore, a not-for-profit firm's fund capital has an opportunity cost that is roughly equivalent to the cost of equity of a similar investor-owned firm, so we would expect the opportunity cost of fund capital to rise as more and more debt financing is used, just as for an investor-owned firm. Finally, not-for-profit firms are subject to the same types of financial distress costs that are borne by investor-owned firms, so these costs are equally applicable. Thus, we would expect the trade-off theories to be applicable to not-for-profit firms and hence for such firms to have optimal capital structures that are defined, as least in theory, as a trade-off between the costs and benefits of debt financing. Note, however, that the asymmetric information theory is not applicable to not-for-profit firms because such firms do not issue common stock.

Although the trade-off theory may be conceptually correct for not-for-profit firms, a problem arises when applying the theory. Not-for-profit firms do not have access to the equity markets—their sources of "equity" capital are government payments, private contributions, and excess revenues. Thus, managers of not-for-profit organizations do not have the same degree of flexibility in either capital investment or capital structure decisions as do their proprietary counterparts.

10–4   Here are some of the more important judgmental issues that should be taken into account:

    (1) Long-run viability.

    (2) Managerial conservatism.

    (3) Lender and rating agency attitudes.

    (4) Reserve borrowing capacity.

    (5) Industry averages.

    (6) Control of investor-owned corporations.

    (7) Asset structure.

    (8) Growth rate.

    (9) Profitability.

    (10) Taxes.

10–5 a. Here is the completed table:

	All Equity			50 Percent Debt		
Probability	0.25	0.50	0.25	0.25	0.50	0.25
EBIT	$1,000,000	$3,000,000	$5,000,000	$1,000,000	$3,000,000	$5,000,000
Interest	0	0	0	720,000	720,000	720,000
EBT	$1,000,000	$3,000,000	$5,000,000	$ 280,000	$2,280,000	$4,280,000
Taxes	400,000	1,200,000	2,000,000	112,000	912,000	1,712,000
Net income	$ 600,000	$1,800,000	$3,000,000	$ 168,000	$1,368,000	$2,568,000
ROE	5.0%	15.0%	25.0%	2.8%	22.8%	42.8%
TIE	n.a.	n.a.	n.a.	1.39	4.17	6.94
E(ROE)		15.0%			22.8%	
Std dev ROE		7.1%			14.1%	

b. See the table above.

c. If Superior Care uses only equity financing, its expected ROE is 15 percent, and σ_{ROE} is 7.1 percent. When 50 percent debt financing is used, expected ROE increases to 22.8 percent. However, this leveraging up of expected return is not without costs: The standard deviation doubles to 14.1 percent. (It seems as if the standard deviation has not quite doubled, but that is because the figures are rounded to the nearest 10th percent.) Thus, the use of financial leverage has both benefits and costs.

Chapter 11

11–1 The two parties are the user of the leased asset (the lessee) and the owner of the asset, usually the manufacturer or a leasing company (the lessor).

11–2 Leases fall roughly into two categories: operating leases and financial leases.

Operating Leases Operating, or service, leases generally provide for both financing and maintenance. Ordinarily, operating leases require the lessor to maintain and service the leased equipment, and the cost of the maintenance is built into the lease payments. Also, operating leases are not fully amortized. A final feature of operating leases is that they frequently contain a cancellation clause, which gives the lessee the right to cancel the lease and to return the equipment before the expiration of the basic lease agreement. This is an important consideration to the lessee, for it means that the equipment can be returned if it is rendered obsolete by technological developments or if it is no longer needed because of a decline in the lessee's business.

Financial Leases Financial, or capital, leases are differentiated from operating leases in that (1) they typically do not provide for maintenance service, (2) they typically are not cancelable, (3) they are generally for a period that approximates the economic life of the asset, and hence (4) they are fully amortized (that is, the lessor receives rental payments equal to the full cost of the leased asset plus a return on the funds employed).

11–3 a. The Internal Revenue Service (IRS) classifies leases as guideline and nonguideline. In a guideline lease, ownership benefits (depreciation tax deductions) accrue to the lessor, but the lessee's lease (rental) payments are fully tax deductible. A lease that does not meet the tax guidelines is called a nonguideline, or non-tax-oriented, lease. For this type of lease, the lessee can only deduct the interest portion of each lease payment. However, the lessee is effectively the owner of the leased equipment; thus, the lessee can take the tax depreciation.

b. Leases are classified by accountants as either capital leases or operating leases. Accounting rules require firms that enter into capital leases to restate their balance sheets to report the leased asset as a fixed asset and the present value of the future lease payments as a liability. This process is called capitalizing the lease, and the net effect is to create a balance sheet similar to the one that would result if the leased asset were purchased with debt financing. Operating leases are not shown directly on the balance sheet, but long-term operating leases must be disclosed in the footnotes to the balance sheet.

11–4   a. If the basic lease parameters are identical between the lessee and the lessor, any positive value that accrues to one party must come at the expense of the other party. Thus, under symmetrical conditions, leasing is a zero-sum game. Leasing becomes advantageous to both parties when differences exist between the parties.

b. One of the primary motivations for leasing is tax differentials. If the lessee and lessor are facing different tax situations, it may be possible to structure a lease that is beneficial to both parties.

Leasing is an attractive financing alternative for many high-technology items that are subject to rapid and unpredictable technological obsolescence. A lessor that specializes in state-of-the-art equipment might be exposed to significantly less risk than the user of the equipment.

A type of lease that is gaining popularity among healthcare providers is the per-procedure lease. Since a per-procedure lease changes the payment for the equipment from fixed to variable, the lessee's risk is reduced.

Leasing can also be attractive when a firm is uncertain about how long an asset will be needed. A lease with a cancellation clause would permit the lessee to simply return the equipment if it is no longer needed.

Also, some companies find leasing attractive because the lessor is able to provide maintenance or other services on favorable terms.

Finally, leasing may be financially attractive for smaller firms that have limited access to debt markets. Specialized leasing companies might be more willing to provide financing, and charge lower rates, than conventional lenders because specialized leasing companies may be able to more easily assess the credit risk of the lessee.

11–5 a. Place the cash flows associated with ownership on a time line:

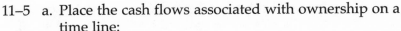

	0	1	2	3	4	5
Cost	($1,000,000)					
Tax savings		$40,000[a]	$64,000[a]	$38,000[a]	$24,000[a]	$ 22,000[a]
Maintenance	(8,000)[b]	(8,000)[b]	(8,000)[b]	(8,000)[b]	(8,000)[b]	
Res value						92,000c
	($1,008,000)	$32,000	$56,000	$30,000	$16,000	$114,000

[a] Depreciation schedule:

Year	Factor	Depreciation Expense	Tax Savings
1	0.20	$ 200,000	$ 40,000
2	0.32	320,000	64,000
3	0.19	190,000	38,000
4	0.12	120,000	24,000
5	0.11	110,000	22,000
6	0.06	60,000	12,000
Total		$1,000,000	$200,000

b After-tax maintenance cash flow = $10,000(1 − 0.20) = $8,000.
c Net residual value = $100,000 − ($100,000 − $60,000)(0.20) = $92,000.

The present value cost of owning at the firm's 8 percent after-tax cost of debt is $817,197.

b. Place the cash flows associated with leasing on a time line:

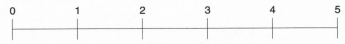

0	1	2	3	4	5
Lease pmts ($164,000)[a]	($164,000)[a]	($164,000)[a]	($164,000)[a]	($164,000)[a]	

[a] $205,000(1 − 0.20) = $164,000.

The present value cost of leasing at the firm's 8 percent after-tax cost of debt is $707,189.

c. The net advantage to leasing (NAL) is $817,197 − $707,189 = $110,008, and hence the MRI system should be leased.

d. Place the lessor's cash flows on a time line:

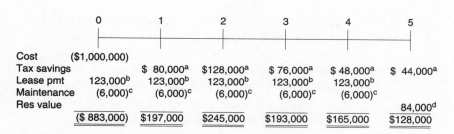

	0	1	2	3	4	5
Cost	($1,000,000)					
Tax savings		$ 80,000[a]	$128,000[a]	$ 76,000[a]	$ 48,000[a]	$ 44,000[a]
Lease pmt	123,000[b]	123,000[b]	123,000[b]	123,000[b]	123,000[b]	
Maintenance	(6,000)[c]	(6,000)[c]	(6,000)[c]	(6,000)[c]	(6,000)[c]	
Res value						84,000[d]
	($ 883,000)	$197,000	$245,000	$193,000	$165,000	$128,000

[a] This is each year's depreciation expense as calculated above times the lessor's tax rate of 40 percent.
[b] After-tax lease payment = $205,000(1 − 0.40) = $123,000.
[c] After-tax maintenance payment = $10,000(1 − 0.40) = $6,000.
[d] After-tax residual value = $100,000 − ($100,000 − $60,000)(0.40) = $84,000.

The lessor's NPV of the lease investment is the present value of the net cash flows when discounted at the after-tax opportunity cost of capital or 9%(1 − T) = 9%(0.6) = 5.4%. NPV = −$78,625. Thus, the lessor should not write the lease.

Chapter 12

12–1 a. Capitation is a flat periodic payment per enrollee to a healthcare provider that is the sole reimbursement for providing defined services to a defined population. The word *capitation* is derived from the term *per capita,* which means per person. Generally, capitation payments are expressed as some dollar amount per member per month (PMPM), where the word *member* typically means enrollee in a managed care plan, usually a health maintenance organization (HMO). For example, a primary care physician may receive a capitated payment of $14 PMPM for attending to the healthcare needs of 250 HMO enrollees. Under this contract, the physician would receive $14(250)(12) = $42,000 in total capitation payments over the year, and this amount must cover all of the primary care services specified in the contract that are provided to the covered population. Capitated payments often are adjusted for age and gender, but no other adjustments are typically made.

b. Under conventional reimbursement systems, the greater the utilization, the greater the revenues. All volumes to the left of breakeven (in a graph such as Figure 12–1) produce a loss for the provider, while all volumes to the right of breakeven produce a profit. Thus, the incentive for providers is to increase utilization because increased volume leads to increased profits. Under capitation, all volumes to the left of breakeven produce a profit, whereas all volumes to the right of breakeven result in a loss. Under capitation, providers have the incentive to decrease utilization because decreased volume leads to increased profits. The only way to increase revenues under capitation is to increase the number of covered lives (enrollees).

Capitation completely reverses the actions that providers must take to assure financial success, and many providers will find it difficult to adjust to the new, perverse (by conventional reimbursement standards) incentive system. Under conventional reimbursement, the keys to success are to work harder, increase volume, and hence increase profits; while under capitation, the keys to profitability are to work smarter and decrease volume. Since the primary means to profitability with conventional reimbursement is increased volume, increased reimbursement rates, or both, the primary task of managers is to maximize utilization and reimbursement rates. Furthermore, any deficiencies in cost control often can be overcome by higher volume. Under capitation, the primary path to profitability is through cost control, so the key to success is lower volume and cost-effective treatment plans.

12–2 Experience to date suggests two powerful trends: fewer hospital beds and a physician mix that contains a greater proportion of primary care physicians. Most importantly, the data tell us that historical utilization rates based on conventional reimbursement methodologies are not good predictors of future utilization when the payment system is capitation.

12–3 If the costs at a provider are mostly fixed, financial risk is actually reduced under capitation because the fixed revenue stream better matches the fixed cost structure. On the other hand, if the cost structure is predominantly variable, moving to capitation from one of the conventional reimbursement methods will increase financial risk since the fixed revenue stream is a poor match for a cost structure that is highly correlated to volume.

12–4 a. Risk pools are pools of money that are initially withheld from providers but then later allocated on the basis of how well a set of predefined financial goals are met. Risk pools can be used with any type of reimbursement system, such as the use of withholds in a per diem system, whereby the hospital is rewarded if utilization is less than expected and, in effect, penalized by not getting some portion or all of the amount withheld if utilization exceeds targets.

b. Risk pools are designed to reward those providers that are most able to control costs through better utilization management, better cost control, or both. Risk-sharing arrangements can occur among physicians only, among physicians and institutions, or among all providers. Furthermore, risk pools can be established to promote only financial goals or some combination of financial and nonfinancial goals.

Note that if a system is fully integrated and all subsidiary providers are owned by, and hence directly responsible to, the same parent, there is only one bottom line (and only one boss), so there is no need for risk-sharing arrangements. Proper incentives are created by managerial control. However, in most systems today, providers are loosely affiliated in some way rather than part of the same corporation, and hence risk-sharing arrangements are needed to align the incentives of the diverse parties involved.

Typically, risk-sharing arrangements allocate 10 to 20 percent of each reimbursement dollar to one or more risk pools, often for primary care, specialty (referral) care, and institutional care. Then, throughout the year, expenses are charged against the applicable pools, and at year-end, each pool's expenses are reconciled, that is, compared with those budgeted. Any surpluses are distributed to the participating providers on the basis of a pre-arranged formula. Any deficits are typically funded from network reserves, which are established specifically to cover system cost overruns.

12–5   Capitated payments expose providers to financial risks that differ from those associated with conventional reimbursement systems. As with all financial risks, there are actions that can be taken to reduce the impact of capitation-induced risks. The two most commonly used risk management techniques are (1) the establishment of reserves and (2) stop-loss provisions (reinsurance).

The first line of defense against financial risk by any organization is the maintenance of adequate reserves. When healthcare providers accept capitated rates, they agree to provide whatever services are required for a fixed monthly fee. If all goes well, that is, if utilization and costs are controlled, the provider will end the year with a profit. But, if realized utilization and costs exceed estimates, the losses have to be covered in some way, and hence the need for reserves becomes apparent.

Rather than establishing reserves to cover every conceivable cost situation, many providers elect to "reinsure" the risk. Such insurance, which is now offered by dozens of insurance companies, is called reinsurance or medical stop-loss insurance. (The term *reinsurance* has traditionally been used to mean insurance bought by insurance companies from other insurance companies to limit the risk assumed by the first insurer in covering potential losses. However, the term is now being used in the healthcare industry when a provider seeks insurance to limit capitation risk.)

Stop-loss insurance is written to protect providers from losses on individual patients rather than from aggregate losses on a contract. The idea is to insure the provider against catastrophic "budget buster" patients, not to guarantee a certain level of overall profitability. For example, a hospital might purchase stop-loss insurance with a deductible, or threshold, of $100,000 per patient. The insurer might agree to pay 80 percent of billed charges in excess of this threshold amount. Of course, the lower the threshold and the higher the percentage of any excess paid by the insurer, the higher the stop-loss insurance premium.

Using Spreadsheets to Make Better Financial Decisions

To be truly effective in today's highly competitive healthcare industry, managers need to be proficient in computer modeling because spreadsheet models permit managers to gain insights into financial decision making they would simply miss in the old pencil-and-calculator environment. As an introduction to the power and usefulness of spreadsheets, this book contains a diskette with models that illustrate five financial applications:

1. Discounted cash flow (DCF) analysis.
2. Capital investment decisions.
3. Merger valuation.
4. Capital structure decisions.
5. Leasing decisions.

There are four different versions of each of the five models on the diskette:

1. Lotus for DOS version.
2. Lotus for Windows version.
3. Excel version.
4. Baler version.

Lotus 1-2-3 and Excel models are provided for those readers who have access to an IBM-compatible personal computer (PC) with Lotus, Excel, or compatible spreadsheet software. Note that the diskette contains two versions of the Lotus models: one version for DOS users and another for Windows users. The spreadsheet models are also provided in a "stand-alone" version created by Baler software, and these models can be accessed and run on any IBM-compatible personal computer under DOS without special spreadsheet software.

MODEL FILE NAMES

Lotus for DOS models on the diskette have file names CHAPXX.WK1 where XX is the chapter number, for example, CHAP04.WK1. The Lotus for Windows models have file names CHAPXX.WK4 where XX is the chapter number, for example, CHAP04.WK4. Finally, the Excel models have file names CHAPXX.XLW where XX is the chapter number, for example, CHAP04.XLW.

MODEL STRUCTURE

All models are organized vertically into three sections divided by double dashed lines. The first section briefly describes the concept of the model and any graphics associated with it. The second section contains INPUT DATA and KEY OUTPUT, while the bottom section contains the body of the model. The models are designed so that input data changes feed into the MODEL-GENERATED DATA section for recalculation, and the new output data is automatically displayed both in the body and in the KEY OUTPUT section. The KEY OUTPUT section was created so that the results of input data changes can be seen without having to move to a different screen location.

The models are protected so that only certain cells in the INPUT DATA section can be changed. With the protection mode on, it is impossible to make changes, either inadvertent or deliberate, that would destroy the model. If you try to change one of the protected cells, your computer will "beep" and an error message will be displayed. Press the escape (ESC) key to start over. If you want to modify the model for other uses, you must first disable the protection feature.

MODEL GRAPHICS

Each model contains one or more graphs. However, the manner in which the graphs are displayed varies with the software used.

If you are using the Baler or Lotus for DOS versions, the graphs can be viewed by pressing the F10 key or by following the instructions given with the model. Once a graph is displayed, you can return to the spreadsheet by pressing any key.

If you are using the Lotus for Windows version, click on EDIT, then click on GO TO on the pull-down menu. Then select CHART from the TYPE OF ITEM menu that appears, and one or more graph names will be displayed. Click on the desired graph name, then click on the OK button to display the graph.

If you are using Excel, the graph name will appear on a tab at the bottom of the screen. Click on that tab, and the graph will be displayed.

USING THE BALER MODELS

If you do not have any spreadsheet software on your computer, but do have DOS, you can still access the Baler versions of the models. The Baler software models on the diskette have file names CHAPXX.WKB where XX is the chapter number, for example, CHAP04.WKB. However, to run the models, the diskette contains an accompanying .OVR file plus the Baler run engine with file name RUN.EXE. All required Baler files are contained on the diskette supplied with the book.

To retrieve a Baler model, place the diskette in the computer's diskette drive, usually designated either A or B. Then, enter a: or b:, depending on the drive being used, and the A or B prompt will appear. Next, enter RUN CHAPXX to retrieve the model. For example, enter RUN CHAP04 to retrieve the model for Chapter 4. After a few moments, the spreadsheet will appear on your screen.

INSTRUCTIONS FOR EACH MODEL

Chapter 4: Discounted Cash Flow (DCF) Analysis

To begin, spend a few minutes looking through the model to get a feel for its structure. (The arrow keys are used to move around the spreadsheet.) Note that the model contains separate subsections for dealing with lump-sum cash flows, annuities, and a six-period (Periods 0 through 5) uneven cash flow stream. The uneven cash flow stream can accommodate fewer than six cash flows by merely placing zeros as input in the unwanted periods, but the model cannot deal with more than six cash flows without modification.

Place the pointer on Cell G54, which calculates the future value of a lump sum. Note in the control panel at the top of the screen that the formula uses the input data from Cells D25 (the present value), D27 (the interest rate), and D28 (the number of periods), to calculate the future value, $161.05 with the existing data, which is then displayed in Cells G54 and H25. (In spreadsheet notation, * is the multiplication sign and ^ raises a value to a power.)

Now, move the pointer to Cell G62 and note that it contains the @RATE function, which is a spreadsheet built-in financial @function. The @RATE function calculates the interest rate for two lump sums given the future value, present value, and number of periods. Note that some of the output cells scattered from G54 to G96 contain formulas, while others contain @functions. Between the two techniques, all discounted cash flow calculations can be incorporated directly into the spreadsheet.

Now, look back at the Chapter 4 self-assessment exercises. Rework Exercises 4–1 through 4–5a, but this time use the spreadsheet model instead of a financial calculator to find the solutions. Check your model answers against the solutions given in Appendix A.

When changing the input data in the INPUT SECTION, note the following points:

1. The input data are contained in Cells D25–D28, D32–D36, and D41–D47. These are the only cells that can be changed.

2. Dollar amounts (values or numbers) must be entered without commas or other formatting conventions such as dollar signs. Only decimal points (periods) and signs (minus sign when necessary) are permitted. For example, $1,000.50 would be entered as 1000.5 or 1000.50. The dollar cells automatically display the values entered to two decimal places (dollars and cents) with commas and dollar signs.

3. Interest rates (percentages) must be entered as decimals. Thus, 10 percent is entered as .1 or 0.1 or 0.10. The percent cells automatically display the values entered as percentages with one decimal place.

Also, note that the spreadsheet contains a graphical display of the compounding process. (If you are using the Baler or Lotus for DOS version, press the F10 key to view the graph. If you are using one of the other models, use the applicable procedure for that software to view the graph.)

Chapter 7: Capital Investment Decisions

To begin the spreadsheet exercise, note that spreadsheet CHAP07 models a capital investment analysis for a project that has a five-year life. Spend a few minutes looking through the model to get a feel for its structure. The key output from the model is the project's NPV, IRR, and payback.

To better understand the usefulness of the model in making capital budgeting decisions, refer to the self-assessment exercises in Chapter 7. Specifically, rework Exercise 7–5, but this time use the spreadsheet model instead of a financial calculator to find the solution. Note the following points:

1. The input data are contained in Cells D22 through D33. These are the only cells that need to be changed.

2. Dollar amounts (values or numbers) must be entered without commas or other formatting conventions such as dollar signs. Only decimal points (periods) and signs (minus sign when necessary) are permitted. For example, $1,000.50 would be entered as 1000.5 or 1000.50. The dollar cells automatically display the values entered to the nearest dollar, with commas and dollar signs as needed.

3. Interest rates (percentages) must be entered as decimals. Thus, 10 percent is entered as .1 or 0.1 or 0.10. The percent cells automatically display the values entered as percentages with one decimal place.

Once you are satisfied with the solution to Exercise 7–5, use the model to complete Exercise 8–5 in the Chapter 8 self-assessment exercises. This exercise uses the same example but extends the analysis to include risk analysis. Note the following points:

1. This model has a data table, a spreadsheet feature that simplifies sensitivity analyses. The entire data table, which is in the range C87 to D94, must be unprotected to recalculate, so it shows up on the spreadsheet in green (or bright white). The data table works like this:
   a. The spreadsheet takes each value from C88 to C94 and uses it as input data in Cell D24.
   b. The resulting NPV, which first appears in Cell E77, is written into the appropriate cell in Column D (for

example, the NPV that results when procedures per day is 10.5 appears in Cell D88). Once the data table is set up, the sensitivity analysis can be completed almost instantaneously.

One problem with data tables is that they do not automatically recalculate when input data is changed. However, when the F8 key is pressed (Baler or Lotus for DOS), the last data table accessed manually is recalculated. Since this spreadsheet has only one data table, pressing F8 causes the data table to recalculate, and hence its output will reflect any input data changes since the last data table recalculation.

2. The spreadsheet contains a graphical display of the data table.

3. The bottom section of the module contains a completed scenario analysis for the project detailed in Exercises 7–5 and 8–5. Note that most of the data is protected and cannot be changed. However, you can change the probabilities of occurrence of the three scenarios to see the effect on the expected NPV, standard deviation of NPV, and coefficient of variation of NPV.

Chapter 9: Merger Valuation

To begin, retrieve the spreadsheet CHAP09, which models a merger valuation using DCF analysis. Use the arrow keys to move the highlighter around the model. Spend a few minutes looking through the model to get a feel for its structure. Note that all dollar amounts are in millions. The key output of the model consists of the value of the proposed acquisition, along with the discount rate used and the new beta coefficient.

To better understand the model, refer to the self-assessment exercises in Chapter 9. Specifically, rework Exercises 9–5a and 9–5b, but this time use the spreadsheet model instead of a financial calculator to find the solutions. Note the following points:

1. The input data are contained in Cells D21–D24, D26–D28, D30–D31, and D33–D34. These are the only cells that can be changed.

2. Dollar amounts (values or numbers) must be entered without commas or other formatting conventions such as dollar signs. The dollar cells automatically display the values entered to the nearest dollar (nearest million) with commas (if needed) and dollar signs.

3. Interest rates and tax rates (percentages) must be entered as decimals. Thus, 10 percent is entered as .1 or 0.1 or 0.10. The percent cells automatically display the values entered as percentages with one decimal place.

4. This model has a data table, which is a spreadsheet feature that simplifies sensitivity analyses. The entire data table, which is in the range B60 to C67, must be unprotected to recalculate, so it shows up on the spreadsheet in green. The data table works like this:

   a. The spreadsheet takes each beta value from B61 to B67 and uses it as input data in Cell D26.

   b. The resulting values are written into the appropriate cells in Column C. Once the data table is set up, the sensitivity analysis can be completed almost instantaneously.

   One problem with data tables is that they do not automatically recalculate when input data is changed. However, if using the Baler or Lotus for DOS, pressing the F8 key will recalculate the last data table accessed manually. Since this spreadsheet has only one data table, pressing F8 causes the data table to recalculate, and hence its output will reflect any input data changes since the last data table recalculation.

5. The spreadsheet contains a graphical display of the data table.

Chapter 10: Capital Structure Decisions

To begin, note that spreadsheet CHAP10 models the capital structure decision for a firm that is assumed to have perpetual cash flows. (Perpetual cash flows are constant-value cash flows that last forever.) However, for your use of the module, the most important part of the spreadsheet is the MODEL-GENERATED DATA section titled ROE Analysis. Use the arrow keys to move the highlighter around this section of the model. Spend a few minutes looking through the section to get a feel for its structure. The key output for this section is the expected ROE and standard deviation of ROE.

To understand the usefulness of the model, refer to the self-assessment exercises contained in Chapter 10. Specifically, rework Exercises 10–5a and 10–5b, but this time use the spreadsheet model instead of a financial calculator to find the solutions. Note the following points:

1. The input data for the ROE analysis are contained in Cells B28, B29, and B31, and Cells C61 through E62. These are the only cells that need to be changed.

2. Dollar amounts (values or numbers) must be entered without commas or other formatting conventions such as dollar signs. Only decimal points (periods) and signs (minus sign when necessary) are permitted. For example, $1,000.50 would be entered as 1000.5 or 1000.50. The dollar cells automatically display the values entered to two decimal places (dollars and cents) with commas and dollar signs.

3. Interest rates (percentages) must be entered as decimals. Thus, 10 percent is entered as .1 or 0.1 or 0.10. The percent cells automatically display the values entered as percentages with one decimal place.

4. The CV in Row 74 stands for coefficient of variation, which is defined as the standard deviation divided by the expected value. CV is a standardized measure of risk (risk per unit of return) and is often a better measure of risk than is the standard deviation.

5. The spreadsheet contains a graphical display.

Chapter 11: Leasing Decisions

To begin, retrieve the spreadsheet CHAP11, which models lease analysis. Use the arrow keys to move the highlighter around the model. Spend a few minutes looking through the model to get a feel for its structure. Note that the model has separate input sections for general data, for the lessee, and for the lessor. The key output of the model consists of NAL (NPV) and IRR for both the lessee and lessor.

To better understand the model, refer to the self-assessment exercises contained in Chapter 11. Specifically, rework Exercises 11-5a through 11-5d, but this time use the spreadsheet model instead of a financial calculator to find the solutions. Note the following points:

1. The input data are contained in Cells D22–D23, D27–D30, and D34–D37. These are the only cells that can be changed.

2. Dollar amounts (values or numbers) must be entered without commas or other formatting convention such as dollar signs. Only decimal points (periods) and signs (minus sign when necessary) are permitted. For example, $1,000.50 would be entered as 1000.5 or 1000.50. The dollar cells automatically display the values entered to two decimal places (dollars and cents) with commas and dollar signs.

3. Interest rates and tax rates (percentages) must be entered as decimals. Thus, 10 percent is entered as .1 or 0.1 or 0.10. The percent cells automatically display the values entered as percentages with one decimal place.

4. This model has a data table, which is a spreadsheet feature that simplifies sensitivity analyses. The entire data table, which is in the range B135 to E142, must be unprotected to recalculate, so it shows up on the spreadsheet in green. The data table works like this:

   a. The spreadsheet takes each value from B136 to B142 and uses it as input data in Cell D23.

   b. The resulting lessee's NAL and lessor's NPV are written into the appropriate cells in Columns C and D. Once the data table is set up, the sensitivity analysis can be completed almost instantaneously.

   One problem with data tables is that they do not automatically recalculate when input data is changed. However, when using the Baler or Lotus for DOS model, when the F8 key is pressed, the last data table accessed manually is recalculated. Since this spreadsheet has only one data table, pressing F8 causes the data table to recalculate, and hence its output will reflect any input data changes since the last data table recalculation.

5. The spreadsheet contains a graphical display of the data table.

INDEX